LIBRARY

Direct Line: 020 7290 2940   Direct Fax: 020 7290 2939
email: library@rsm.ac.uk

LOAN PERIODS

Thoracic Anaesthesia: principles and practice

Thoracic Anaesthesia: principles and practice

Edited by:

S Ghosh BSc MBBS FRCA

R D Latimer MA MBBS FRCA

Department of Cardiothoracic Anaesthesia and Intensive Care,
Papworth Hospital, Cambridge University Teaching Hospitals Trust,
Cambridge, UK

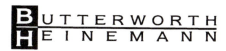

BUTTERWORTH
HEINEMANN

OXFORD AUCKLAND BOSTON JOHANNESBURG MELBOURNE NEW DELHI

1999

Butterworth-Heinemann
Linacre House, Jordan Hill, Oxford OX2 8DP
225 Wildwood Avenue, Woburn, MA 01801-2041
A division of Reed Educational and Professional Publishing Ltd

 A member of the Reed Elsevier plc group

First published 1999

© Reed Educational and Professional Publishing Ltd 1999

British Library Cataloguing in Publication Data
A catalogue record for this book is available from the British Library

Library of Congress Cataloguing in Publication Data
A catalogue record for this book is available from the Library of Congress

ISBN 0 7506 4062 6

Typeset by BC Typesetting, Keynsham, Bristol
Printed and bound in Great Britain by MPG Books Ltd, Bodmin, Cornwall

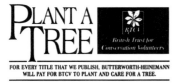

Contents

Contributors

S. Ahmed, Department of Anaesthesia, Papworth Hospital, Cambridge, UK

C. J. Bateman, Department of Anaesthesia, Royal Brompton Hospital, London, UK

K. J. Benson, Department of Anaesthesia, Queen's Medical Centre, Nottingham, UK

R. Bingham, Department of Anaesthesia, Great Ormond Street Hospital, London, UK

P. Clarke, Department of Thoracic Surgery, Austin and Repatriation Medical Centre, Melbourne, Australia

I. D. Conacher, Department of Anaesthesia, Freeman Hospital, Newcastle Upon Tyne, UK

L. Doolan, Department of Anaesthesia, Austin and Repatriation Medical Centre, Melbourne, Australia

R. O. Feneck, Department of Anaesthesia, St. Thomas' Hospital, London, UK

J. Gothard, Department of Anaesthesia, Royal Brompton Hospital, London, UK

M. Gressier, Department d'Anesthesie-Reanimation, Hôpital Cardiologique, Lyon, France

I. Hardy, Department of Anaesthesia, Papworth Hospital, Cambridge, UK

B. F. Keogh, Department of Anaesthesia, Royal Brompton Hospital, London, UK

J. D. Kneeshaw, Department of Anaesthesia, Papworth Hospital, Cambridge, UK

G. Lee, Department of Anaesthesia, Wythenshawe Hospital, Manchester, UK

E. Mackson, Department of Anaesthesia, Papworth Hospital, Cambridge, UK

R. P. Mahajan, Department of Anaesthesia, Queen's Medical Centre, Nottingham, UK

W. T. McBride, Department of Anaesthesia, Queen's University of Belfast, Belfast, Northern Ireland

K. McNeil, Department of Chest Medicine, Papworth Hospital, Cambridge, UK

R. Mills, Department of Anaesthesia, Papworth Hospital, Cambridge, UK

J. Neidecker, Department d'Anesthesie-Reanimation, Hôpital Cardiologique, Lyon, France

S. J. B. Nicoll, Department of Anaesthesia, Great Ormond Street Hospital, London, UK

V. Piriou, Department d'Anesthesie-Reanimation, Hôpital Cardiologique, Lyon, France

H. Porter, Department of Anaesthesia, Royal Brompton Hospital, London, UK

A. Schweizer, Department d' Anesthesie-Reanimation, Hôpital Cardiologique, Lyon, France

D. Smith, Department of Anaesthesia, Southampton General Hospital, Southampton, UK

Sir Keith Sykes, Emeritus Professor of Anaesthesia, University of Oxford, Oxford, UK

A. Vuylsteke, Department of Anaesthesia, Papworth Hospital, Cambridge, UK

W. C. Wilson, Department of Anesthesiology, University of California San Diego Medical Center, California, USA

I. G. Wright, Department of Anaesthesia, Harefield Hospital, Harefield, UK

M. Zammit, Department of Anaesthesia, Papworth Hospital, Cambridge, UK

Preface

This book is intended to provide an easily readable source of information for the everyday practice of thoracic anaesthesia. It is aimed at anaesthetists of all levels involved in the care of thoracic surgical patients. We hope that the newcomer to the specialty will find it useful both in the clinical setting and in preparing for examinations, and that the experienced thoracic anaesthetist will be able to use it to prepare lectures and tutorials, as well as to refer to it for guidance.

We would like to thank the friends whom we have the luck to work with, and our families for their support and encouragement during the many hours spent in editing chapters. Most of all, those who contributed their expertise by writing for this book deserve special mention.

Sunit Ghosh
Ray Latimer
Cambridge, 1999

Acknowledgements

The illustrations for Chapter 1 were produced by the Medical Illustration Department, Wythenshawe Hospital, Manchester.

The illustrations for Chapters 3 and 4 are by J. Higson, West Cambridge Anaesthetics Group, Cambridge.

The illustrations for Chapter 16 are by Beth Croce, Cardiac Surgery Publishing Office, AUSTIN and Repatriation Medical Centre, Victoria, Australia.

History and equipment: the evolution of endobronchial apparatus for one-lung ventilation and anaesthesia

G. Lee

And the Lord God caused a deep sleep to fall upon Adam, and he slept: and He took one of his ribs, and closed up the flesh instead thereof.

(Genesis Ch. 2 v. 21)

Whilst the first anaesthetic may have been for a thoracic operation, safe anaesthesia specifically for thoracic surgery is a relatively new development in the history of modern anaesthetic practice. This chapter aims to describe and explain the evolution of endobronchial apparatus for one-lung ventilation from 1920 to the present day in roughly chronological order, since that is the area of specific interest to the student of thoracic anaesthesia. Some critical and comparative appraisal of the pieces of apparatus is included, and some knowledge of basic bronchial anatomy and thoracic surgery is assumed.

Early anaesthesia

Prior to 1900, surgeons rarely ventured into the chest. Thoracotomy was an uncommon and hazardous operation. It had been recognized for centuries that respiration rapidly became ineffective once the chest was open, although the reasons for this were not understood. It had also been known since 1550 that animals could be kept alive with an open chest using positive pressure ventilation, but it was not known how to achieve this effectively in humans. It had been realized that maintenance of a differential pressure across the lungs during thoracotomy helped to delay respiratory failure. This led to the development of ingenious positive pressure headboxes and negative pressure operating chambers with an airtight seal around the patient's neck; the airways remained at a constant positive pressure with respect to the open thoracic cavity while the patient breathed spontaneously under anaesthesia. Positive pressure ventilation by insufflation of air using bellows and tracheal intubation with various designs of metal tube had been advocated for resuscitation for drowning and asphyxia in the eighteenth and early nineteenth centuries, but artificial respiration was not widely used in anaesthesia until the mid-twentieth century.

Inhalational anaesthesia had been successfully administered through tracheal tubes by 1900, although the techniques were difficult and it was not widely used by the medical profession of the day. The tracheal tubes available were difficult to insert, and even though laryngoscopes had been described, they were not in common use. Both tracheal and bronchial insufflation of anaesthetic gas under pressure had been tried for thoracic work. Anaesthesia had even been performed for successful thoracotomy, using a combination of a metal resuscitation tube and bellows ventilation with the Fell–O'Dwyer apparatus, in 1899. None of these techniques were widely accepted at the time, although they all contained the roots of modern thoracic anaesthesia.

The prerequisites for modern anaesthesia

Simultaneous advances in several areas were necessary for modern thoracic anaesthesia to develop. The development of safe anaesthetic agents and apparatus for their delivery was vital. An understanding of the anatomy of the lower airway, the mechanism of normal and pathological pulmonary gas exchange and lung ventilation was necessary. The concept of modern 'balanced anaesthesia', using a muscle relaxant, was invaluable. The advances in materials science and technology that allowed the development of rubber endotracheal and endobronchial tubes, reliable and safe mechanical ventilators and, more recently, plastic tubes and fibre optics, were crucial. It should also be remembered that concomitant medical advances in areas such as asepsis, antibiosis and public health were also of great significance, as the focus of chest disease gradually changed during the period under consideration from chronic infective lung disease towards mostly malignant disease. Surgical techniques were advancing rapidly at the same time, and increasingly challenging operations frequently highlighted the inadequacy of the available anaesthetic apparatus. While all these medical advances should be borne in mind, this chapter will concentrate on the apparatus for controlling the airway during thoracotomy, mentioning other developments only when necessary for contextual reasons.

Tracheal intubation

The first necessary advance was easy and reliable tracheal intubation. While there are many claims to early successes in this field, the accepted pioneers of tracheal intubation were Ivan Magill and Stanley Rowbotham. Magill and Rowbotham were officers in the Royal Army Medical Corps during the First World War, and were posted after the war to the Queen's Hospital for Facial and Jaw Injuries at Sidcup, Kent (now Queen Mary's Hospital). With a little anaesthetic experience between them, they anaesthetized war casualties with horrendous facial injuries for procedures in the new field of plastic surgery in the early 1920s under Major, later Sir, Harold Gillies. Tracheal insufflation of ether and air using a gum-elastic catheter was already available, but was limited by the risk of aspiration of blood and debris in this type of surgery and the need for an escape route for the expiratory gas. They initially added a second tube to allow the escape of expiratory gas, with a throat pack to protect the airway, and finally developed to-and-fro breathing through a single rubber tracheal tube. The anaesthetist could thus control the airway with tube and throat pack, while the surgeon could work unhindered on the face and jaw.

Magill was particularly inventive during this decade, and described a number of developments in anaesthetic apparatus and technique. These included his famous intubating forceps, his breathing attachment, blind nasal intubation, the incorporation of Seibe–Gorman flowmeters (the first 'rotameters') into his anaesthetic apparatus and the first rubber tracheal tubes to be 'armoured' with a wire spiral in their wall, which he named 'surgeon-proof tubes'!

As was the normal custom at the time, both Magill and Rowbotham took up various other part-time positions as anaesthetists at hospitals in and around London. Amongst other posts, in 1923 Magill was appointed 'chloro-formist to the Brompton Hospital for Consumption and Diseases of the Chest', where he turned his mind to anaesthesia for thoracic surgery.

The cuffed tube

During the same period, following the First World War, American anaes-thetists were developing techniques for tracheal intubation. The idea of attaching an inflatable balloon or cuff to the tracheal tube was not new, having been described several times since 1871, but Arthur Guedel and Ralph Waters in the United States were the first formally to describe the 'closed endotracheal technique for the administration of anaesthesia', in 1928. To make their point, they proved that they were able to anaesthetize a dog and completely immerse both dog and anaesthetic apparatus in a tank of water with no ill effect!

Early thoracic surgery

Thoracic surgery in the 1920s consisted primarily of surgery for tuberculosis, which was treated by collapsing the affected lung, or for empyema, which required rib resection and drainage of the infected cavity. The patients were in poor health, continually producing copious quantities of purulent sputum. The lung disease would remain unilateral as long as the patient could cough effectively, but one of the risks of surgery was the spread of the pus into the 'good' lung as the cough reflex was inhibited and the patient positioned for the operation. Anaesthesia was either local or inhalational, with spontaneous respiration throughout, although anaesthetic circuits were beginning to incorporate a reservoir bag that could be squeezed.

Magill's first contribution was the design of a wide-mouthed tracheal tube connector (Magill's 'suction union'), which facilitated suction through the tube with a fairly large suction catheter. However, in 1928 he was still advo-cating local anaesthesia or light general anaesthesia using nitrous oxide and oxygen with a tight-fitting facemask for thoracoplasty or decortication. Essentially he was maintaining the patient's cough reflex throughout the operation to remove tracheal secretions, which couldn't have made for a 'quiet' surgical field, but Magill insisted that this gave the best results at the time. Tracheal intubation alone was not the answer to the secretion problem, but further developments were limited by anatomy, the lung pathology and the materials available to manufacture tubes capable of occluding a bronchus safely whilst maintaining a route for ventilation.

Endobronchial intubation and one-lung anaesthesia

The concept of endobronchial intubation had its roots in the late nineteenth century. Experimental physiology work on dogs published by Head in 1889 described endobronchial intubation using a long, cuffed metal bronchial tube, attached to a short tracheal tube. However, the first description of 'closed endobronchial anaesthesia', or true one-lung anaesthesia, came from Joseph Gale and Ralph Waters of Madison, Wisconsin, USA, as a direct extension of earlier cuffed endotracheal tube work (Gale and Waters, 1932). Their tube incorporated a large single cuff, and was intended for blind passage under deep spontaneous breathing anaesthesia. With the tip bent to one side by moulding in warm water, they found that it could be passed into either main bronchus by directing the tip to right or left as required and advancing it until resistance was encountered. The cuff would then be inflated to straddle the carina, successfully isolating the opposite lung (Fig. 1.1). This gave one-lung anaesthesia immediately at the start of the procedure. They also described how spontaneous respiration could be assisted manually if breathing was inadequate. The tube had to be withdrawn into the trachea at the end of the surgery to inflate both lungs, and could be advanced back down the bronchus if the operative lung needed to be collapsed again. Whilst this provided adequate one-lung anaesthesia, it had several drawbacks: the tube was easily dislodged during the surgery; collapse of the lung was slow as it relied on gas absorption; the right upper lobe bronchus could be obstructed with a right-sided cannulation; clearance of secretions from the collapsed lung had to be done by the surgeon; and the tube had to be moved to allow reinflation or further collapse of the lung. Furthermore, blind positioning could be made difficult by anatomical distortion in the patient.

A second tracheal cuff was soon added by Rovenstine, in 1936, his tube being made of woven silk. This immediately allowed the option of one- or two-lung ventilation without moving the tube, since both lungs could be ventilated with the tracheal cuff inflated and the bronchial cuff deflated, providing that the tube itself was not a tight fit in the main bronchus. However, all the other limitations of the Gale and Waters tube were still present, particularly the lack of suction down the operative side.

Magill's thoracic apparatus

Magill was working on the problem at the same time in London. He described both his endobronchial tubes and his bronchus blocker in 1935, but he believed in accurate placement of both tube and blocker under

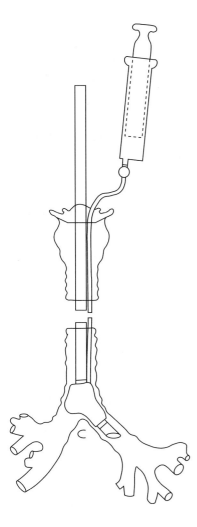

Figure 1.1 Gale and Waters' endobronchial intubation.

direct vision and also devised the necessary rigid intubating bronchoscope and tracheoscope respectively for their insertion. Magill's tubes (Fig. 1.2) were not unlike more modern armoured latex tubes in principle, consisting of a wire spiral covered with a thin rubber tube (making them kink-resistant), with a single, smooth cuff. The wire spiral was allowed to protrude from the distal end of the right-sided tube, preventing too deep an insertion, in an attempt to ensure maintenance of ventilation to the right upper lobe.

Magill's bronchus blocker was a smooth rubber balloon on the tip of a suction catheter, which could be stiffened with a wire stilette, if necessary. The tubes were inserted under direct vision into the appropriate main bronchus by 'railroading' over a lubricated intubating bronchoscope. The blocker was also passed under direct vision, using a specially devised split-sided straight tracheoscope (although it could also be passed down an

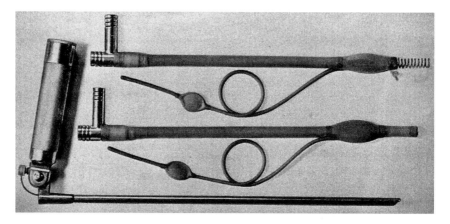

Figure 1.2 Magill's endobronchial tubes and intubating bronchoscope. Note the right-sided tube at the top.

8 mm diameter rigid bronchoscope). The blocker was then inflated and a cuffed tracheal tube was inserted in the trachea alongside the stalk of the blocker.

The endobronchial tubes had similar problems to those of Gale and Waters': instability, slow lung collapse, lack of flexibility and lack of a suction channel. There was at least some recognition of the problem of the short right main bronchus, with the early take-off of the right upper lobe bronchus, and a more accurate mechanism for placement. The bronchus blocker similarly had problems of instability and lack of flexibility when it came to inflating and deflating the lung, and it was in the way during a pneumonectomy, but it did allow suction and quicker lung collapse. Magill's intubating bronchoscope was small enough to pass inside adult-size tracheal tubes, with a small illuminating bulb at the tip and batteries in the handle. The view was fairly limited, particularly in comparison to modern fibre-optic bronchoscopes; thus both tube and blocker required considerable expertise for accurate placement, and they remained the province of specialized units and anaesthetists.

Other bronchus blockers

Throughout the 1930s and 1940s, the principles of endobronchial intubation advanced little further. Various attempts were made to improve on Magill's bronchus blocker during this time. Crafoord, a Swedish surgeon, in 1938 advocated packing the bronchus to be blocked with a ribbon gauze pack using rigid bronchoscopy – his 'tampon' technique. Other materials were tried in an attempt to make a blocker that was less prone to movement, and the most successful blocker ever developed was that of Vernon Thompson (Fig. 1.3), although it was never formally described in the literature. It was larger than Magill's and hence could only be placed through the larger adult Negus rigid bronchoscopes, but it incorporated a nylon mesh bag

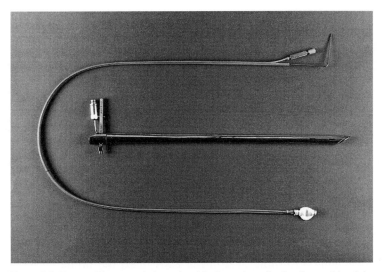

Figure 1.3 Vernon Thompson's bronchus blocker, wire stilet in place, with adult Negus bronchoscope. Note the length. It is bent double for photographic purposes, but is over twice the length of the bronchoscope when straight to allow the 'scope to be withdrawn without disturbing the blocker once in place.

over the rubber cuff, which 'gripped' the bronchial wall and made it less easy to dislodge.

New bronchus blockers were still being described in the early 1950s – Pinson (of ether bomb fame) published his blocker as late as 1952. This consisted of a wire-stiffened plastic tube tipped with a conical perspex plug, which was held in position by constant suction – an old principle, but using new materials and constant suction apparatus. Endobronchial apparatus was about to change radically, however.

Medical advances of the 1940s

By the 1940s, there was significant progress in various areas of medicine that impacted on thoracic anaesthesia. Safer anaesthetic agents such as trichloro-ethylene and intravenous agents such as thiopentone became available. Cyclopropane was manufactured, and the use of positive pressure ventilation with this agent to suppress spontaneous respiratory effort during a thorac-otomy was remarkable when described in 1941. The problem with it was that patients became 'light' very quickly if any leak appeared in the circuit and allowed dilution of inspired gas; for example, as a result of the endo-bronchial apparatus becoming dislodged during the thoracotomy. The first crude mechanical ventilators had become commercially available, but were not in widespread use. Accurate surgical dissection of the lung and ligation of hilar structures for lobectomy became standard practice. Streptomycin, penicillin and anti-tuberculous drugs were available.

Thoracic surgeons were also beginning to diversify into other thoracic surgical areas – for instance, the first successful repair of a tracheo-oesophageal fistula took place in 1941, the first palliative shunt for Fallot's tetralogy was developed by Blalock and Taussig in 1945, and Ivor Lewis described his two-stage oesophagectomy operation in 1946. These advances in surgery must have presented a considerable challenge to the thoracic anaesthetists of the day, with the apparatus available at the time. There is plenty of evidence to suggest that the available anaesthesia was not ideal. There was still debate amongst anaesthetists and surgeons about the need to conserve patient cough effort during 'wet lung' cases and to operate under local anaesthesia. It was eventually realized that coughing in the lateral position with the chest open was ineffective, and more likely to spread the pus than control it. A number of surgeons in the 1940s even described various operative approaches to the chest involving positioning the patient in such a way as to control the lung secretions using gravity. Beecher, in the USA, advocated operating with the patient in a steep head-down lateral position, to favour drainage of secretions up the trachea rather than down into the dependent lung. Overholt, also in the USA, used the prone position with the operative side slightly down to keep secretions within the diseased lung. Parry-Brown popularized lung resection in a similar prone position in the UK. The operative technique for the posterior approach is quite different from the familiar lateral approach, and would now be considered more difficult. That surgeons developed these approaches at all suggests that the anaesthetists' control of the lungs was far from perfect. There was a need for better apparatus.

Bronchoscopic spirometry

The first successful pneumonectomies had taken place from 1931 to 1933, and survival with one lung had been proved possible. Unilateral lung collapse for tuberculosis was both well established and quite successful. Physicians at the time were also investigating techniques for isolating the airway to one or other lung, for the purposes of measuring individual lung function and administering drugs in liquid or gaseous form to one lung only while preventing asphyxia.

In 1932, Jacobaeus and colleagues from Stockholm, Sweden, published a paper describing experiments on bronchoscopic spirometry (or 'broncho-spirometry', as they named it), which included a description of a cuffed rigid bronchoscope that could cannulate either main bronchus. This was followed by a description of a coaxial, double-lumen, rigid metal broncho-scope with tracheal and bronchial cuffs for endobronchial intubation (Fig. 1.4). The two lumens, while concentric, were designed to contain the same volume of air and offer the same resistance to gas flow. The apparatus was passed into either main bronchus, the cuffs were inflated and spirometric and gas exchange measurements could be obtained for each lung independently. While anaesthesia is mentioned, the degree of sedation or anaesthesia used is not clear in the paper. The authors do refer to the effects that anaesthesia, insertion of the bronchoscope and the resistance of the apparatus

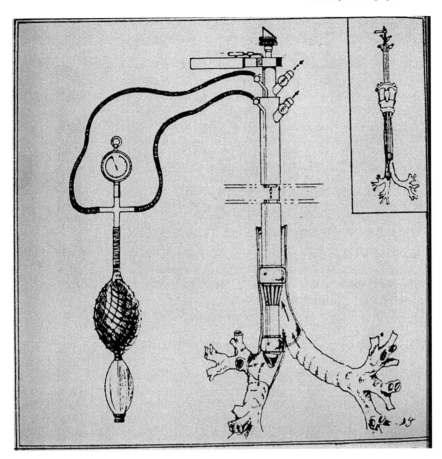

Figure 1.4 Frenckner's coaxial double-lumen rigid bronchoscope for bronchospirometry.

could have on any measurements made. This is the first apparatus described using the principles of the double-lumen tube.

Rubber tubes for bronchospirometry

The rigid Swedish apparatus obviously had limitations. Various workers realized that the apparatus required was a flexible, double-lumen rubber tube with tracheal and bronchial cuffs, which could be passed blindly down the trachea and reliably into a main bronchus of a patient under minimal sedation and topical anaesthesia only.

The first of these was developed by Paul Gebauer in Cleveland, Ohio, in 1938; it was a left-sided rubber double-lumen tube that would certainly be recognized by a modern anaesthetist, although the lumens were small by current standards. Available in three adult sizes, it incorporated a fine steel spring in its wall for rigidity and had a preformed shape that helped it to pass into the left main bronchus. It was, however, not easy to position, and required X-ray control. William Zavod of New York described a similar rubber tube in 1940, which also incorporated a small steel plate in its tip that would show up clearly on X-ray. Positioning was still a problem. A metal stilette with a distal curve was passed down the bronchial lumen of this tube to direct it through the larynx and into the left main bronchus under fluoroscopic control. In an attempt to reduce inaccuracies in bronchospirometric measurements produced by the high resistance of these tubes, Norris and colleagues, in 1948, even cannulated the left main bronchus with a single-lumen tube and allowed right lung ventilation via the larynx and mouth. However, accurate positioning of the tube remained the fundamental problem, particularly in the presence of anatomical distortion due to lung disease.

Carlens' tube – the breakthrough

The breakthrough again came from Sweden, in 1949, when Eric Carlens (from the same Ear, Nose and Throat department as Frenckner in Stockholm) invented his now familiar double-lumen tube (Fig. 1.5). Initially this was described for bronchospirometry.

Carlens' tube was made of moderately rigid rubber to a preformed shape; the cuffs and pilot tubes were added, and the tube finished by dipping in latex solution. The bevel at the tip was cut at the optimum angle for entering the left main bronchus when it reached the carina. He also recommended the use of a shaped stilet to assist placement and, of course, he designed the carinal hook to ensure that the tube was unlikely to pass too far down the bronchus. The hook was to be tied down during insertion using thread with a slipknot, which could be released once the tube was past the vocal cords. Reliable cannulation of the left main bronchus could be obtained without X-ray screening, the lumens were certainly larger and gave much lower resistance than those of Gebauer's and Zavod's tubes, and patients could even exercise

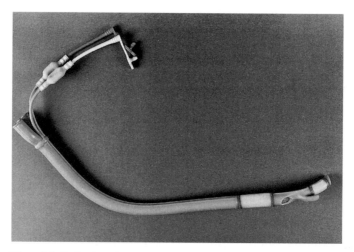

Figure 1.5 Carlens' 'catheter'.

on a cycle ergometer with the tube in place! This was a major breakthrough, and its anaesthetic potential was immediately seen – its successful use in thoracic anaesthesia was described just the following year (1950) by Viking Bjork, the Swedish surgeon, and Carlens. (The patient was intubated when awake by Carlens himself, and then anaesthetized for the thoracotomy!) This tube is still readily available, and remains the most reliable for entering the left main bronchus on blind passage. This is probably due to the rigidity of the tube, the angle of bevel at the tip of the bronchial lumen, and the fact that the carinal hook pushes against the opposite wall of the trachea as the tip enters the left main bronchus.

Progress in the 1950s

The 1950s represented a period of tremendous development in anaesthesia. Many techniques routinely used today became accepted practice during that period, such as the use of muscle relaxants, positive pressure ventilation and modern halogenated volatile anaesthetic agents. Surgeons were embarking on increasingly complex surgery, more for lung cancer than for infective lung disease. Radical pneumonectomy for tumour was described by Brock and Whytehead in 1955, and bronchoplastic surgery had started. Between 1951 and 1956, several surgeons described 'sleeve resection'. This involved resecting an upper lobe, together with a part of the main bronchus, anastomosing the remaining bronchus end-to-end or to the lower trachea, and reconstructing the carina. The thoracic surgeon's expectations of the anaesthetist's apparatus must have increased accordingly.

Although acclaimed as a major advance in the field, the Carlens catheter had its limitations given the advances in surgery at the time. It was not universally accepted in thoracic anaesthesia, and a proliferation of attempts to improve on the apparatus ensued. The carinal hook could be awkward, and wasn't to every anaesthetist's liking. It was inconvenient to the surgeon when closing the bronchial stump during a right pneumonectomy or operating at the carina, and the lumens were still relatively small when it came to passing the largest possible suction catheter to clear viscous secretions. Mechanical ventilators were coming into routine use, and the resistance to both inspiration and expiration was still fairly high. The tube also had to be pulled back into the trachea during a period of apnoea while the surgeon closed the bronchus during a left pneumonectomy. The search was on for an endobronchial tube with the largest possible internal bore and the lowest possible resistance, which could be used to cannulate either main bronchus safely, and that would allow the surgeon the best possible access to the main bronchus and carina from the operative side without the tube obstructing the operative field. In addition, it had to be easy to position both blindly and accurately. This was not to be achieved for another 10 years. The anatomy of the short right main bronchus and the right upper lobe bronchus remained the principal bar to the invention of a successful right endobronchial tube.

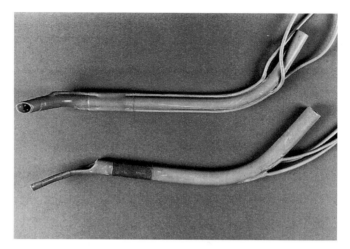

Figure 1.6 Macintosh–Leatherdale bronchial tube (top) and tracheal tube with bronchus blocker (bottom).

Combined single-lumen tubes and bronchus blockers

The idea of fixing a bronchus blocker onto the end of a tracheal tube appealed to some workers, since this combined a low resistance tube for ventilation with control of the operative lung. Sturtzbecker was the first to describe such tubes in 1953. He devised two types, both being rubber tracheal tubes with an inflatable blocker extending from the tip, which also contained a suction lumen. One had a blocker of 7 cm length for insertion into either main bronchus; the other was of 9 cm length for insertion into a lower lobe bronchus for lobectomy only. A wire stilet was used to direct the blocker into the side required, and secretions could be drained through the suction lumen. The whole tube still had to be withdrawn to allow the surgeon to close the bronchus, since the blocker was in the way.

In 1955, Macintosh and Leatherdale of Oxford described a pair of tubes of preformed shape for cannulation of the left main bronchus (Fig. 1.6), which were simple to use, easy to position blindly and allowed collapse of one lung and reventilation of both lungs without the tube being moved. One was a simple left-sided single-lumen endobronchial tube with tracheal and bronchial cuffs and a suction lumen opening just below the tracheal cuff. This gave good ventilation of the left lung and some control of secretions from the right. By choosing a size of tube that was not a tight fit in the left main bronchus, both lungs could be ventilated again without moving the tube if the tracheal cuff was inflated and the bronchial deflated. The other was a tracheal tube with a left-sided bronchus blocker at the end, which contained a suction lumen. This allowed good ventilation of the right lung while the left was collapsed, some control of secretions and easy reventilation of both lungs without moving the tube; however, it still posed the problem of having to pull the tube back during a period of apnoea while the surgeon closed the bronchial stump during a left pneumonectomy. The suction lumens for the collapsed lung were small in both the Sturtzbecker and Macintosh–Leatherdale apparatus, and proved inadequate for cases with gross secretions.

Intubation of the right main bronchus – the slotted cuff

The left pneumonectomy still posed a problem. The only right-sided tube so far was the Vellacott tube (1954), which was an ingenious tube specifically for right upper lobectomy. A single-lumen tube, it had tracheal and bronchial cuffs and openings at the tip for ventilation of the right middle and lower lobes, and between the cuffs at the carina for ventilation of the left lung. The bronchial cuff was intended to obstruct the right upper lobe bronchus, controlling secretions in the lobe during surgery on it, and prevent loss of ventilation through any bronchopleural fistula in the upper lobe. It certainly did not allow ventilation of the upper lobe – quite the opposite.

The next breakthrough came in 1955. Wally Gordon, a surgeon, and Ronald Green, an anaesthetist, working together at St George's Hospital in London, saw the need for a right-sided endobronchial tube that would reliably allow ventilation of all three lobes of the right lung, giving free surgical access to the left main bronchus and lower left tracheal wall. They realized that closer study of the bronchial anatomy of the area was the key to successful design of a tube, so they examined bronchograms of 80 adults with normal bronchi (40 of each sex) and made accurate measurements of the right upper lobe take-off and tracheo-bronchial angle. From their measurements, they were able to design a range of tube sizes with correct relative dimensions and angles. The resultant tube, described initially in 1955 and later modified, was the first to incorporate the 'slotted cuff' – a right-sided endobronchial cuff with an aperture which, when positioned,

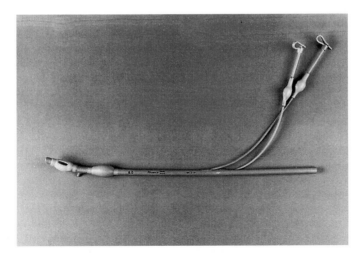

Figure 1.7 Modern version of the Gordon–Green single-lumen endobronchial tube.

opened opposite the upper lobe bronchus (Fig. 1.7). They also used a carinal hook, slightly shorter than Carlens' hook, to prevent the tube from passing too far down because, like the Macintosh–Leatherdale, it was intended for passing blindly – although an intubating bronchoscope could be used. The correct tube size was again one that was not a tight fit in the bronchus, allowing both lungs to be reventilated easily by deflation of the bronchial cuff.

There has always been some mild controversy over whether the tube should be named the 'Gordon–Green' or the 'Green–Gordon', anaesthetists naturally favouring the latter. In fact, Gordon was the first author of the first description of the tube in *The Lancet* in 1955, while Green's paper, although giving a much better description of their work, did not appear in *Anaesthesia* until 1957 (Green and Gordon, 1957). Therefore, by convention, it should probably be the surgeon first!

It is now realized that the rubber tube with the slotted cuff was, in fact, a much cleverer idea than the original inventors thought at the time. During manufacture, the slot was cut out of the tube and the edges of the cuff were glued by hand to the *inside* edge of the slot. This made the narrow slot actually open up and become wider as the cuff was inflated because of tension in the rubber of the cuff. A short portion of bronchial cuff proximal to the slot engaged the upper surface of the main bronchus, but most of the cuff inflation occurred on the opposite side to the slot, which had the effect of pushing the widened slot up towards the upper lobe bronchus origin. Although Gordon and Green did not realize it, these manoeuvres had the net effect of improving the margin of error for position of the tube with respect to the upper lobe bronchus, and of allowing for some anatomical variation. While this did not have a major impact on the use of their tube, it was one of the factors that accounted for the success of the right-sided Robertshaw tube some years later, which uses an identical cuff, and for the failure of some other right-sided tubes that used a different design. It is a property of rubber tubes, which still cannot be emulated by the manufacturers of plastic double-lumen tubes using high-volume, low-pressure cuffs.

The problem of sleeve resection

As mentioned above, the 1950s represented a particularly inventive period in anaesthesia, many of the advances being stimulated by progress in surgery. For example, Sir Clement Price Thomas was one of the pioneers of the increasingly aggressive lung and bronchial sleeve resection of the time at the Brompton Hospital. William Pallister, having to anaesthetize many such cases there, was vexed by the frequent damage done to his left endobronchial tube cuff by the surgeon during these operations. He was already using Machray's tubes, which were modified Magill single-lumen rubber tubes with a much smaller cuff for the left main bronchus to avoid obstructing the surgeon's access. However, he still found that the surgeon would puncture the cuff, causing him to lose control of the ventilation and anaesthesia. His response was to design a single-lumen left-sided endobronchial tube with tracheal and bronchial cuffs which, like the Magill and Machray tubes, had to be positioned using an intubating bronchoscope, but which incorporated a second bronchial cuff inside the outer one. When the surgeon punctured the outer cuff during the operation, the anaesthetist could simply inflate the second cuff, preventing loss of ventilation or disruption of the surgery. The 'Brompton Pallister' tube was described in 1959, although it had been in use for some time before that. It was certainly a superb example of the anaesthetist's ingenuity in rising to meet the needs of the surgery of the day.

Modifications of the Carlens tube

As might be expected, modification of the Carlens tube was inevitable during this period. Whilst it was a major advance, it had its limitations. The carinal hook was considered unnecessary by some and even hazardous by others, the lumens were small, the resistance to gas flow was still quite high, and the material of manufacture (a stiff rubber tube with thin cuffs coated with latex) was not durable.

The first of the modified Carlens tubes was that developed by Roger Bryce-Smith of Oxford and described in 1959. Shaped rubber extrusion manufacturing was available by that time, particularly from the Leyland and Birmingham Rubber Company, which helped to develop many anaesthetic products. Bryce-Smith's left-sided double-lumen tube was made of cured, extruded rubber, with cuffs made of thin sheet rubber and pilot tubes included within the walls of the tube as part of the extrusion rather than being added on later – a more sleek and durable design than the Carlens. Shaped with the appropriate anatomical curves, its lumens were in the antero-posterior plane rather than left to right, making the tube rather flat from side-to-side. This made it easier to pass through the vocal cords, and allowed slightly larger lumens than the Carlens. The bronchial lumen was posterior, the tracheal anterior, and the carinal hook was dispensed with altogether. Whilst being less damaging to the cords, this configuration meant that the tracheal lumen opened in the midline, directly over the anterior aspect of the carina, rather than over the right main bronchus. This immediately limited the quality of suction access to the right main bronchus. Fenestrations were added at the lower end of the tracheal lumen in an effort to improve the suction, but this aspect of the tube was always its main limitation. Bryce-Smith, working with Richard Salt, the technician in the Nuffield Department of Anaesthetics at Oxford, realized that he could utilize Gordon and Green's slotted right cuff design to make a right-sided version of his left-sided double-lumen tube. This was duly published the following year, 1960, the right-sided version being known as the Bryce-Smith Salt tube (Fig. 1.8). The tube had the same suction problems for the non-intubated bronchus; the slot is similar to that of the Gordon–Green, but is in a slightly different position – a little more proximal and anterior.

A right-sided version of the Carlens tube was also inevitable at this time, and this was published in the same edition of *Anaesthesia* as the Bryce-Smith Salt tube! Again inspired by the Gordon–Green tube, Malcolm White of Middlesborough worked with Rusch Ltd of Stuttgart to produce a right-sided Carlens-type tube, with carinal hook and slotted right bronchial cuff. However, the slot was a little smaller than that of Gordon and Green, and was of necessity manufactured differently because of the latex-dip process used to make the cuffs of the Carlens tube. Instead of being glued to

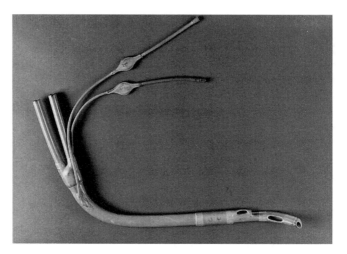

Figure 1.8 Bryce-Smith Salt tube.

the inside edges of the slot, the thin cuff was merely stuck onto the outside edges of the slot. The slot being short, and lacking all the properties of the Gordon and Green design, it was less successful in ensuring right upper lobe ventilation than it might have been.

By 1960 a reasonable range of endobronchial apparatus was available to the anaesthetist, although some of the items required considerable expertise in their use and would not have been used regularly outside the major thoracic units. Various single- and double-lumen endobronchial tubes were on the market for cannulation of either main bronchus, each with its own advantages and disadvantages. A double-lumen tube was still required that incorporated the best features of the Carlens tube, was made with a rubber extrusion similar to the Bryce-Smith, used a slotted cuff identical to the Gordon–Green, and was of the correct size and curvature to allow successful and reliable blind positioning down either side in the majority of patients such that it could be used by the non-specialist anaesthetist.

Frank Leonard Robertshaw

Frank Robertshaw came to Manchester in 1954, and immediately became involved in thoracic anaesthesia, working with John Dark, the thoracic surgeon. Using the Carlens tube extensively, he soon realized its problems and saw the need for major modifications. Although he found no problem in placing the tube, he thought that the narrow lumens were a major drawback by virtue of their high resistance to gas flow and the limited size of suction catheter that could be passed down them. He also considered the imported German tubes to be expensive, and thought a cheaper British alternative could be made. Although ventilators could overcome the inspiratory resistance, he felt that the resistance to passive expiration was significant, especially in cases of emphysema, where it compounded the patient's air trapping. Robertshaw thought that the best solution was to use a double-lumen tube with the largest possible lumens, leading him to develop his tube by

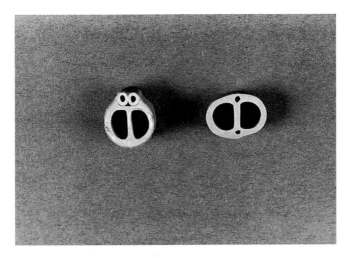

Figure 1.9 Cross-sections showing rubber extrusion patterns for comparable sized tubes. Left: 37G Carlens'. Right: Medium Robertshaw.

a process of trial and error, with the close co-operation of the Leyland and Birmingham Rubber Company of Leyland, Lancashire. The basic rubber extrusion used produced two D-shaped lumens side-by-side (Fig. 1.9). The lumens were rather larger and rounder than the equivalent Carlens tube. The pilot tubes were in the front and back walls, the tube having a flattened appearance from front to back. The enlarged lumens immediately reduced the resistance to gas flow and allowed the passage of a larger suction catheter to deal with viscous secretions. The right bronchial cuff followed accurately the pattern of the Gordon–Green (which was also made at Leyland). The carinal hook was not considered necessary and was omitted altogether.

Robertshaw then experimented clinically to obtain the correct sizes for an adult range of tubes, and the correct relative dimensions and angles for each of the three sizes. On regular visits to Leyland, each slight modification was incorporated into a further prototype, which would be made for him by hand while he took lunch; he would then return to Manchester with the latest specimen tube to try it out. Thus the Robertshaw tube was truly designed to meet clinical needs in a practical manner. After considerable experimentation, Robertshaw published details of his now familiar 'low resistance double-lumen endobronchial tubes' in 1962, and they are still quoted as the gold standard against which other double-lumen tubes are compared.

Like the Gordon–Green, the Robertshaw tube contained features that have proved even more successful than its inventor could possibly have guessed at the time. The style of extrusion, giving a flattened tube with two D-shaped lumens, was intended for low resistance and ease of suction. Robertshaw had no idea that this would also facilitate the passage of a fibre-optic bronchoscope, or that thoracic anaesthetists would ever find themselves having to anaesthetize patients with end-stage emphysema and gross air trapping (requiring the lowest possible expiratory resistance), for lung volume reduction surgery or lung transplantation. This extrusion pattern has since been copied by most of the manufacturers of plastic double-lumen tubes. It has now been demonstrated that the right-sided Leyland rubber Robertshaw still has the best margin of error of all right-sided double-lumen tubes with respect to the right upper lobe bronchus. However, Robertshaw did not patent his tube; he did not consider it sufficiently original, and maintained that he had merely taken the best features of several other tubes and incorporated them into one. He retired in 1979 through ill health, and died in 1992, having received little recognition for his contribution to thoracic anaesthesia.

Plastic double-lumen tubes

The relative merits of rubber and plastic tubes and various types of cuff have been hotly debated in recent years, and the debate continues. Bronchial rupture is certainly well described with both types of tube. When anaesthetizing patients with extremely non-compliant lungs, such as cases of lung fibrosis for single-lung transplantation, the required cuff pressure to make a seal has to approach the very high peak intrapulmonary pressure in the dependent lung. This may well negate the theoretical value of the high-volume, low-pressure cuff. With the increasing profile of environmental issues, the idea of reusable products made from sustainable resources may yet win the day; however, disposable plastic tubes have been developed in profusion in recent years.

The first successful double-lumen tube made of polyvinyl chloride (PVC) was devised by the National Catheter Corporation (NCC) in the USA, who indeed consulted Frank Robertshaw during the development of their Bronchocath. NCC subsequently became part of Mallinckrodt, and the tube has undergone various modifications, such as the blue colour coding of the endobronchial cuff, addition of radio-opaque markers, etc. The tube is very similar to the Robertshaw in cross-section, but the use of extruded PVC allows the walls of the tube to be marginally thinner than that of the equivalent rubber tube, giving slightly larger lumens. The cuffs are of the high-volume, low-pressure type, but the right bronchial cuff has completely different properties from the rubber tube. As with most other plastics (and unlike rubber), PVC is thermoplastic and softens on rising to body temperature, which does not help to promote tube stability. The left-sided Bronchocath is much like the Robertshaw, although the bronchial limb is shorter. If anything, this makes obstruction of the left upper lobe bronchus less likely if the tube is inserted too far. It can also be advantageous during a double-lung transplant, allowing the left bronchial anastomosis to be sutured without having to withdraw the tube. The bevel at the tip, like the Carlens tube, is the reverse of the Robertshaw which, if anything, makes inadvertent intubation of the right main bronchus with the left-sided tube less likely. Accurate placement of the right-sided tube in particular and regular checking of tube position requires more frequent use of a fibre-optic device, although the Bronchocath is also available with a carinal hook.

Plastic double-lumen tubes are also made by several other manufacturers, including Portex, Rusch and Sheridan (Fig. 1.10). The overall profile of the tubes is very similar, and there is little to choose between the types as far as

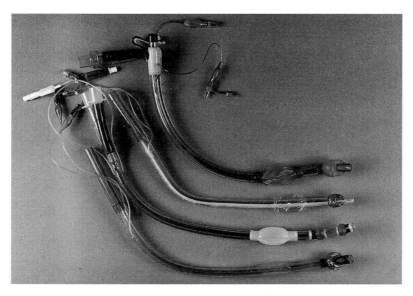

Figure 1.10 Some currently available disposable plastic right-sided double-lumen tubes showing bronchial cuffs. From top down: Portex, Rusch, Sheridan, Mallinckrodt.

the left-sided tubes are concerned. The perennial problem has always been the right bronchial cuff, which doesn't behave like the slotted rubber cuff – as evidenced by the wide variation in design between the manufacturers. They all have a slot in the tube of varying size for the upper lobe orifice, but the cuff design varies. The inflated cuff does not pull on the edge of the slot, so the slot size is fixed. The Sheridan tube has an ingenious pair of cuffs, with one above and one below the slot – an idea that has also been tried in right-sided rubber tubes in the past. There is little evidence that any one of the available plastic right-sided tubes is any better than any other for ventilation of the right upper lobe – the user must be prepared to employ a fibre-optic bronchoscope to be certain of tube position, and the margin of error of position is much less than with the red-rubber Robertshaw.

Other ideas revisited

Some older ideas have been revisited in recent years in plastic, with varying degrees of success. One such was the coaxial double-lumen tube designed by Nazari and colleagues from Pavia, Italy, and described in 1986. In this case, two lungs could be ventilated using a normal large tracheal tube and, when collapse of the operative lung was required, a small, cuffed, shaped inner tube would be passed down through the tracheal tube (blindly) into the required bronchus to allow ventilation of one lung through the inner tube and the other through the remaining annular lumen of the outer tube. The inner tube for the right side incorporated a small sidearm near the tip, which was designed to cannulate the upper lobe bronchus. The whole design was

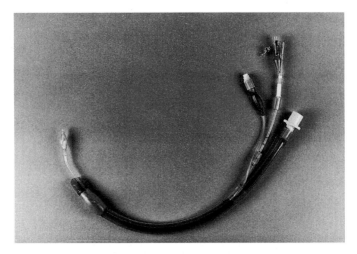

Figure 1.11 Univent endotracheal tube with bronchus blocker.

subsequently found to have a very high resistance, suction was very limited and insertion of the inner tubes was difficult. It really required fibre-optic positioning, but no access to the trachea was possible once the inner tube had been inserted, so it was impossible to view the occluded bronchus from above.

The idea of a tracheal tube with a bronchus blocker has also been revisited, in the form of the Univent tube, manufactured by Fuji Systems of Tokyo, Japan (Fig. 1.11). This device consists of a silicon rubber tracheal tube with a small second lumen, through which a small inflatable balloon on the end of a stiff plastic suction tube can be advanced into the main bronchus of the lung to be collapsed. The blocker can be positioned blindly although fibre-optic positioning is quite simple, using the tracheal lumen to view the advancing blocker from above. Suction down the collapsed side is possible, although the suction lumen is small, as was the case with the old rubber blockers. There have been a number of publications describing the successful use of this device in various circumstances. It certainly gives one-lung ventilation with a low expiratory resistance, and it is easy to use in conjunction with a fibre-optic bronchoscope. Whether it offers any real advantage over modern double-lumen tubes is a matter of debate (see Chapter 19).

Single-lumen endobronchial tubes and simple bronchus blockers have also recently been revisited in plastic. Rusch now manufacture a single-lumen, right-sided PVC endobronchial tube that could, in fact, be used on either side. It has a cuff around a slot for the upper lobe bronchus, but has no carinal hook, making blind positioning difficult. Rusch also market a modern bronchus blocker, which consists of a flexible plastic tube with a cuff at the tip. It has no wire or other device to stiffen it, or any suction lumen. It closely resembles a Fogarty embolectomy catheter – both Fogarty and Swan–Ganz catheters have been used as bronchus blockers in the past.

Short double-lumen tubes intended for one-lung anaesthesia or differential lung ventilation in patients with longstanding tracheostomies can also be obtained from at least two of the manufacturers of plastic tubes.

Paediatric double-lumen tubes

It has always been taught that one-lung anaesthesia is rarely required in children, paediatric double-lumen tubes do not exist, and that the lumens of a paediatric double-lumen tube would present such a high resistance as to be impossible to use safely. A limited number of paediatric Robertshaw tubes, both right and left, have in fact been made by Leyland Rubber in the past, strictly on a bespoke basis for specific children of 6–8 years of age, largely for bronchopulmonary lavage in cases of alveolar proteinosis. Techniques have also been described of using long tracheal tubes advanced into one or other main bronchus to ventilate one lung only, and of using Fogarty catheters as bronchus blockers, placed under bronchoscopic vision. Some plastic double-lumens, including the Bronchocath, are now available in sizes down to 28 French gauge (left side only), which can be used in children from about 10 years onwards, while red-rubber Robertshaw tubes can now be obtained in an extra small (32G) size (right and left). Otherwise, the situation for smaller children has not changed appreciably (see Chapter 12).

Constant positive airway pressure (CPAP) in one-lung anaesthesia

The use of oxygen insufflation to the collapsed lung to reduce the shunt during one-lung anaesthesia has been widely practised for some years. Traditionally, oxygen from a source other than the anaesthetic machine was passed down the lumen of the collapsed side using a suction catheter. The resistance to outflow caused by the occupation of most of the tube lumen by the catheter necessarily led to a slight distending pressure in the collapsed lung, which helped to reduce the hypoxia even further. While many thoracic anaesthetists have probably improvised for years, the first commercially available apparatus for providing oxygen to the collapsed lung with a calibrated constant positive airway pressure valve has been marketed by Mallinckrodt in the last few years, specifically for the Broncho-cath. The manufacturers of anaesthetic machines have yet to catch up by providing the thoracic anaesthetist with a second, flow-calibrated supply of oxygen from the machine.

The current position of the 'Robertshaw' tube

In 1991, Rusch Ltd purchased Leyland Medical Ltd (the modern descendant of the Leyland and Birmingham Rubber Company) and immediately closed its factory in Lancashire. Orders for Leyland Robertshaw tubes were automatically diverted to Rusch, who provided their versions of the tubes. These were manufactured along the same lines, and used the same basic rubber extrusions, as their Carlens tubes, but without the hooks. Initially, the right-sided versions exhibited slots for the right upper lobe similar to

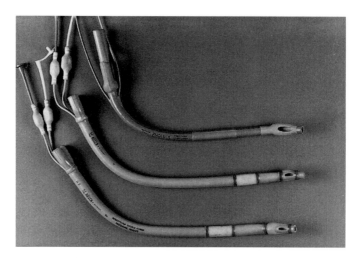

Figure 1.12 Currently available medium sized right-sided red-rubber double-lumen tubes showing bronchial cuffs. Top: Robertshaw (Phoenix); middle: White's (Rusch); bottom: 'Robertshaw' (Rusch).

those of White's tube, which had never behaved in quite the manner of the true Gordon–Green type. Despite modification, these tubes were not perceived by anaesthetists as being equivalent to those developed by Frank Robertshaw himself (Fig. 1.12).

The term 'Robertshaw' now seems to have become a generic name for all double-lumen tubes, made of any material, which resemble in principle his original design. While this may be a fitting tribute to the success of his design, he was quite specific in his design, even down to the exact angles and dimensions of the tubes, and would intermittently check the manufacturers if any significant variation came to light.

Later, in 1991, a group of ex-Leyland workers (including the very same one who had made Robertshaw's prototypes for him 30 years previously) with countless years of experience in the rubber industry between them were able to set up their own factory, naming themselves 'Phoenix Medical'. They swiftly updated and modernized the idea of the rubber double-lumen tube, and sought the approval of the late Frank Robertshaw's executors to manufacture tubes to his pattern, with the addition of new features such as the conventional blue colouring of the bronchial cuff. These tubes are now readily available again, and this company is the only one currently making tubes true to Robertshaw's original specification. The range has been increased with the addition of an extra small size and pre-sterilized, single-use tubes made from rubber.

To complete the picture, Phoenix Medical can now also produce modernized versions of the Gordon–Green style of tube on request, with up-to-date blue bronchial cuffs, still retaining the traditional carinal hook.

> **KEY POINTS**
>
> - The history of endobronchial intubation reflects contemporary progress in other areas of medicine, and in the associated technology.
>
> - The development of new equipment was often stimulated by progress in surgery and other branches of medicine.
>
> - There are few truly original new ideas in the field of thoracic anaesthetic equipment, and much can be learnt from study of past designs.
>
> - The double-lumen tube remains the standard means of producing lung separation in adult anaesthesia.
>
> - While both rubber and plastic have their proponents, rubber tubes may still offer some advantages in this field, since there are differences in the behaviour of the two materials that become clinically significant in tubes of this complexity.

Bibliography

Barry, J.E.S. and Adams, A.P. (1996). The development of thoracic anaesthesia. In *The History of Cardiothoracic Surgery from Early Times* (R. Hurt, ed.). Parthenon Publishing.

Benumof, J.L. (1995). *Anaesthesia for Thoracic Surgery*. Saunders.

Carlens, E. (1949). A new flexible double-lumen catheter for bronchospirometry. *J. Thorac. Surg.*, **18**, 742–6.

Gale, J.W. and Waters, R.M. (1932). Closed endobronchial anesthesia in thoracic surgery. *J. Thorac. Surg.*, **1**, 432–7.

Green, R. and Gordon, W. (1957). Right lung anaesthesia. Anaesthesia for left lung surgery using a new right endobronchial tube. *Anaesthesia*, **12**, 86–93.

Jacobaeus, H.C., Frenckner, P. and Bjorkman, S. (1932). Some attempts at determining the volume and function of each lung separately. *Acta Medica Scand.*, **79**, 174–215.

McKenna, M.J., Wilson, R.S. and Botelho, R.J. (1988). Right upper lobe obstruction with right-sided double-lumen endobronchial tubes: a comparison of two tube types. *J. Cardiothorac. Anesth.*, **2**, 734–40.

Rendell-Baker, L. (1980). History of anesthesia for thoracic surgery: a chronology. *Anesthesiol. Rev.*, **7(10)**, 8–12.

Robertshaw, F.L. (1962). Low resistance double-lumen endobronchial tubes. *Br. J. Anaesth.*, **34**, 576–9.

White, G.M.J. (1960). Evolution of endotracheal and endobronchial intubation. *Br. J. Anaesth.*, **32**, 235–46.

2

Pulmonary physiology during one-lung ventilation

Sir Keith Sykes

Introduction

One-lung ventilation is required to control the distribution of ventilation if the airways to the opposite lung are to be opened, or if the surgical procedure is facilitated by collapse of that lung. The technique is also used to prevent spread of secretions from one lung to the other, and as a route for therapeutic unilateral lung lavage. One-lung ventilation is inevitably associated with gross changes in respiratory physiology. Amongst other factors, the extent of these changes is affected by posture and by the effects of anaesthesia and muscle paralysis. In order to clarify the significance of these effects, the factors that govern the normal distribution of ventilation and blood flow in the lungs will be discussed, and consideration then given to how these distributions are modified by the adoption of the supine and lateral positions. This will be followed by a description of the effects of anaesthesia and muscle paralysis. Finally, how these and other factors may modify the changes produced by one-lung ventilation will be discussed.

Normal distribution of perfusion and ventilation

Distribution of perfusion

Since the pulmonary circulation is a low pressure, low resistance system, the distribution of flow is primarily determined by the effects of gravity and the resistance of the blood vessels in each region of the lung. Approximately 40 per cent of the total pulmonary vascular resistance (PVR) arises in the intra-alveolar vessels (the pulmonary capillaries), which are exposed to alveolar pressure. The remainder is contributed by the extra-alveolar vessels, which are situated in the lung parenchyma. These are held open by the difference in pressure between the interior of the vessel and the pressure in the surrounding interstitial space, which is closely related to regional lung volume. Since the resistance of the smaller extra-alveolar vessels may also be affected by changes in vasomotor tone, they exert a major role in determining the distribution of blood flow.

Intra-alveolar vessels

It is well known that the resistance of the intra-alveolar vessels is governed by the relationship between the pulmonary arterial (P_{PA}), pulmonary venous (P_{PV}) and alveolar pressures (P_{ALV}). In the erect posture, the lung may be divided into three zones as defined by West (Fig. 2.1a):

- Zone 1, in the non-dependent area of the lungs where P_{ALV} is greater than P_{PA} and P_{PV} and the alveolar capillaries are collapsed so that there is no blood flow
- Zone 2, where P_{PA} is greater than P_{ALV} but the latter is greater than P_{PV}, and in which blood flow increases approximately linearly from top to bottom of the zone
- Zone 3, where both P_{PA} and P_{PV} are greater than P_{ALV} and there is less increase in flow than in Zone 2.

Since these zones are determined by the relationship between the three pressures, the magnitude of blood flow to each zone will depend on the height and geometry of the lung and on alveolar pressure. Thus there may be a Zone 1 in the erect or lateral posture, but it is unlikely to be present in the supine posture since the vertical height of the supine lung is less than the P_{PA} (Fig. 2.1b). Zone 1 will be increased if P_{ALV} is increased or if P_{PA} is decreased by vasodilator drugs or a decrease in cardiac output, but will be abolished when P_{PA} is increased by exercise or inotropes.

Although this simple model is still valid, subsequent work has revealed more complex interactions that affect the distribution of flow. For example, there is usually some blood flow in Zone 1. There are three possible reasons.

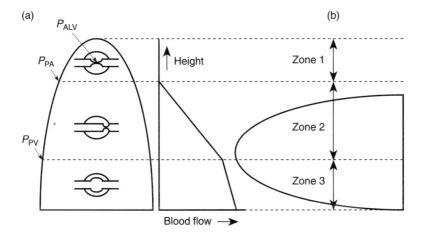

Figure 2.1 The three zone model of the lung showing how the distribution of blood flow from top to bottom of the lung (centre) is determined by the alveolar (P_{ALV}), pulmonary artery (P_{PA}) and pulmonary venous (P_{PV}) pressures. Zone 1, which may be present in the erect lung (a), is not present in the supine position (b) because the vertical height of the lung is less than P_{PA}.

First, the pericapillary pressure (which compresses the capillaries) is less than alveolar pressure, because the latter also has to overcome the surface tension of the fluid lining the alveoli. Second, there are vessels situated in the corners of the alveoli that do not appear to be affected by alveolar pressure, and which can be seen to be perfused under Zone 1 conditions. Third, the size of the zone in the West model is defined by the pulmonary artery mean pressure, which is lower than the pressure existing in the vessels during systole.

The increase in flow in Zone 2 has been explained by the Starling resistor or waterfall effect: the alveolar pressure compresses the capillaries and creates an obstruction to outflow similar to a weir in a river. Flow in this zone is thus governed by the $P_{PA} - P_{ALV}$ difference rather than by the $P_{PA} - P_{PV}$ difference. Since the $P_{PA} - P_{ALV}$ difference increases linearly down the lung, flow also increases linearly. It is still not clear whether the increase in flow in this zone is due mainly to recruitment or distension of vessels, but there is also now some evidence that there may be a more active mechanism that intermittently opens and closes capillary networks to accommodate the changes in flow.

In Zone 3, the driving pressure is $P_{PA} - P_{PV}$. Both pressures increase equally from top to bottom of the zone, so there should be no increase in flow down the zone. Since there is a small increase in flow, it is presumed that the higher intravascular pressures must produce some further distension of vessels in this zone.

Under some circumstances, a Zone 4 of reduced blood flow has been observed in the most dependent parts of the lung. This is probably caused by the increased resistance produced by the long arterial pathway to this part of the lung; however, it may also be due to an increase in interstitial pressure due to transudation of fluid into the interstitial space, to a reduction in regional lung volume associated with airway closure or dependent zone collapse, or to hypoxic pulmonary vasoconstriction induced by regional underventilation (see below).

Extra-alveolar vessels

The extra-alveolar vessels include the large vessels at the hilum and the smaller vessels situated within the lung parenchyma. All these vessels are exposed to variations in pleural pressure, which can alter their diameter and resistance. Changes in pleural pressure around the major vessels produce minimal changes in total PVR since the vessels are large and have a small resistance to flow. However, variations in pleural pressure produce major changes in the resistance of the vessels situated within the lung parenchyma, and so have an important effect on the distribution of pulmonary blood flow. These smaller vessels are held open by the difference between the intravascular pressure and the sub-atmospheric pressure in the interstitial space surrounding the vessels (Fig. 2.2). This pressure is generated by the elastic recoil of surrounding lung tissue, and appears to be closely related to the pressure in the pleural space at the same vertical height as that segment of lung. When the lung is expanded by a spontaneous inspiration,

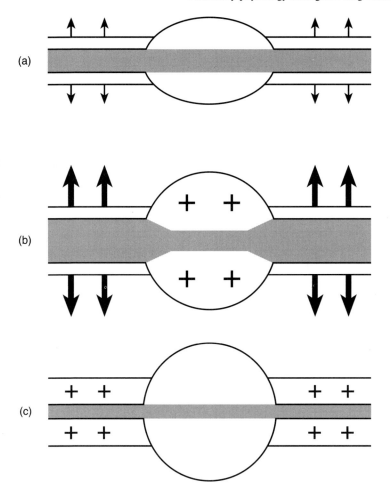

Figure 2.2 Factors determining pulmonary vascular resistance in intra- and extra-alveolar vessels.

(a) The extra-alveolar vessels are held open by the difference between intravascular pressure and the sub-atmospheric pressure in the interstitial space surrounding the vessel. The intra-alveolar vessels are held open by the difference between the pressure in the capillaries and the alveolar pressure.

(b) Inflation of the lung increases lung elastic recoil pressure and so reduces the absolute pressure in the interstitial space. This expands the extra-alveolar vessels and decreases their resistance. The resistance of the intra-alveolar vessels is little changed by spontaneous breathing, since alveolar pressure remains close to atmospheric pressure but is increased when the lungs are inflated by positive pressure. The resulting increase in intra-alveolar resistance may result in a marked increase in total pulmonary vascular resistance when alveolar pressures are high (for example, during the application of positive end-expiratory pressure).

(c) An increase in interstitial pressure due to oedema narrows extra-alveolar vessels and so reduces flow to areas of oedematous lung.

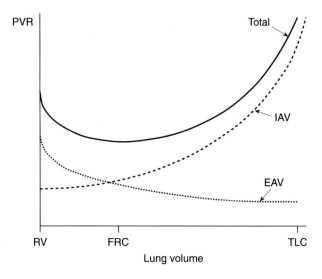

Figure 2.3 Changes of resistance of intra-alveolar (IAV) and extra-alveolar vessels (EAV) with lung volume. Total pulmonary vascular resistance (PVR) is minimal at FRC.

absolute interstitial pressure decreases, so expanding the extra-alveolar vessels and decreasing resistance. Conversely, a decrease in lung volume increases resistance. Inflation of the lung by the application of a positive alveolar pressure produces a similar increase in lung elastic recoil pressure, and so decreases extra-alveolar resistance. However, it also compresses and lengthens the capillaries in the alveolar walls and so increases their resistance. Since the total pulmonary vascular resistance (PVR) is the sum of these two resistances, the plot of PVR against lung volume is U-shaped with the minimum value at functional residual capacity (FRC). As shown in Figure 2.3, high inflation pressures produce a large increase in PVR.

As absolute pleural pressure is least in the non-dependent parts of the pleural space, vessels in these zones should be larger and have a lower resistance than those in dependent zones. The resulting differences in resistance should tend to offset the differences in flow induced by gravity. A decrease in lung volume below FRC tends to narrow vessels in dependent zones, so making the distribution of blood flow more even. An increase in interstitial pressure due to the accumulation of fluid also tends to narrow these vessels, so reducing flow to oedematous areas of lung (Fig. 2.2). Recent studies have shown that regional blood flow per unit volume of lung is greater in the hilar regions than in the periphery of the lung, both in the vertical and horizontal plane. This appears to be due to the increased resistance associated with the increased length of the vessels serving the periphery of the lung, and may be an explanation for the presence of a Zone 4.

Hypoxic pulmonary vasoconstriction

Extra-alveolar vessels are not only affected by lung volume and changes in interstitial pressure, but are also the site of active changes in vessel tone. In the normoxic lung there is little vascular tone. However, when alveolar Po_2 is decreased, the thin walled, smaller pulmonary arterioles ($< 500\ \mu$m) narrow, so reducing flow to the hypoxic area of lung. The mechanism of this hypoxic pulmonary vasoconstrictor response (HPV) is still unknown, but it appears to be a specific characteristic of pulmonary smooth muscle cells. It is believed that the sensitive site lies within the muscle cell of the small arteriole, and that this is able to sense changes in alveolar Po_2 since alveolar gas can diffuse into the vessel wall from the surrounding alveoli. The HPV response curve is S-shaped, with the maximum response occurring between alveolar Po_2 levels of 8 kPa and 4 kPa (60–30 mmHg). The magnitude of the HPV response varies between individuals, but on average there appears to be about a 50 per cent reduction in blood flow when alveolar Po_2 is decreased to mixed venous levels. Decreases in mixed venous Po_2 can also stimulate HPV; these have about one-third of the effect of alveolar Po_2. HPV is usually augmented by an increase in Pco_2. Since a collapsed lung equilibrates with mixed venous Pco_2, which is approximately 1 kPa higher than arterial Pco_2, blood flow is less than it would be if the lung were ventilated with a gas mixture which produced an alveolar Po_2 similar to mixed venous Po_2, but a Pco_2 equal to arterial Pco_2. HPV is most effective when the hypoxic segment is small, for there is a large reservoir of normal lung to receive the diverted flow and the resulting increase in P_{PA} is small. When the hypoxic segment is large, there is less normal lung to receive the diverted blood. As a result, P_{PA} increases and this opposes the increase in vascular tone in the hypoxic segment, so decreasing the efficiency of the mechanism. The administration of vasoconstrictor drugs may preferentially constrict the vessels in the oxygenated areas of lung and so produce a similar effect.

The HPV response is decreased by both an increase in P_{PA} and an increase in left atrial pressure above about 15 mmHg (Fig. 2.4). Handling the lung releases vasodilator prostaglandins, which decrease HPV. Vasodilator drugs such as nitroglycerine and nitroprusside, β-adrenergic drugs such as isoprenaline, dobutamine, ritodrine, orciprenaline and salbutamol, and several calcium channel blockers also depress the mechanism. Inhalational anaesthetics have a similar action, but the effect appears to be unimportant in the concentrations used clinically. Vasoconstrictor drugs such as dopamine, adrenaline and phenylephrine may produce constriction in normoxic areas of lung and increase P_{PA}, so decreasing the efficiency of the mechanism.

Distribution of ventilation

Regional differences in ventilation may be due to regional differences in airway resistance or to regional differences in compliance. Regional differences in airway resistance have little influence on the distribution of

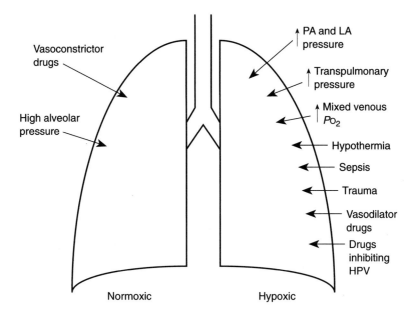

Figure 2.4 Factors that tend to increase blood flow to a hypoxic lung.

ventilation in the normal lung when the patient inspires from FRC and airflow rates are normal, but may tend to divert ventilation to the non-dependent zones when high inspiratory flow rates are used or when dependent zone airway resistance is increased by a reduction in FRC. However, variations in regional resistance in patients with severe airway disease may cause major regional differences in gas distribution.

In the normal lung, the distribution of ventilation during spontaneous respiration is governed mainly by the pressure/volume (P/V) characteristics of the lungs, though distribution may be modified by the paralysis of chest wall muscles or by ribcage distortion due to disease. The pressure difference governing lung expansion is the transpulmonary pressure (alveolus to pleural space). This varies with the vertical height of the lung, since pleural pressure (with respect to atmospheric pressure) is approximately $-10\,cmH_2O$ at the apex of an erect (30 cm high) lung and about $-2.5\,cmH_2O$ at the base. This difference in pressure of about $0.25\,cmH_2O$ per cm height is mainly due to the gravitationally induced difference in shape between the lungs and chest wall. As shown in Figure 2.5, the lungs are most compliant in the normal range of tidal volume and become less compliant at high lung volumes. Since the volume of any given alveolus (expressed as a percentage of the volume it would occupy at total lung capacity) is determined by the transpulmonary pressure, it can be seen that alveoli in the non-dependent parts of the lung have a larger resting volume than those in the dependent zones. During inspiration from FRC absolute pleural pressure decreases, so increasing alveolar volume. However, a given increase in transpulmonary pressure produces a greater expansion in

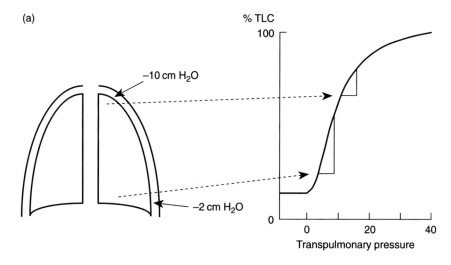

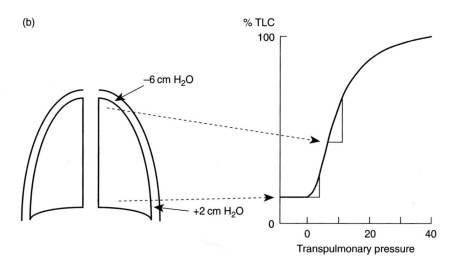

Figure 2.5 Distribution of ventilation. Alveolar volume is expressed as a percentage of the volume at total lung capacity (TLC) plotted against the transpulmonary pressure.

(a) The non-dependent alveoli are subjected to a high transpulmonary pressure due to the gravitationally induced gradient of pleural pressure, and so have a relatively larger volume than the dependent alveoli at the normal resting end-expiratory position (FRC). Because the dependent alveoli lie on the lower, steeper part of the lung P/V curve, they receive more ventilation during a spontaneous inspiration.

(b) A decrease in transpulmonary pressures due to loss of lung elastic recoil leads to dependent airway closure. This increases ventilation in non-dependent zones.

the dependent alveoli than in non-dependent alveoli because the former are on a steeper part of the P/V curve.

Airway closure

The small airways are also influenced by transpulmonary pressure, and expand and contract with the alveoli. The dependent airways are narrower than those in non-dependent zones and have a higher resistance to airflow, particularly at low lung volumes. Expiration towards residual volume causes the transpulmonary pressure difference to become negative in dependent lung regions so that the airways in these regions narrow to such an extent that gas exchange between the alveoli and main bronchi is prevented, so creating alveoli with a low ventilation/perfusion ratio. This phenomenon is known as airway closure. There are still a number of unanswered questions concerning the significance of airway closure and, in particular, its importance as a cause of hypoxaemia. It is also not clear why airway closure does not lead to atelectasis, though collateral ventilation may help to prevent this.

Increasing age results in a decrease in the elastic recoil of the lungs so that absolute pleural pressure increases and transpulmonary pressure decreases. This causes the lung volume at which airway closure occurs, the closing capacity, to increase with increasing age (Fig. 2.6). FRC also increases with age, but to a lesser extent. In many patients aged 60 years or above, closing capacity exceeds FRC when they are in the erect posture; airway closure could thus account for the decrease in arterial Po_2 seen in such

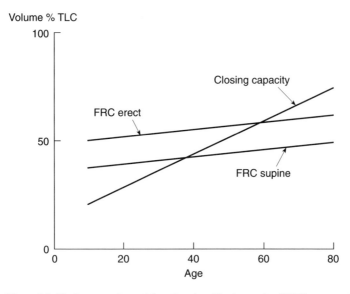

Figure 2.6 Closing capacity and functional residual capacity (FRC) expressed as a percentage of TLC, plotted against age in erect and supine positions.

patients. Younger patients with a closing capacity less than FRC in the erect posture may display airway closure when the supine posture is adopted since this decreases FRC by 0.5–0.8 l. Such patients may have a normal arterial Po_2 when standing, but a decreased Po_2 when supine. If airway closure is present in dependent zones, lung inflation from FRC will result in gas initially being distributed to non-dependent zones, ventilation of dependent zones only occurring when the transpulmonary pressure difference becomes positive enough to open the closed airways (Fig. 2.5). When these airways are open, ventilation is once again distributed mainly to dependent zones. Thus, the overall distribution will depend on the tidal volume and the extent of airway closure.

It is apparent that the regional distribution of ventilation during spontaneous respiration depends on the shape of the lung P/V curve, the initial lung volume, and the regional transpulmonary pressure (which is determined by the vertical height of each part of the lung). Although ventilation increases about two-fold from top to bottom of the erect lung, and blood flow increases four-fold, these mechanisms ensure reasonable matching of ventilation to perfusion.

Effects of posture

Blood flow

The gravitational distribution of blood flow is maintained in the supine and prone positions, but there will usually be no Zone 1 because of the reduced vertical height of the lung (Fig. 2.1). If a positive end-expiratory pressure (PEEP) is applied, the alveolar vessels in the non-dependent parts of the lung are compressed and this results in a shift of blood flow from non-dependent to dependent lung regions, so increasing alveolar dead space. In the lateral position the heart is situated between the two lungs, so that the dependent lung is subject to Zone 3 conditions. Again, a Zone 1 will only appear in the non-dependent lung if P_{PA} is decreased or PEEP is applied to both lungs. If PEEP is applied only to the dependent lung, it shifts blood flow towards the non-dependent lung.

Ventilation

The regional distribution of ventilation will again depend on the shape of the lung P/V curve, the initial lung volume and the vertical height of each part of the lung. However, in the supine or lateral positions the chest wall modifies the distribution of ventilation because the weight of the liquid abdominal contents exerts a lateral pressure of approximately 1 cmH$_2$O per cm height on the caudal side of the diaphragm. This pressure forces the diaphragm up into the chest, so decreasing FRC, and causes the shape of the diaphragm to become more convex in the dependent zone. The increased curvature increases the efficiency of contraction in this area, thus augmenting dependent zone ventilation (Fig. 2.7).

(a)

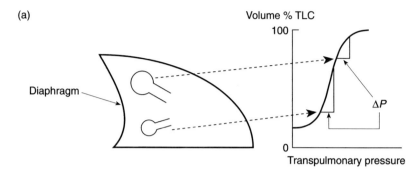

(b)

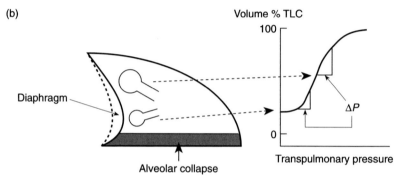

(c)

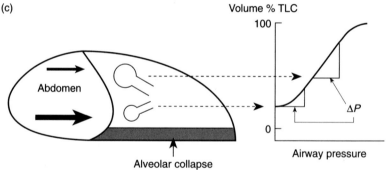

Figure 2.7 Distribution of ventilation in supine position.

(a) Awake, breathing spontaneously.

(b) Induction of anaesthesia with spontaneous respiration results in a decrease in inspiratory muscle tone. FRC is decreased, due to cranial movement of the diaphragm and change in shape of the ribcage, and alveolar collapse appears in the dependent lung regions. This results in a reduction in TLC. Dependent alveoli are now on the knee of the lung P/V curve so that distribution favours the non-dependent zones.

(c) Anaesthesia with muscle paralysis allows the abdominal pressure to be transmitted to the diaphragmatic areas of the lungs so that distribution is now governed by the P/V curve of the total respiratory system. Since abdominal pressure is greatest in dependent zones, there is a further shift of ventilation to non-dependent zones.

ΔP, change in pressure during inspiration.

Effects of anaesthesia and muscle paralysis

Blood flow

The induction of anaesthesia usually results in an increase in alveolar dead space; this is probably caused by a decrease in P_{PA} and a zone of reduced flow in non-dependent areas. Anaesthesia may also result in dependent zone atelectasis. This produces a reduction in blood flow in the affected areas, probably mainly due to HPV. The addition of muscle paralysis has little further effect on blood flow.

Ventilation

General anaesthesia with spontaneous respiration appears to reduce inspiratory muscle tone in the diaphragm and other respiratory muscles so that, in the supine position, FRC is further reduced by about 500 ml. This brings FRC close to residual volume. The ribcage moves inward and the diaphragm moves cranially, but diaphragmatic activity is maintained (Fig. 2.7). The decrease in FRC results in the development of crescentic areas of atelectasis in the most dependent zones of the lung in about 90 per cent of patients who have been pre-oxygenated or who are breathing oxygen-rich mixtures. Patients who have not received more than 30 per cent oxygen do not appear to develop these changes. The atelectasis occurs with intravenous agents (such as the barbiturates or propofol) and with inhalational agents (such as halothane, enflurane or isoflurane). The only anaesthetic agent so far tested that does not produce atelectasis is ketamine. However, atelectasis does occur with this agent if muscle paralysis is induced. The presence of atelectatic areas has been documented in anaesthetized neonates as well as adults, and the magnitude of the changes in adults does not seem to be related to age. There appears to be more atelectasis in the obese, but atelectasis has not been observed in patients with chronic obstructive airways disease. The atelectasis can be reduced by the application of hyperinflations and high levels of PEEP, but reappears within 1 minute if PEEP is removed. In patients who develop atelectasis, there is an increased spread of ventilation/perfusion ratios and an increase in right-to-left shunt to 6–8 per cent of the cardiac output. Distribution in the ventilated parts of the lung depends on the position of the alveoli on the lung P/V curve.

Paralysis of the diaphragm by the administration of muscle relaxant drugs permits the lateral abdominal pressure of the abdominal contents to be transmitted directly to the pleural space, so causing a further reduction in dependent zone ventilation (Fig. 2.7). The distribution of ventilation is now determined by the combined lung–chest wall P/V curve. Ventilation is thus directed into the more compliant non-dependent zones, so reversing the normal distribution and causing a gross mismatch between ventilation and perfusion (Fig. 2.8).

In the lateral position a similar pattern of changes occurs (Fig. 2.9). The dependent lung is compressed by the weight of the heart and mediastinum, by the lateral pressure exerted by the abdominal contents and, possibly, by pads used for positioning. Atelectasis is likely to occur in dependent zones. The lower compliance of the dependent lung causes ventilation to be greater

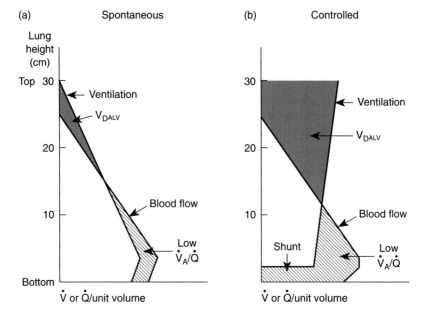

Figure 2.8 Magnitude of ventilation (V) and perfusion (Q) plotted against lung height in erect lung.

(a) Conscious, spontaneous ventilation. The increase in blood flow down the lung is greater than the increase in ventilation, and there may be areas with a low ventilation/perfusion ration (low V_A/Q) due to dependent airway closure.

(b) Anaesthesia and muscle paralysis increase both alveolar dead space (V_{DALV}) and areas with a low ventilation/perfusion ratio ($\dot{V}_A/\dot{Q}$); compression atelectasis increases right to left shunt.

in the non-dependent lung both during spontaneous and controlled ventilation, and opening the chest widely removes the constraints imposed by the chest wall and further increases upper lung compliance, so accentuating the distribution to the non-dependent lung.

There is evidence to suggest that the distribution of ventilation during controlled ventilation is more uniform in the prone position. This may explain why arterial Po_2 may be increased when patients with the adult respiratory distress syndrome are turned into this position.

One-lung anaesthesia

The passage of a double-lumen endotracheal tube enables each lung to be ventilated independently. Usually both lungs are ventilated from a common source until the chest is open, and then all the ventilation is directed into the lung on the opposite side to the operation. The bronchus on the operated side is usually opened to atmosphere via one lumen of the tube so that this lung collapses. Since most operations are performed in the lateral position, the situation when the non-ventilated lung is uppermost and the pleural space is open to atmosphere will be discussed first. There will then

(a) Lung
height

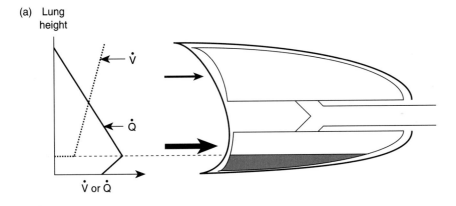

(b)

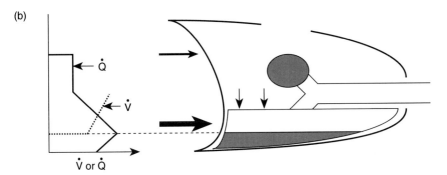

Figure 2.9 Distribution of ventilation ($\dot{V}$) and perfusion ($\dot{Q}$) in lateral position.

(a) Closed chest.
(b) Open chest. One-lung anaesthesia.

Shading shows collapsed areas of lung.

be discussion of the differences when one-lung anaesthesia is used in the lateral or supine positions for thoracoscopic surgery and, finally, of the possible methods of minimizing shunt through the non-ventilated lung.

Open chest

CO₂ elimination

If both lungs have relatively normal function before operation, it is usually found that the minute volume required to maintain a normal arterial P_{CO_2} during bilateral ventilation produces similar P_{CO_2} levels when delivered to one lung. This is only possible if the ventilated lung can accept double the ventilation without an undue increase in inflation pressure (since an increase in pressure would increase its alveolar dead space), and if there is a significant diversion of blood flow from the non-ventilated to the ventilated lung (since any continued shunt through the non-ventilated lung would contribute mixed venous blood, which has a higher P_{CO_2} than arterial P_{CO_2} and so would increase the CO_2 load on the ventilated lung). The situation may be different if one or both lungs have pre-existing ventilation/perfusion abnormalities due to disease. For example, arterial P_{CO_2} may decrease if ventilation is directed away from a diseased lung that has a large alveolar dead space. On the other hand, if both lungs are diseased it may not be possible for the remaining lung to cope with the whole body CO_2 production, so the arterial P_{CO_2} will rise.

Oxygen transfer

Unilateral ventilation inevitably results in an increase in right-to-left shunt due to continuing blood flow through the collapsed lung. The magnitude of the shunt is slightly greater if it is the larger right lung that is non-ventilated, but depends mainly on the P_{PA}, the vertical height of the lung, the effectiveness of the HPV mechanism, and conditions in the ventilated, dependent lung. The effect of the shunt on arterial P_{O_2} depends on the mixed venous P_{O_2}, which in turn depends on the relationship between cardiac output and oxygen consumption.

The distribution of ventilation and blood flow in the anaesthetized, paralysed patient during one-lung ventilation is shown in Figure 2.9. After stopping ventilation to the upper lung, there is a gradual decrease in arterial P_{O_2} due to continuing blood flow through the non-ventilated lung, the rate of decrease being governed by the volume of oxygen in the alveoli and the magnitude of blood flow. When the alveolar P_{O_2} falls to about 8 kPa (60 mmHg), the HPV mechanism comes into play, so reducing blood flow by increasing the extra-alveolar vessel resistance. The reduction in blood flow is usually complete within about 10 minutes, and thereafter the shunt should be unchanged at around 20–30 per cent instead of the 40–50 per cent that would have been expected in the absence of HPV.

If the lower lung is normal and is ventilated with a high percentage of oxygen, a shunt of 20–30 per cent should result in an arterial P_{O_2} of more than 10 kPa. If the arterial P_{O_2} is less than this, the situation must be reviewed. One possible cause of hypoxia is that there may be a decrease in alveolar P_{O_2} in the lower lung due to the delivery of a gas mixture with a low oxygen concentration or to inadvertent underventilation. There may also be an increase in shunt in the dependent lung due to malpositioning of the double-lumen tube, pre-existing disease, atelectasis or the retention of secretions. A tension pneumothorax may produce a similar effect. Alternatively, there may be an increased shunt due to persistent blood flow through the upper lung. This may occur if P_{PA} is increased by the application of PEEP to the lower lung, or by the administration of vaso-constrictor or inotropic drugs. Upper lung blood flow may also be increased by handling the lung (which releases vasodilator prostaglandins), or by the administration of vasodilator drugs or drugs that inhibit HPV (Fig. 2.10). An increase in transpulmonary pressure due to the presence of adhesions, or an increase in left atrial pressure, may also decrease the effectiveness of the HPV mechanism. A not infrequent cause of a low arterial P_{O_2} is a

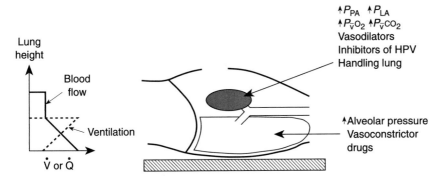

Figure 2.10 Factors affecting blood flow to non-ventilated lung during one-lung anaesthesia. P_{PA}, P_{LA}, pulmonary artery and left atrial pressures; $P_{\bar{v}}O_2$, $P_{\bar{v}}CO_2$, mixed venous Po_2 and Pco_2.

decrease in cardiac output. This may be caused by a decreased venous return due to vasodilation or inadequate fluid replacement, the application of excessive airway pressure to the ventilated lung or cardiac failure.

It has now been demonstrated that one-lung ventilation through a double-lumen tube frequently results in the development of intrinsic PEEP of 3–8 cmH$_2$O in the ventilated lung. This phenomenon is caused by incomplete emptying of the lung in the time available for expiration. It is not usually present when both lungs are being ventilated through such a tube, since the tidal volumes and airflow rates are then halved. However, the resistance of all endobronchial tubes is non-linear, so high pressure differences are generated when all the tidal volume is directed through one lumen of the tube, especially when the smaller sizes of tube are being used. Variations in intrinsic PEEP may explain why the application of a set level of extrinsic PEEP to the dependent lung produces variable changes in arterial Po_2.

Closed chest

When one-lung anaesthesia is being used for thoracoscopic procedures in the closed chest, it is necessary to consider the influence of pleural pressure on blood flow through the non-ventilated lung. If the lung were to be collapsed by occluding the airway when the chest wall was intact, it would produce a marked decrease in absolute pleural pressure. This would increase the transpulmonary pressure difference, which would tend to distend the extra-alveolar vessels, so opposing the increase in vasomotor tone produced by HPV. Blood flow would thus be higher than in a lung collapsed in a similar manner but with the chest open. If the bronchus is open to atmosphere via one lumen of a double-lumen tube, and there are no adhesions between the lung and pleura, the lung collapses and blood flow is reduced by the usual mechanisms. If, however, lung collapse is prevented by adhesions between lung and pleura, so increasing transpulmonary pressure and decreasing the effectiveness of HPV in the underlying areas of lung, the reduction in blood flow to the non-ventilated lung may be impeded. Thus, in the presence of adhesions, shunt may be greater than in the completely collapsed lung. High intrapleural pressure will also tend to reduce cardiac output, which further reduces arterial Po_2.

In some thoracoscopic procedures the surgeon requires the patient to be in the supine position. Collapse of one lung with the patient in this position usually results in a larger shunt than in the lateral position, because the collapsed lung tends to fall into the dependent part of the thorax. It is thus exposed to Zone 3 conditions, which tend to reduce the efficiency of the HPV mechanism.

KEY POINTS

- The distribution of pulmonary blood flow is predominantly influenced by gravity, the alveolar pressure and pulmonary vascular pressures. Blood flow thus increases from non-dependent to dependent zones in all body positions, though there may be an area of reduced blood flow in the most dependent part of the lungs due to airway closure or atelectasis. When alveolar pressure is increased or P_{PA} is decreased, there may be a zone of reduced blood flow in the non-dependent area of the lung; this will result in an increase in alveolar dead space.

- Ventilation also increases from non-dependent to dependent zones during spontaneous ventilation, but to a lesser degree than perfusion. However, when FRC is reduced by the supine posture and general anaesthesia, the alveoli move onto different parts of the P/V curve and there may be airway closure and dependent zone atelectasis, so that ventilation may be delivered preferentially to the non-dependent zones of the lung. When the diaphragm is paralysed by muscle relaxants, it is forced up into the chest by the lateral pressure exerted by the abdominal contents. Since this pressure is greatest in dependent zones, ventilation is directed mainly into non-dependent zones. In the lateral position, the weight of the mediastinum and contents further compresses the dependent lung, so accentuating the ventilation/perfusion mismatch. The pattern of these changes is similar whether the patient is in the supine, prone or lateral positions. However, in the lateral position there is a greater vertical distance between the top and bottom of the lungs, so the zones are more clearly differentiated.

- During one-lung ventilation there is a decrease in arterial Po_2. This is due mainly to an increase in right-to-left shunt due to continuing blood flow through the non-ventilated lung, though it may be accentuated by a decrease in mixed venous Po_2 secondary to a decrease in cardiac output. The shunt through the non-dependent lung may be increased by an increase in P_{PA}, or by other factors that decrease the efficiency of the HPV mechanism. Atelectasis, retention of secretions and pulmonary oedema in the dependent lung may also contribute to the increase in shunt. All these factors may be affected by pre-existing lung disease.

Bibliography

Bindslev, L., Santesson, J. and Hedenstierna, G. (1981). Distribution of inspired gas to each lung in anesthetized human subjects. *Acta Anaesth. Scand.*, **25**, 297–302.

Bindslev, L., Hedenstierna, G., Santesson, J. *et al.* (1980). Airway closure during anaesthesia, and its prevention by positive end expiratory pressure. *Acta Anaesth. Scand.*, **24**, 199–205.

Eisenkraft, J.B. (1990). Effect of anaesthetics on the pulmonary circulation. *Br. J. Anaesth.*, **65**, 63–78.

Hambraeus-Jonzon, K., Bindslev, L., Mellgard, A.J. and Hedenstierna, G. (1997). Hypoxic pulmonary vasoconstriction in human lungs. A stimulus–response study. *Anesthesiology*, **86**, 308–15.

Hedenstierna, G. (1996). Effects of anaesthesia on respiratory function. In *Baillière's Clinical Anaesthesiology: The Lung in Anaesthesia and Intensive Care* (R.G. Pearl, ed.), pp. 1–16. Baillière Tindall.

Inomata, S., Nishikawa, T., Saito, S. and Kihara, S. (1997). Best PEEP during one-lung ventilation. *Br. J. Anaesth.*, **78**, 754–6.

Marshall, B.E., Marshall, C., Frasch, F. and Hanson, C.W. (1994a). Role of hypoxic vasoconstriction in pulmonary gas exchange and blood flow distribution. 1. Physiological concepts. *Intens. Care Med.*, **20**, 291–7.

Marshall, B.E., Marshall, C., Frasch, F. and Hanson, C.W. (1994b). Role of hypoxic vasoconstriction in pulmonary gas exchange and blood flow distribution. 2. Pathophysiology. *Intens. Care Med.*, **20**, 379–89.

Morrell, N.W., Nijran, K.S., Biggs, T. and Seed, W.A. (1995). Magnitude and time course of acute hypoxic vasoconstriction in man. *Resp. Physiol.*, **100**, 271–81.

Rothen, H.U., Sporre, B., Engberg, G. *et al.* (1995). Prevention of atelectasis during general anaesthesia. *Lancet*, **345**, 1387–91.

Sykes, K. (1995). The pulmonary circulation. In *Cardiovascular Physiology* (H.-J. Priebe and K. Skarvan, eds), pp. 139–72. BMJ Publishing Group.

West, J.B. (1977). *Regional Differences in the Lung*. Academic Press.

3

Anatomy of the lungs and pleura

R. Mills and K. McNeil

Introduction

The lungs are responsible for a multitude of functions, ranging from their integral role in respiration and gas exchange to diverse metabolic and immunological activities. The role of the lungs and airways as the organs responsible for the provision of oxygen and disposal of carbon dioxide makes them pivotal to the practice of anaesthesia.

Macroscopic anatomy

Despite being paired organs, the lungs and major airways are not anatomically symmetrical. The following sections describe the major airway divisions and pulmonary anatomy down to segmental level.

Airways

The trachea extends from the larynx to the carina. The length of the trachea varies depending on the age and height of the individual, but in the adult is usually 10–12 cm long. The trachea is mobile, and lengthens and shortens during respiration. The luminal diameter ranges in adults from approximately 1–2 cm. During childhood, this diameter is roughly equal in millimetres to the age of the child in years.

At the carina, the trachea divides into the right and left main bronchi. The right main bronchus (RMB), at approximately 2.5 cm long (mean ± s.d.: 2.3 ± 0.7 cm in men, 2.1 ± 0.7 cm in women), is wider and shorter than the left main bronchus (LMB). Importantly, it sits more vertically than the LMB and, combined with its greater width, this creates a tendency for foreign bodies (including endotracheal tubes) to pass more easily into the right side. This difference can be further accentuated by mediastinal pathology, which may cause either widening of the carina (e.g. enlarged subcarinal lymph nodes) or a superior shift of the LMB itself (as occurs with enlargement of the left atrium).

The RMB gives off the right upper lobe bronchus from its lateral wall, and continues as the bronchus intermedius. This runs for approximately

2 cm before giving off the middle lobe bronchus from its anterior wall and continuing as the right lower lobe airway.

In contrast, the LMB is usually 5.4 ± 0.7 cm in men and 5.0 ± 0.7 cm in women (mean $\pm$ s.d.), and divides into upper and lower lobe bronchi. The left upper lobe airway usually arises more anteriorly than its right-sided counterpart. These subtle differences in the anatomy of the main bronchi have obvious implications for the design and placement of double-lumen tubes.

The airways continue to branch into segmental and sub-segmental divisions, and these follow the pulmonary segments of the same names, discussed in the next section.

Pulmonary anatomy

The lungs are separated by fissures into lobes, three on the right (upper, middle and lower) and two on the left (upper and lower). The oblique fissures on both sides separate the upper and lower lobes. The right middle lobe is bordered superiorly by the horizontal fissure separating it from the upper lobe, and infero-laterally by the right oblique fissure separating it from the lower lobe (Fig. 3.1).

All of the primary branches of the major (lobar) airways are termed segmental bronchi, because each is responsible for airways supplying the functionally independent units of lung called broncho-pulmonary segments.

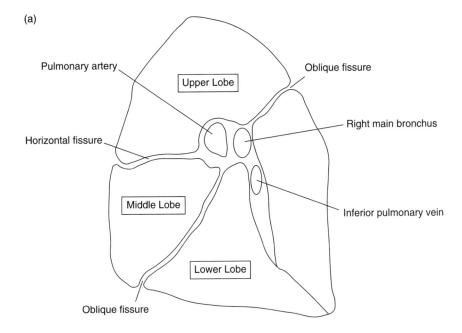

(a)

Pulmonary artery

Upper Lobe

Oblique fissure

Horizontal fissure

Right main bronchus

Middle Lobe

Inferior pulmonary vein

Lower Lobe

Oblique fissure

Figure 3.1

(a) Fissures and lobes of medial surface of right lung.

(b)

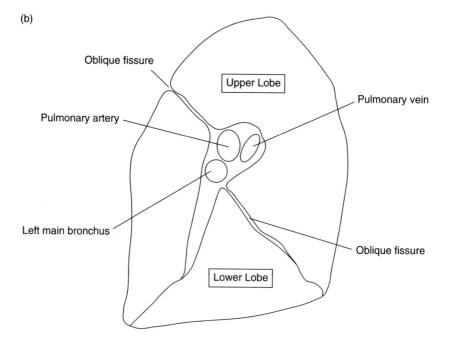

Figure 3.1 *continued*

(b) Fissures and lobes of medial surface of left lung.

Again, subtle differences exist between the right and left sides. The lobar structure and main segments of the lungs are described below (Fig. 3.2).

Right lung
Upper lobe: apical, posterior and anterior segments
Middle lobe: medial and lateral segments
Lower lobe: apical (superior) segment and basal segments (anterior, posterior, medial and lateral).

Left lung
Upper lobe: apico-posterior and anterior segments, lingula segments (superior and inferior)
Lower lobe: apical (superior) segment, basal segments (anterior, posterior, medial and lateral).

Surface anatomy

It is useful to know the surface markings of the pulmonary lobes and major fissures as an aid to correct orientation during the physical examination and correlation of signs with changes on the chest radiograph.

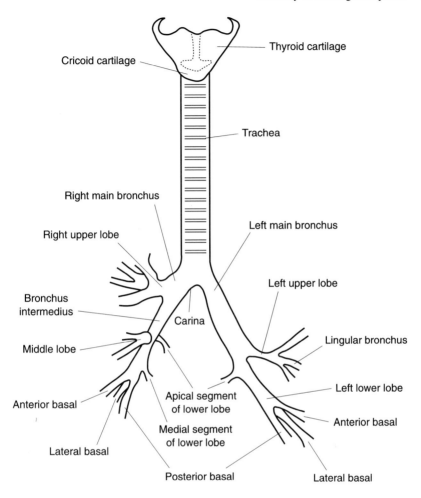

Figure 3.2 Anterior aspect of tracheobronchial anatomy.

The oblique fissure on both sides runs posteriorly from the fourth thoracic vertebra to the sixth intercostal space anteriorly, ending at the costochondral junction. On the right side, the additional horizontal fissure runs in the fourth intercostal space from the right oblique fissure posteriorly to the midpoint of the sternum anteriorly (Fig. 3.3).

Bronchoscopic anatomy

An understanding of the segmental anatomy of the lung and airways is necessary during bronchoscopy. The normal anatomical relationship of the segmental airways is detailed in Figure 3.2.

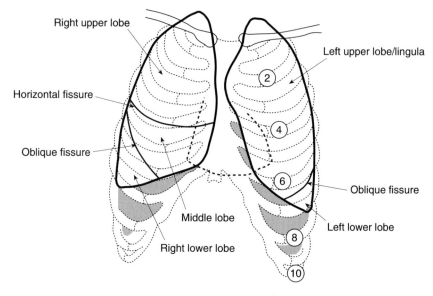

Figure 3.3 Surface anatomy of fissures and lobes in relation to intercostal spaces.

Radiographic anatomy

Knowledge of the gross and surface anatomical relationships of the lungs is directly applicable to the radiographic appearance of the lungs on plain postero-anterior (PA) and lateral chest X-rays (Fig. 3.4). The radiology of the lungs as seen on computerized tomography (CT) scanning is outlined in Figure 3.5.

Several points are worth discussion. On the PA film, the heart is bordered on the right side by the middle lobe, and on the left by the lingula (Fig. 3.3). This means that shadowing obscuring the heart borders must lie in either of these two 'lobes'. Similarly, on the lateral film the diaphragm lies in contact with the lower lobes along its entire length.

Pleura: function and reflexions

The pleura consists of a membrane of fibrous tissue that covers each lung and lines the thoracic cavity. The parietal pleura lines the thoracic wall and thoracic surface of the diaphragm, from which it ascends over the pericardium to cover the mediastinum as a continuous sheet. The visceral pleura is projected from around the root of the lung, and tracks into the depths of the interlobular clefts.

Under normal conditions, the visceral layer on the lung is in contact with the parietal layer, but the anterior and inferior reflexions extend further than the lung edge (Fig. 3.6).

The primary function of the pleura is to provide a frictionless interface between the mobile lung and its cavity. In addition, this potential space

(a)

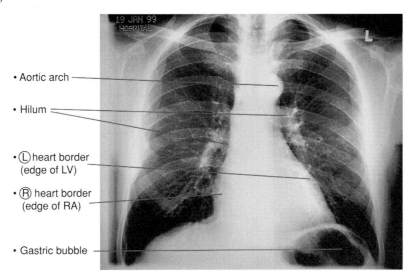

- Aortic arch
- Hilum
- Ⓛ heart border
  (edge of LV)
- Ⓡ heart border
  (edge of RA)
- Gastric bubble

(b)

Ⓡ lateral CXR

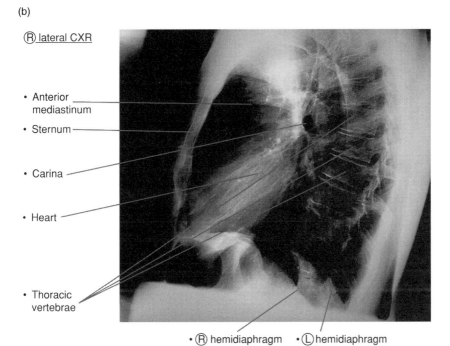

- Anterior
  mediastinum
- Sternum
- Carina
- Heart
- Thoracic
  vertebrae

- Ⓡ hemidiaphragm   • Ⓛ hemidiaphragm

Figure 3.4

(a) Normal postero-anterior chest X-ray.
(b) Normal lateral chest X-ray.

- Sternum
- Ascending aorta
- S.V.C.
- Pulmonary trunk
- (R) main bronchus
- (L) main bronchus
- Oesophagus
- Vertebral body

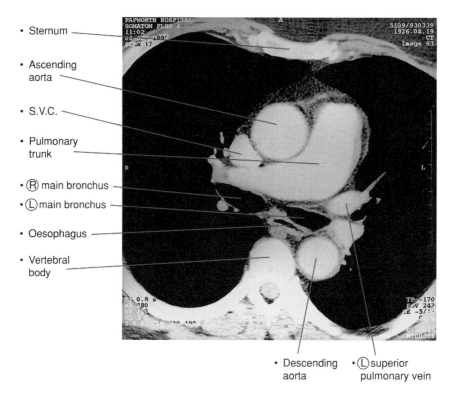

- Descending aorta
- (L) superior pulmonary vein

Figure 3.5 Normal CT scan (T4/5 level).

allows room for the lung to expand during maximum inspiration. The cuff of pleura at the hilum (pulmonary ligament) permits descent of the hilum with diaphragmatic movement on deep inspiration, as well as distension of the pulmonary veins during episodes of increased vascular activity.

The pleura ascends as far as the neck of the first rib. Right and left sternocostal reflexions meet behind the sternum at the level of the second ribs, and both descend to the level of the fourth ribs. At this point the left pleura deviates variably to the sixth or seventh rib. Both right and left reflexions cross the mid-clavicular line at the eighth rib, and mid-axillary line at the tenth. From here the vertebral reflexion ascends on the vertebral bodies (T12–T1).

Conclusion

Knowledge of the anatomy of the lungs and airways is essential for assessment of the patient with pulmonary pathology and for accurate interpretation of the chest X-ray. A basic understanding of the internal anatomy of the major airways and the subtle differences between the right and left sides allows observational bronchoscopy and one-lung anaesthesia to be performed effectively and safely.

(a)

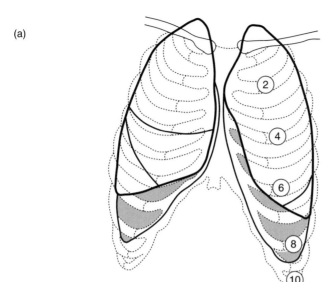

(b)

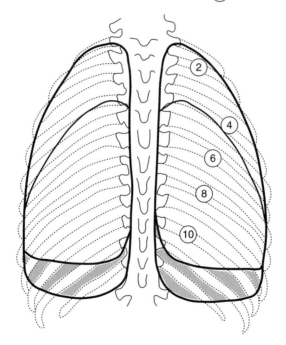

Figure 3.6

(a) Pleural reflexions (anterior).
(b) Pleural reflexions (posterior).

4

Indications and techniques for one-lung ventilation

J. D. Kneeshaw

Introduction

The practice of thoracic anaesthesia requires the anaesthetist to be skilled in establishing and safely maintaining one-lung anaesthesia in patients with compromised lung function and limited respiratory reserve.

The indications for one-lung anaesthesia can appear confusing, and this confusion is compounded by the numerous devices available for isolation of one lung. In order to achieve this relatively simple goal, a double-lumen endobronchial tube, a single-lumen endobronchial tube or a bronchus blocker may be used. The equipment available is described in detail in Chapter 1, and the pros and cons of the different means of attaining one-lung ventilation are also discussed in Chapter 19. The aim of this chapter is to discuss the indications for one-lung ventilation, and to describe the practical conduct of one-lung anaesthesia.

One-lung ventilation and anaesthesia

In general terms, one-lung ventilation is required for the following reasons:

- Prevention of soiling of one lung by spillage of material from the other.
- Control of the distribution of ventilation.
- Facilitation of surgical access for operations on the lung or other structures within the hemithorax.

The indications for one-lung ventilation are often described either in terms of absolute or relative in conjunction with specific procedures. It may be more practical to consider the indications in terms of a continuum ranging from those that would be virtually impossible without one-lung ventilation to those for which one-lung ventilation renders the surgery less difficult. Factors relating to the patient and the anaesthetist can then be taken into account before deciding whether one-lung ventilation is appropriate in any particular case. This is discussed in more detail in the following sections, and summarized in Table 4.1.

Table 4.1 Indications and contraindications for one-lung anaesthesia

Indications		Contraindications
	Strong	
Bronchopleural fistula		
Pulmonary abscess		
Endobronchial haemorrhage		Large airway obstruction
Bronchiectasis		
Bronchial disruption		
Lavage for alveolar proteinosis		Difficult intubation
Bullous lung disease		
Undrained pneumothorax		Occasional thoracic anaesthetist
Trauma		
Lobectomy (upper lobes)		Limited movement/ instability of cervical spine
Pneumonectomy		
Access to pericardium and the left atrium		
Lobectomy (either lower or right middle lobes)		Young children
Thoracoscopic surgery		
Oesophageal surgery		Small adults
Surgery of aortic arch and descending aorta		
Spinal surgery		Full stomach
Transmyocardial laser revascularization	Weak	
Internal mammary artery harvest		

Spillage of material from one lung to the other

Historically, endobronchial intubation, or the blocking of a main bronchus and the conduct of anaesthesia using one lung, was introduced to prevent the spillage of material from one lung to the other. This material was either of an infective or corrosive nature, or was present in such volume that its passage into the normal lung would render ventilation impossible. The patients were usually suffering from pulmonary abscesses (often tuberculous) or severe bronchiectatic disease.

The number of patients for whom the prevention of spillage of material from one lung into the other presents a significant problem has reduced in recent years, and the majority of one-lung anaesthesia is now conducted for reasons of ease of surgical access. Despite the decreased number of patients who are at a high risk from spillage from one lung to the other, this group still presents a significant risk for anaesthesia. Such patients will therefore usually be near the top of lists of indications for one-lung anaesthesia. Two special circumstances in which patients are at risk from the spillage of material into the lung should be noted. One is the patient with alveolar proteinosis, in whom a double-lumen tube is used to isolate each lung in turn for bronchial lavage, and the other is the patient in whom endobronchial intubation and one-lung ventilation is used to control endobronchial haemorrhage.

Patients with an abnormal distribution of ventilation

High on most lists of patients for whom one-lung anaesthesia is indicated are those in whom bronchial intubation and ventilation allow the control of what would otherwise be an abnormal distribution of ventilation. These are patients with bronchial disruption, a bronchopleural fistula, unilateral bullous lung disease or an undrained pneumothorax. In patients with bronchial disruption or a bronchopleural fistula, much of the ventilation will be ineffective unless ventilation to the abnormal lung is occluded, resulting in gross alveolar hypoventilation. In those with bullous disease or an undrained pneumothorax, there will be gas trapping leading to a unilateral increase in intrathoracic pressure and mediastinal shift; this in turn may cause a loss of systemic venous return and circulatory collapse.

It should be noted that patients with a large bronchopleural fistula in the early post-operative period following pulmonary surgery (usually pneumonectomy) are also at risk from spillage of large quantities of fluid from the pleural space through the fistula into the normal lung. These patients with post-operative broncho pulmonary fistulae are therefore at risk for two reasons, and present one of the strongest cases for endobronchial intubation and one-lung anaesthesia.

Surgical access

Lung resection

Patients undergoing surgery for lung resection may require bronchial intubation and one-lung anaesthesia in order to facilitate surgery. In these patients, the requirement for one-lung anaesthesia is less pressing than above and relates to the ease with which pulmonary dissection can be undertaken. Resection of either lower lobe or the right middle lobe is usually perfectly feasible without one-lung anaesthesia, the surgeon utilizing lung retractors to obtain access. Surgery involving the upper lobes is said to be more difficult without one-lung anaesthesia. Surgery at the hilum (for example, pneumonectomy) and surgery involving the pericardium and the left atrium is certainly more challenging if one-lung anaesthesia is not possible.

Non-pulmonary surgery

Surgical access for oesophageal surgery, thoracic spinal surgery and vascular surgery involving the aortic arch, ductus arteriosus and the descending aorta is often made much easier by one-lung anaesthesia. These procedures may be more difficult, but are not impossible if, for some reason, one-lung anaesthesia cannot be provided.

Transmyocardial laser revascularization of the heart (TMR) is under evaluation in Europe and Asia, although trials in the USA and UK have shown increased mortality and little symptomatic benefit in comparison to medical therapy for angina. When not combined with another cardiac procedure, this is performed through a left anterior or lateral thoracotomy. One-lung anaesthesia may be required for the procedure, although retraction of the left lung often suffices.

Thoracoscopic surgery

An increasingly wide variety of surgical activity is being undertaken thoracoscopically in many centres. This ranges from uncomplicated pleural biopsy to video-assisted lobectomy. Indeed, as discussed in Chapter 10, the whole spectrum of intrathoracic surgical procedures seems to have been reported as being achievable with thoracoscopic techniques in the recent surgical literature. The importance of one-lung anaesthesia in this area of work varies with the type of surgery undertaken. Patients with large pleural effusions and those in whom thoracoscopic surgery is undertaken for diagnostic purposes or for the treatment of pleural lesions do not essentially require one-lung anaesthesia. For patients undergoing more complicated pulmonary surgery or surgery on other intrathoracic structures, one-lung anaesthesia provides a great surgical advantage, maintaining a still and easily accessible operating field. One-lung anaesthesia may also reduce the risk of lung trauma when thoracoscopic ports and cannulae are introduced into the thorax.

Where it is not immediately obvious, the decision to perform any particular procedure with one-lung anaesthesia should be made jointly between the surgeon and the anaesthetist, remembering that most surgeons who have been trained in the last 10 years have come to expect one-lung anaesthesia for almost all thoracoscopic procedures.

The use of video-assisted thoracoscopy to harvest the left, right or both internal mammary arteries with a closed chest for minimally invasive coronary artery surgery (MICAS) is a particular case in point. One-lung anaesthesia may be of benefit in hastening the procedure by providing a better view for the surgeon. However, the potential hazard of hypoxia associated with one-lung anaesthesia in patients with severe ischaemic heart disease tends to mitigate against this as an indication for single-lung ventilation. Many centres are now undertaking similar procedures in which access to the mammary artery is gained via a limited anterior thoracotomy. In general, one-lung anaesthesia is not essential for minimally invasive cardiac surgery if the surgical access is open rather than thoracoscopic.

Trauma surgery

Patients needing urgent thoracotomy following trauma should be managed with endobronchial intubation if circumstances permit. This is particularly important if there is a suspicion of damage to structures around the hilum or if there is evidence of airway disruption or unilateral pulmonary haemorrhage.

General considerations for one-lung ventilation

Factors relating to the patient's clinical condition must be taken into consideration. The presence of large airway obstruction, either from extrinsic compression or from lesions within the airway, which may prevent the placement of endobronchial equipment, will tend to mitigate against one-lung anaesthesia.

The presence of diffuse lung disease may indicate insufficient respiratory reserve for the tolerance one-lung ventilation, and requires investigation pre-operatively.

It has been said that endobronchial intubation is best avoided in patients with a full stomach, where a standard rapid sequence induction and endotracheal intubation may be safer. However, patients presenting for urgent thoracotomy following trauma will frequently need one-lung anaesthesia. A technique of rapid sequence endobronchial intubation should be considered.

Care should be taken in patients in whom endotracheal intubation has previously been difficult or may be predicted. The passage of endobronchial devices is more challenging than endotracheal intubation.

Small adults pose specific technical difficulties. Small double-lumen endobronchial tubes are often difficult to place, they have a high internal resistance to gas flow and are very susceptible to kinking. Even with the aid of the fibre-optic bronchoscope, accurate placement of tubes in these small patients is difficult. The problems are further exacerbated if the patient has arthritic or traumatic limitation of movement, or instability of the cervical spine.

As discussed in Chapters 1 and 12, children present similar problems to small adults, and it is difficult to find endobronchial equipment suitable for use in children below 12 years of age. Fortunately, in small children undergoing thoracic surgery it is usually quite easy to retract the lung on the operative side to provide adequate surgical exposure; the retracted lung tends to collapse quickly. Where it is essential to provide one-lung anaesthesia in children, it is possible to insert an endotracheal tube into the appropriate bronchus under fibre-optic guidance. Care is needed to ensure that the tube does not obstruct an upper lobe bronchus, and in these circumstances it may help to cut the bevel off the tube before insertion. An alternative approach to the protection of normal lung from spillage or to control endobronchial haemorrhage in children and very small adults is the use of a small balloon catheter, such as a Fogarty embolectomy catheter, inserted under bronchoscopic control to act as a bronchus blocker. In emergency situations, a balloon-tipped pulmonary artery catheter may be easier to find and will perform the same function.

Despite the ever-lengthening list of procedures for which one-lung anaesthesia seems to be indicated, it should always be remembered that one-lung anaesthesia adds considerably to the complexity of the anaesthetic technique and also to the associated level of risk. Placement of an endobronchial tube should not be pursued at all costs. Prolonged attempts at endobronchial intubation may put the patient at risk – at best from damage caused by trauma, and at worst from hypoxia. It is all too easy to be so distracted by the technology of one-lung anaesthesia or its complexity that a falling blood pressure or profound bradycardia goes unnoticed.

The occasional thoracic anaesthetist would be well advised to have a very low threshold for abandoning one-lung anaesthesia in favour of a more familiar and perhaps safer technique. One-lung anaesthesia should not be attempted if the anaesthetist is not familiar with, or does not have access to, fibre-optic bronchoscopy to confirm the tube position. There are very few surgical procedures that a competent thoracic surgeon cannot perform, albeit with some difficulty, with positive pressure ventilation through a single-lumen endotracheal tube.

Techniques for one-lung ventilation

One-lung ventilation is currently most commonly achieved by using a double-lumen endobronchial tube. The most widely used devices are the ranges of plastic endobronchial tubes. The more traditional resterilizable rubber tubes, often of the Robertshaw pattern, are mainly in use in specialist centres. Left- and right-sided single-lumen endobronchial tubes are occasionally of use in particular circumstances, such as patients with small major airways or those with abnormal endobronchial anatomy. Bronchial blockers are not in general use, however. In a few centres, Fogarty embolectomy catheters are used in specific circumstances: for example in children, as mentioned above, or when endobronchial intubation cannot be achieved, but isolation of a lung or area of lung is crucial. A combined endotracheal tube and bronchus blocker, the Univent tube, is available, but has yet to gain widespread acceptance.

Choice of side of tube (left vs. right)

The primary choice between a left- or right-sided endobronchial tube is determined by the surgical procedure being undertaken. Secondary factors include patient pathology and the anaesthetist's preference. In general, safe one-lung anaesthesia with adequate protection of the ventilated lung from aspiration or spillage is more reliably produced by intubation of the main bronchus of the ventilated lung – that is, the bronchus of the non-operated side. Although it has been argued that lower lobectomy is easy to accomplish with ipsilateral bronchial intubation, it is impossible to guarantee before the chest is open that the patient will require only lower lobectomy, and not more extensive resection or even pneumonectomy.

Pathological factors that may influence the choice of a specific side of tube include narrowing, distortion or friability of the main bronchus arising as a result of tumour, infection or inflammation. Rarely, anatomical anomalies such as a congenitally narrow or sharply angled bronchus or early origin of the left or right upper lobe bronchus may influence the choice of tube. The frequency with which the right upper lobe bronchus is found to be abnormally close to the carina or even above it appears to have been over-emphasized. Information about these pathological or anatomical abnormalities should be sought from radiographs and CT scans, or from information from previous bronchoscopy. Indeed, it would be foolish to attempt elective endobronchial intubation without at least looking at a plain chest radiograph.

Many anaesthetists express quite strongly held preferences for the use of either left- or right-sided endobronchial tubes. This is usually based on the dogma handed down from the 1950s that it is easier to place a left-sided tube than a right. As discussed in Chapter 3, the right main bronchus favours intubation because of its more linear relationship to the trachea and its greater width. The shorter length of bronchus proximal to the upper lobe orifice is said to be associated with a greater risk of collapse of the right upper lobe from a poorly positioned endobronchial cuff occluding the upper lobe bronchus. Fortunately, as early as 1955 the Gordon–Green single-lumen endobronchial tube was designed with an orifice in the endobronchial part of the tube to allow ventilation of the right upper lobe bronchus. This design feature was continued in the Robertshaw tube, and is now seen (with some modification) in newer designs of right-sided endobronchial tubes. Checking and adjusting the placement of a right-sided endobronchial tube with the aid of a fibre-optic bronchoscope prevents occlusion of the upper lobe bronchus. If a right-sided endobronchial tube is correctly placed, the bronchoscope can be manipulated through the orifice in the bronchial lumen to view the upper lobe segmental bronchi.

It should be noted that occlusion of the left upper lobe bronchus by a poorly positioned left-sided tube can also occur. This is seen less frequently, because the greater length of the left main bronchus proximal to the origin of the left upper lobe bronchus makes it more difficult for a tube of correct size to be passed far enough into the bronchus for the cuff to obstruct the upper lobe bronchial orifice. Some endobronchial tubes have carinal hooks designed to prevent the tube from advancing too far into the bronchus. These hooks generally hinder the passage of tubes through the glottis, and may produce mucosal damage.

Choice of size of tube

Single-use plastic tube sizes are quoted as Charriere (Ch) gauge, which is equivalent to French (Fr) gauge. Multi-use rubber Robertshaw type tubes are supplied in three sizes; small, medium and large. The large size corresponds approximately to 39 Ch and the medium to 37 Ch. Many of the older designs of single-lumen endobronchial tube are sized by the internal diameter in millimetres. It should be noted that tubes of the same apparent size from different manufacturers often have different luminal diameters because of variations in tube wall thickness. This has implications for the passage of fibre-optic bronchoscopes or suction catheters when using small tubes.

In general, the largest tube that will pass easily through the larynx and into the bronchus should be used. Larger tubes minimize the resistance to gas flow, present a smaller risk of kinking and increase the likelihood of

(a)

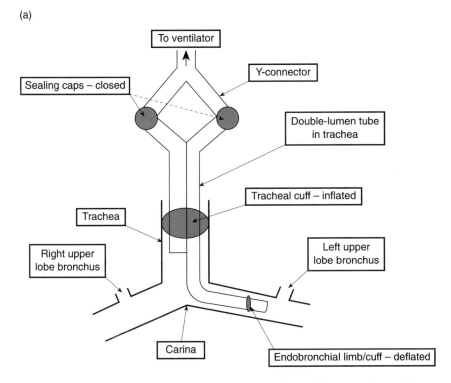

Figure 4.1 Establishing one-lung ventilation and checking the double-lumen tube position clinically.

(a) After placing the double-lumen tube, the tracheal cuff is inflated until there is no audible gas leak and breath sounds can be auscultated bilaterally. Airway pressure and end-tidal CO_2 are monitored.

(b)

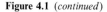

Figure 4.1 (*continued*)

(b) Following inflation of the tracheal cuff, the limb of the Y-connector connected to the tracheal lumen is clamped and the sealing cap of that limb opened to release gas to the atmosphere. The endobronchial cuff is gradually inflated until no breath sounds can be auscultated over the deflated lung, and the audible leak from the open lumen of the tube ceases on application of positive pressure ventilation. There should be a good air entry to the ventilated lung. The peak airway pressure during one-lung ventilation should be less than 40 cmH$_2$O. When using a right-sided tube, adequate ventilation of the right upper lobe should specifically be sought by auscultation of the apex of the lung superior to the clavicle.

successfully isolating one lung without having to over-inflate the endo-bronchial cuff. Adult males can usually accommodate a large (39 or 41 Ch gauge) right-sided tube or a medium (37 Ch gauge) left-sided tube. Small males and average-sized females require medium (37 Ch gauge) tubes. The smallest sizes of endobronchial tubes are very difficult to use because of their propensity to kink, and because it is difficult to pass suction catheters or bronchoscopes through their internal lumina.

Placement of double-lumen tubes

Laryngoscopy is performed in the standard manner, and the tube passed through the larynx with the concavity of the endobronchial limb facing upwards. Once through the larynx, the tube is rotated to the appropriate side so that the endobronchial limb slides into the correct bronchus. It may be helpful to rotate the patient's head to the opposite side to the lung to be intubated, so that the bronchus is brought more into line with the trachea.

If difficulty is encountered in passing the tube through the larynx, first check that the patient's head is in the optimum position with the neck well flexed and the head extended on the neck. If it is still difficult to pass the tube, a malleable stilet or bougie may be used to adjust the shape of the tube and guide it into the trachea. Magill's forceps may be used to pick up the tip of the tube in the pharynx and place it in line with the larynx. Occasionally, a fibre-optic bronchoscope may be required to guide the endobronchial limb into the correct position.

Following passage of the tube and checking of its position (see below), both the tracheal and bronchial cuffs should be maintained inflated throughout the procedure to help stabilize the tube and prevent spillage of material from one lung to the other.

Checking the tube position

The procedure for clinically checking the correct placement of a double-lumen tube is shown in Figure 4.1. The correct position of the tube should be confirmed using a fibre-optic bronchoscope (Fig. 4.2). This is

(a)

Figure 4.2 Checking tube position by fibre-optic bronchoscopy.

    (a)   On passing the bronchoscope through the tracheal lumen, the carina should be visible with the main bronchus to one side and the endobronchial limb of the tube seated in the opposite bronchus. The outermost acceptable position of the endobronchial limb is with a small crescent of its bronchial cuff visible above the carina.

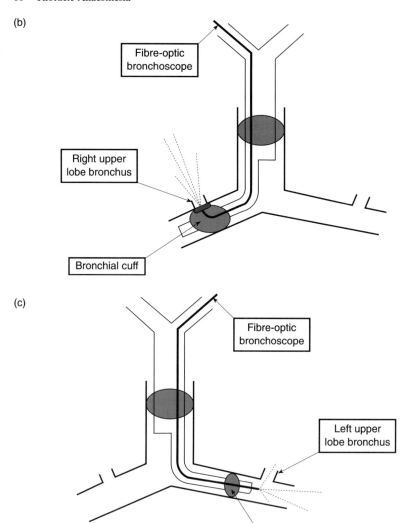

Figure 4.2 (*continued*)

(b) and (c) Bronchoscope passed through bronchial lumens of right-
and left-sided tubes respectively to view the orifice of the
upper lobe bronchus. With a correctly placed right-sided
tube, the orifice of the upper lobe bronchus will be
visible through the slot in the endobronchial limb, and it
should be possible to manipulate the bronchoscope into
the upper lobe bronchus to visualize its division into
segmental bronchi. With a left-sided tube, the orifice of
the upper lobe bronchus should be seen distal to the tip
of the tube.

discussed in Chapter 19, and is particularly relevant to the use of right-sided tubes. The tube position should be re-checked, both functionally and bronchoscopically, after the patient has been placed in the lateral thoracotomy position.

Single-lumen endobronchial tubes

Multi-use rubber single-lumen endobronchial tubes are still available (see Chapter 1), but their use tends to be confined to specialist thoracic centres.

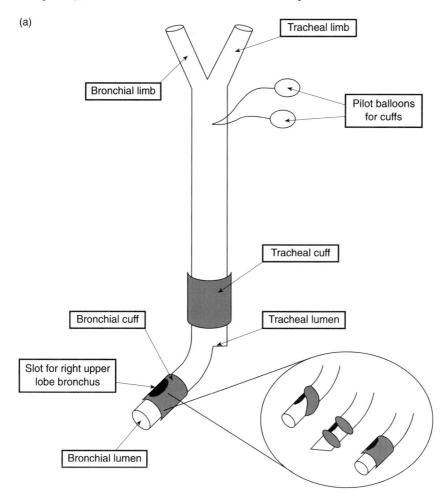

(a)

Figure 4.3 Diagram of double- and single-lumen endobronchial tubes and Univent tube.

(a) Right-sided double-lumen endobronchial tube with inset showing different available designs of the bronchial cuff. The width and length of the slot for the right upper lobe bronchus and the size of the cuff vary with differing manufacturers and designs. Left-sided tubes have cuffs of a cylindrical design, with little significant variation between manufacturers.

(b)

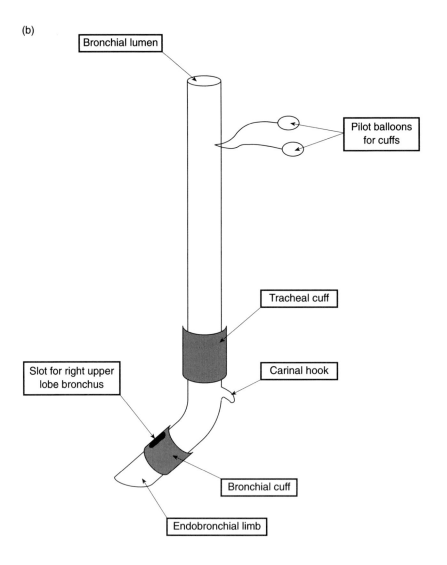

Figure 4.3 (*continued*)

(b) Single-lumen endobronchial tube.

The Gordon–Green tube is less bulky than an equivalent double-lumen tube, and is therefore easier to pass into the trachea. Although originally designed with a slotted bronchial cuff for right-sided use, it can be placed in either main bronchus, over a bronchoscope or blindly. A modified Macintosh–Leatherdale single-lumen left endobronchial tube is now avail-

(c)

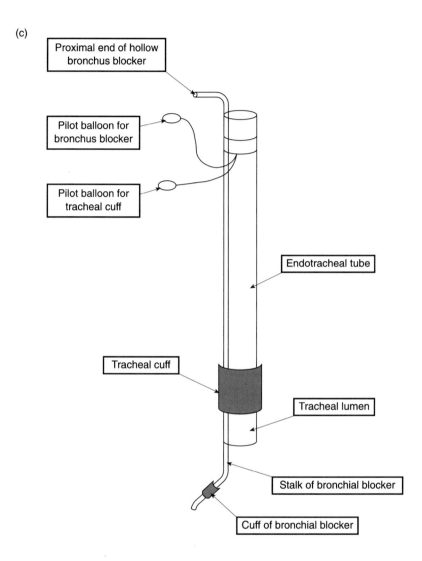

Proximal end of hollow
bronchus blocker

Pilot balloon for
bronchus blocker

Pilot balloon for
tracheal cuff

Endotracheal tube

Tracheal cuff

Tracheal lumen

Stalk of bronchial blocker

Cuff of bronchial blocker

Figure 4.3 (*continued*)

(c) Univent tube.

able, which has the advantage of ease of passage into the trachea combined with excellent moulded curves for both the pharynx and the left main bronchus. Single-lumen endobronchial tubes are sized, like endotracheal tubes, by internal diameter in millimetres. The external diameter of these tubes may be slightly greater than that of the equivalent endotracheal tube because of the thickness of the rubber wall.

Following passage of a single-lumen tube into the appropriate bronchus, the tracheal cuff is inflated. Ventilation of the opposite lung continues by overspill of gas around the deflated bronchial cuff. When one-lung ventilation is required, the bronchial cuff is inflated and the tracheal cuff deflated to allow collapse of the non-ventilated lung. Some authorities prefer to keep both cuffs inflated and to allow the lung to collapse by absorption of alveolar gases. This may reduce the possibility of aspiration of gastric contents.

The drawbacks of using a single-lumen endobronchial tube are as follows:

- Ventilation of the non-intubated lung relies on overspill of gas and may be poor
- Collapse and re-inflation of the non-intubated lung are slow
- There is no access for suctioning the non-intubated lung.

Bronchial blockade

In the absence of commercially manufactured alternatives, bronchial blockade is achieved by placement of an embolectomy catheter alongside, or through, an endotracheal tube. The bronchus to be occluded is identified by fibre-optic bronchoscopy, and the 'blocker' positioned under direct vision. The Univent tube, which has achieved some popularity in the United States and parts of Europe, comprises an endotracheal tube with a narrow channel in its anterior internal wall that holds a moveable bronchus blocker. The blocker has a low-pressure, high-volume cuff, and a central lumen for suctioning.

The general design of double- and single-lumen endobronchial tubes and the Univent tube is diagrammatically represented in Figure 4.3.

Aims of the ideal technique of ventilation for one-lung anaesthesia

One-lung anaesthesia should aim to produce normocapnia and normoxia. The non-dependent, non-ventilated lung should be completely collapsed and the dependent, ventilated lung should not be atelectatic. However, a ventilatory technique that produces full expansion of the dependent lung and maintains it free of atelectasis may well produce a mean intra-alveolar pressure high enough to increase the mean pulmonary vascular resistance for that lung. This will divert some blood flow to the non-dependent, non-ventilated lung, increasing the shunt through that lung. The increased intrapulmonary pressure will also tend to reduce cardiac output. Both of these factors will tend to worsen hypoxia.

It has been argued that volume controlled ventilation delivers a more consistent tidal and minute volume than pressure controlled ventilation in the presence of surgical manipulation of the lung and mediastinum. However, there is some experimental evidence suggesting that mean intrapulmonary pressures are lower and arterial oxygenation is better maintained with pressure controlled ventilation.

The gases used for ventilation during one-lung anaesthesia should be warmed and 100 per cent humidified. In practice this may lead to unnecessarily complicated anaesthetic circuits and, in most cases, an efficient heat and moisture exchanger attached to the catheter mount of the patient circuit suffices.

Manual ventilation versus mechanical ventilation

A period of manual ventilation may be helpful during the initial opening of the pleura; a pause in ventilation during expiration may prevent damage to the underlying lung. Manual ventilation is also useful during re-inflation of the non-dependent lung (or remaining lobes) at the end of the period of one-lung anaesthesia. It is very helpful to directly visualize lung re-expansion whilst 'squeezing the bag'. Manual ventilation is used to test the integrity of pulmonary and bronchial suture lines; the suture line is held under water and the lung manually inflated to a pressure of 25–30 cmH$_2$O.

Ventilator settings

The minute volume should be set to maintain alveolar ventilation sufficient to produce normocapnia. The respiratory rate and tidal volume selected should minimize peak and mean airway pressures. This minimization of the intrapulmonary pressure tends to prevent the diversion of perfusion to the non-dependent, non-ventilated lung, and may also limit any fall in cardiac output associated with one-lung ventilation. Consequently it has become customary to use lower tidal volumes and more rapid respiratory rates than would be usual in two-lung ventilation. The use of small tidal volumes at high rates is often dictated by the reduced total ventilatory compliance ensuing from the change to one-lung ventilation.

The use of a larger than usual ratio of inspiration to expiration (I : E ratio) during a period of one-lung ventilation should result in a lower peak intrapulmonary pressure, and may allow for better gas exchange by recruiting slow alveoli. However, this strategy may increase the mean intrapulmonary pressure and may not allow a respiratory rate rapid enough to maintain adequate minute ventilation. In practice, an I : E ratio of 1 : 1.5 is usual.

It is impossible to recommend ventilator settings that are appropriate to all patients for one-lung anaesthesia. The following settings provide a suitable starting point for one-lung ventilation in many patients:

Tidal volume	8–10 ml per kg
Respiratory rate	15 breaths per min
FiO$_2$	0.5
I : E ratio	1 : 1.5

Some authorities have recommended the use of 5 cmH$_2$O of positive end expiratory pressure (PEEP) from the onset of one-lung ventilation. This may, however, reduce cardiac output. Others recommend that PEEP should be reserved until the pulmonary physiology has reached some stability following the change from two-lung ventilation to one, and should only be used if hypoxia develops at an FiO$_2$ greater than 0.6.

Initiating one-lung anaesthesia

The following routine is suggested as a practical way of managing the onset of one-lung anaesthesia.

1. Whilst still ventilating both lungs, change the ventilator settings to those anticipated for one-lung anaesthesia.
2. Continuously monitor and record arterial oxygen saturation, end-tidal carbon dioxide (CO_2) concentration, peak inflation pressure and, if possible, the expired tidal or minute volume. This needs to be done some minutes before the start of one-lung ventilation to allow the measured variables to stabilize.
3. Clamp the limb of the Y-shaped catheter mount connected to the non-dependent lung and disconnect that limb from the double-lumen tube (this is usually the tracheal lumen). Only the dependent lung should now be ventilating, and the non-dependent lung should be open to the atmosphere and able to collapse.
4. a. Observe for any change in end-tidal CO_2 concentration, airway pressure and expired tidal volume. If the transition to one-lung ventilation has been correctly accomplished, there will be an increase in peak ventilator pressure (assuming the ventilator is not pressure controlled). The mean inflation pressure when one lung is ventilated has been shown in some studies to be 40–50 per cent higher than when both lungs are ventilated. If the ventilator generates a higher than expected airway pressure and there is still an expired CO_2 trace, the preset inspired tidal volume is too large for the compliance of the ventilated lung. If the peak inspiratory pressure is very high, rapidly reached, and the expiratory CO_2 trace is lost, then either there has been a technical error in the way the double-lumen tube has been set up (see (3) above), the tube has been misplaced or it has become dislodged. If the peak airway pressure is lower than expected, check that the preset tidal volume is being delivered. A small reduction in tidal volume is acceptable, but the loss of more than 15 per cent of the ventilation would suggest that there is a significant leak somewhere in the circuit.
   b. Once the adequacy of ventilation has been established in terms of satisfactory airway pressure and end-tidal CO_2, attention should be focused on the arterial oxygen saturation. A significant decrease in the saturation related to the onset of one-lung ventilation will only occur after several minutes. If the arterial oxygen saturation remains within normal limits, it may be possible to reduce the FiO_2 to less than 0.5. If, however, saturation falls significantly, it is necessary to take action to correct hypoxia (see below).
5. When the pleura is open, visually check that the non-dependent lung is not being ventilated and has collapsed, or is collapsing.

Common ventilatory problems

The non-dependent lung is still being ventilated

The commonest cause for this problem is that the wrong side of the Y connector to the double-lumen tube has been clamped and disconnected. If the connections are correct and the lung is still being ventilated, then the next most likely cause is that the bronchial cuff of the double-lumen tube is either inadequately inflated or may have ruptured. If the cuff is correctly inflated, then the tube may either be in the wrong bronchus or have become proximally displaced so that the bronchial lumen is lying in the trachea.

Check the connections to the tube and check that the bronchial cuff is still inflated. If these are correct, re-check the placement of the tube with a fibre-optic bronchoscope (Fig. 4.2).

The non-dependent lung is not being ventilated, but fails to collapse

This may result either from factors related to the patient and the disease process or from mechanical problems with the endobronchial tube. In either case, there is some obstruction to the airways of the non-dependent lung.

Patient factors

Slow or non-collapse of the lung is commonly seen in patients with asthma or emphysema in whom expiration to atmosphere is delayed. In these patients the lung will collapse, but it may take 5–15 minutes. The problem may also be seen where there is an obstructing lesion (usually tumour) in a large bronchus, which prevents rapid collapse of the lung. If this is the case, the obstructing tumour may have been seen at pre-operative bronchoscopy. Again, the lung will collapse in time as residual gas is absorbed from the alveoli. In both of the above situations the surgeon should be encouraged to be patient. Provided the situation has been correctly assessed, the lung will collapse. In inflamed or infected lungs, the lung may be adherent to the chest wall and may totally or partially fail to collapse.

Mechanical factors

If the tube is placed too proximally, it is possible that the bronchial cuff has herniated across the carina – that is, the cuff is correctly sealing the bronchus to the ventilated lung, but it is also obstructing the non-ventilated lung and preventing it collapsing. This obstruction can also be produced by over-inflation of the bronchial cuff of a correctly placed tube in some of the older designs of red-rubber endobronchial equipment.

The only sure way to check this is to visualize the tube placement and cuff inflation with the fibre-optic bronchoscope (Fig. 4.2).

The capnometer reading indicates a low end-tidal CO_2 but an arterial blood gas shows a high arterial CO_2 tension

The non-ventilated lung has collapsed and the dependent lung appears to be ventilating properly.

In this situation, it is likely that the expired minute ventilation is low and there may be a high airway pressure. This is a common circumstance in one-lung anaesthesia, and may be accompanied by hypoxia (see below). The apparently low end-tidal CO_2 reading is probably anomalous and does not reflect the true alveolar CO_2. This may be because the expiratory time is too short to allow complete expiration. The simple solution is to lengthen the expiratory time and reduce the respiratory rate. This may be difficult to accomplish without a reduction in total minute ventilation. If the tidal volume is increased in an attempt to maintain the minute volume, there will be a further increase in the already high airway pressure because of the relatively low compliance of the dependent, ventilated lung. Alternatively, there may be an air leak around the endobronchial cuff. This can be eliminated by further inflating the cuff or manipulating the tube into a better position.

Adjust the respiratory rate and tidal volume to maintain the best possible minute volume.

Although hypercapnia is best avoided, moderate elevation of the arterial CO_2 tension is not catastrophic, and indeed permissive hypercapnia is an acceptable technique when dealing with patients with severe ventilatory difficulty. This is discussed further in Chapter 15.

Persistent hypoxia

Hypoxia is a frequent complication during the conduct of one-lung anaesthesia. It often develops insidiously, and manoeuvres to correct it should be instituted as soon as it becomes manifest. Readings from all too frequently unreliable pulse oximeters should be checked by arterial blood gas analysis.

It is, to some extent, possible to predict which patients will become hypoxic. These can be briefly summarized as those who have a reduced arterial oxygen saturation either pre-operatively or during ventilation of both lungs, and those with a lower than predicted FEV_1. Hypoxia is also more common in right than in left thoracotomy.

The following strategies may help when dealing with hypoxia during one-lung anaesthesia. They are summarized in Table 4.2.

1. Increase the FiO_2 to 1, check that the delivered gas is 100 per cent oxygen and that the anaesthetic machine and the ventilator are functioning correctly.
2. Check the breathing circuit and the double-lumen tube connectors for disconnection or major leaks. Check that the preset minute ventilation is being delivered (there should be an adequate end-tidal CO_2 trace and there should be a means of directly monitoring the expired tidal or minute ventilation).

Table 4.2. The management of hypoxia

Increase FiO_2 to 1

Check anaesthetic machine and ventilator

Check end-tidal CO_2 trace and expired tidal or minute volume

Check breathing circuit and double-lumen tube for disconnections or leaks

Auscultate dependent lung and suction out debris/sputum

Check tube position with fibre-optic bronchoscope

Assess cardiac output
    maintain or restore circulating blood volume
    consider inotropic agents
    consider TOE

Insufflate O_2 to non-ventilated lung

PEEP the dependent lung

CPAP the non-ventilated lung

Intermittently inflate the non-ventilated lung with oxygen (needs teamwork between the anaesthetist and surgeon)

Pulmonary artery occlusion (if appropriate)

---

3. Ensure the adequacy of ventilation by auscultating the dependent lung, and suction to remove any debris or sputum.
4. Assess the cardiac output initially in terms of blood pressure, pulse rate and the adequacy of the replacement of circulating blood volume. It should be borne in mind that surgical manipulation in and around the hilum may restrict systemic venous return, or may directly compress the heart. If it is felt that the cardiac output is low, then attempts should be made to improve it either by the use of appropriate volume to maintain left ventricular filling or by the judicious use of inotropic agents. If there is any doubt about how best to optimize the cardiac output, it may be advisable to use trans-oesophageal echocardiography to assess left heart filling and myocardial contractility. It is difficult to pass a pulmonary artery catheter with the patient in the thoracotomy position.
5. If there is persistent hypoxia in one-lung anaesthesia which is not related to a low cardiac output or to a mechanical or technical failure, it is likely to be due either to a large shunt through the non-ventilated lung or to worsening ventilation–perfusion matching in the dependent, ventilated lung. The following manoeuvres have been found to be helpful:
   a. *PEEP to the dependent lung.* Ventilation–perfusion mismatch in the ventilated lung is likely to be produced by atelectatic changes caused by the weight of the mediastinum and by ventilating the lung with low tidal volumes. The addition of PEEP to this lung has been shown to be beneficial in the management of hypoxia during one-lung anaesthesia. This effect is produced by recruiting alveoli, increasing the end expiratory volume, and thereby improving gas exchange in the lung. However, this advantageous effect of PEEP may be offset by the increase in the mean intrapulmonary pressure that occurs. This may increase the vascular resistance of the lung, and tend to divert more shunt blood to the non-ventilated lung. Thus, whilst improving the conditions in the ventilated lung, PEEP may occasionally worsen

the shunt through the non-ventilated lung. PEEP may also make hypoxia worse by reducing the cardiac output. PEEP must therefore be used with caution. Experimentally, the correct amount of PEEP to apply has been found to be the same as the measured intrinsic PEEP (PEEPi) for that patient under conditions of one-lung ventilation. Clinically, the best PEEP should be sought empirically, starting with 5 cmH$_2$O and increasing in steps of 2.5 cmH$_2$O until a satisfactory arterial oxygen tension or saturation is reached.

b. *Insufflation of oxygen.* Oxygen at a low flow rate (2–4 l/min) can be insufflated into the non-ventilated lung via a narrow bore tube. Blood flowing through the non-ventilated lung can be oxygenated adequately to alleviate hypoxia using this technique.

c. *Continuous positive airway pressure (CPAP) to the non-ventilated lung.* The application of 5–10 cmH$_2$O of CPAP from a suitable circuit to the non-ventilated lung has been shown by some workers to improve arterial oxygenation. CPAP allows some oxygenation of the shunt blood in the non-ventilated lung. CPAP, like PEEP, has potential disadvantages. CPAP will tend to re-expand the non-ventilated lung, and therefore reduce its vascular resistance. This may worsen the shunt. Partial re-expansion of the lung may also hinder surgical activity and slow the progress of the procedure. CPAP, like PEEP, should be applied cautiously. Start with 5 cmH$_2$O, and gradually increase it until the arterial oxygenation is improved.

d. *Intermittent re-inflation and differential lung ventilation.* Where hypoxia persists despite all attempts to optimize the situation, the arterial oxygenation will usually be improved by intermittent inflation of the non-ventilated lung with oxygen. This can only take place with surgical agreement, and its application requires considerable teamwork between the anaesthetist and the surgeon. It should be noted that when the anaesthetist is having difficulty in maintaining oxygenation, the surgeon is often having difficulty with the surgery. The lung is manually inflated with oxygen, and then allowed to collapse immediately. If this procedure is repeated at 5–10 minute intervals, all but a few patients can be kept reasonably well oxygenated. A similar technique has been described in which, instead of completely ceasing ventilation to the non-dependent lung after it has been collapsed, ventilation is allowed to continue with the Y connector to that lung partially occluded. This allows the lung to be ventilated at low pressure and low volume, and has been reported to improve oxygenation without resorting to full re-inflation.

e. *High frequency jet ventilation (HFJV).* HFJV has been used to alleviate hypoxia whilst providing partially deflated lungs to facilitate surgical access. Some anaesthetists routinely employ HFJV for cases in which soiling of the dependent lung is not an issue.

f. *Pulmonary artery occlusion.* Where it is not possible either to re-inflate or partially ventilate the non-dependent lung, oxygenation can be rapidly improved if the surgeon can occlude the ipsilateral pulmonary artery. This is particularly applicable in patients undergoing lung resection, where the hilar vessels will be identified, but can only be a permanent solution in pneumonectomy.

When severe hypoxia complicates the conduct of one-lung anaesthesia, for whatever reason, the anaesthetist should make the surgeon aware of the problem as soon as possible. Both lungs should be ventilated or the pulmonary artery should be occluded as soon as possible before the patient suffers permanent neurological or myocardial damage. There is no point in providing ideal operating conditions for surgery if the patient sustains a peri-operative myocardial infarction or a debilitating stroke.

Re-establishing two-lung ventilation

With the exception of patients undergoing pneumonectomy, it will be necessary to re-establish two-lung ventilation after a period of one-lung anaesthesia. Simple reconnection of the non-ventilated lung to the breathing circuit will not, in most cases, result in full and complete re-inflation of the lung. It is necessary to apply a greater than usual inspiratory pressure to the previously non-ventilated lung to aid inflation. This is best accomplished by gentle manual ventilation whilst the re-expansion of the lung is directly observed. Both lungs should be suctioned clear of debris/sputum at the termination of one-lung ventilation.

Unilateral pulmonary oedema following re-inflation of the non-ventilated lung after one-lung anaesthesia has been described many times, and its occurrence may relate to the surgical procedure involved and the duration of one-lung ventilation, and to barotrauma inflicted during re-inflation. It is recommended that re-inflation of the lung should take 1 minute rather than one breath, and that a pressure of 45 cmH$_2$O should not be exceeded.

Arterial oxygenation, end-tidal CO$_2$ and expired ventilatory volumes should be closely observed to ensure that two-lung ventilation has been safely and correctly re-established.

KEY POINTS

- The indications for one-lung anaesthesia are seldom absolute, but patients at risk of spilling material from one lung to the other or who have an abnormal distribution of ventilation should usually be managed in this way.

- If one-lung anaesthesia is not possible, most thoracic surgery can be completed with endotracheal intubation utilizing conventional ventilation or HFJV.

- The change from two- to one-lung ventilation should be carefully monitored.

- The anaesthetist should have a logical plan for dealing with ventilatory problems and hypoxia during one-lung anaesthesia.

- One-lung anaesthesia adds to the technical complexity of anaesthesia. It should not be pursued at all cost, and never justifies making patients hypoxic.

- Care should be taken in managing the resumption of two-lung ventilation.

Bibliography

Baraka, A. (1994). Differential lung ventilation as an alternative to one-lung ventilation during thoracotomy. *Anaesth.*, **49**, 881–2.

Bardoczky, G.I., Levarlet, M., Engelman, E. *et al.* (1993). Continuous spirometry for detection of double-lumen endobronchial tube displacement. *Br. J. Anaesth.*, **70**, 499–502.

Brodsky, J.B., Benumof, J.L., Ehrenwerth, J. *et al.* (1991). Depth of placement of left double-lumen endobronchial tubes. *Anesth. Analg.*, **73**, 570–2.

Brodsky, J.B., Macario, A. and Mark, B.D. (1996). Tracheal diameter predicts double-lumen tube size: a method for selecting left double-lumen tubes. *Anesth. Analg.*, **82**, 861–4.

Cohen, E. and Eisenkraft, J.B. (1996). Positive end-expiratory pressure during one-lung ventilation improves oxygenation in patients with low arterial oxygen tensions. *J. Cardiothorac. Vasc. Anesth.*, **10**, 578–82.

Hogue, C.W. Jr (1994). Effectiveness of low levels of non-ventilated lung continuous positive airway pressure in improving arterial oxygenation during one-lung ventilation. *Anesth. Analg.*, **79**, 364–7.

Hughes, S.A. and Benumof, J.L. (1990). Operative lung continuous positive airway pressure to minimize FiO_2 during one-lung ventilation. *Anesth. Analg.*, **71**, 92–5.

Inomata, S., Nishikawa, T., Saito, S. and Kihara, S. (1997). 'Best' PEEP during one-lung ventilation. *Br. J. Anaesth.*, **78**, 754–6.

Inouhe, H., Shotsu, A., Ogowa, J. *et al.* (1982). New device for one-lung anaesthesia: endotracheal tube with moveable blocker. *J. Thorac. Cardiovasc. Surg.*, **83**, 940–1.

Malmkvist, G. (1989). Maintenance of oxygenation during one-lung ventilation. Effect of intermittent re-inflation of the collapsed lung with oxygen. *Anesth. Analg.*, **68**, 763–6.

Obara, H., Tanaka, O., Hoshino, Y. *et al.* (1986). One-lung ventilation. The effect of positive end expiratory pressure to the non-dependent and dependent lung. *Anaesthesia*, **41**, 1007–10.

Rees, D.I. and Wansbrough, S.R. (1982). One-lung anesthesia: percent shunt and arterial oxygen tension during continuous insufflation of oxygen to the non-ventilated lung. *Anesth. Analg.*, **61**, 507–12.

Simon, B.A., Hurford, W.E., Alfille, P.H. *et al.* (1992). An aid to the diagnosis of malpositioned double-lumen tubes. *Anesthesiology*, **76**, 845–9.

Slinger, P., Suissa, S. and Triolet, W. (1992). Predicting arterial oxygenation during one-lung anaesthesia. *Can. J. Anaesth.*, **39**, 1030–5.

Szegedi, L.L., Bardoczky, G.I., Engelman, E.E. and d'Hollander, A.A. (1997). Airway pressure changes during one-lung ventilation. *Anesth. Analg.*, **84**, 1034–7.

Tugrul, M., Camci, E., Karadeniz, H. *et al.* (1997). Comparison of volume-controlled with pressure-controlled ventilation during one-lung anaesthesia. *Br. J. Anaesth.*, **79**, 306–10.

5

Surgery on the lungs

I. G. Wright

Introduction

Therapeutic resection of pulmonary tissue may be carried out for malignancy (primary lung cancer or isolated secondaries), benign tumours (e.g. carcinoid tumours, haemangiomas) or infective processes (e.g. bronchiectasis, tuberculosis, mycetoma, hydatid disease), or for bullous disease of the lung. Surgery for lung trauma and volume reduction surgery for emphysema are covered in Chapters 11 and 13, respectively.

Diagnostic biopsy is usually required prior to definitive resection for lesions susceptible to surgery, or prior to commencement of medical regimens for diffuse disease processes (e.g. fibrosing alveolitis). Cancer is the commonest indication for lung resection, and the pathophysiology of lung cancer is described below. This is followed by a discussion of assessment of pulmonary function prior to surgery.

The chapter concludes with a description of the management of specific operations and other relevant disease processes.

Cancer of the lung

Lung cancer ranks highest on the list of newly diagnosed cancers per year, with a frequency of 13 per cent of all new cancer cases annually on a worldwide basis.

Amongst the common malignant carcinomas of the lung, the current basic distinction is between small cell (oat cell) and non-small cell tumours (squamous cell carcinoma, adenocarcinoma and large cell carcinomas). Small cell tumours behave very aggressively and are usually not curable by surgical resection by the time of presentation, as a result of metastatic disease. Non-small cell lung carcinomas (NSCLC) are more amenable to cure by resection, but between 70 and 90 per cent of even these cases present too late for surgical treatment.

There are three initial stages in determining whether surgery is appropriate for an individual patient; identifying tumour type, staging (determining the degree of tumour spread), and assessing the patient's fitness for surgery. The latter includes an estimation of whether the extent of lung resection required to effect a cure will leave the patient with sufficient respiratory function post-operatively to survive with a reasonable quality of life.

Identifying tumour type

Obtaining tumour tissue for analysis and identification of cell type is usually initially by bronchoscopy with biopsy of visible lesions, or by obtaining bronchial brushings for cytological analysis if no lesion is visible. Cytological analysis of expectorated sputum is positive in 50–60 per cent of lung cancers, with cell type identifiable in 80 per cent of these, though cytological analysis of bronchial lavage fluid obtained at the time of bronchoscopy is more frequently successful. More peripheral lesions are often not seen bronchoscopically and tissue can be obtained by computerized tomographic (CT) guided needle biopsy, with a low rate of complications (e.g. significant pneumothorax or haemorrhage) in skilled hands. Biopsy of affected lymph nodes at mediastinoscopy may provide histology, as well as information for staging. If all of these fail, it will be necessary to obtain tissue by thorocoscopic or open biopsy of the affected lung tissue.

Staging

Staging (the determination of the extent of tumour spread) for lung cancer is by identification of tumour size and location (T), degree of spread to lymph nodes (N), and the presence or absence of distant metastases (M). The required information is obtained by chest X-ray (CXR), more sophisticated radiological investigations such as a CT scan, magnetic resonance imaging (MRI) and positron emission tomography (PET), and by biopsy of lung tissue and mediastinal nodes.

The TNM categorization of the cancer is used to determine operability and the need for adjuvant therapy, and to predict mortality. The 5-year post-operative survival for smaller localized tumours with no lymphatic spread (or spread only to the ipsilateral local lymph nodes) and no metastases is between 50 and 70 per cent. The role of adjuvant chemotherapy or radiotherapy is under constant evaluation, especially as new drugs and regimens undergo clinical trials. Historically, chemotherapy probably added 5 per cent to the 5-year survival. The boundaries of operability are constantly being tested, and case reports of long-term survival in 'non-operable' situations exist. The median survival time from the time of presentation of inoperable carcinoma of the lung is dependent on cell type, but even in the best category (squamous cell) it is only 14 weeks. It seems likely that most tumours are between 8 months and 3 years old by the time the patient presents for treatment.

The challenge for the future is illustrated by the sobering fact that, of 100 patients with cancer of the lung, only eight will be alive 5 years after presentation and only four after 10 years.

Assessing fitness for surgery

Of prime concern is the estimation of whether the patient will have sufficient residual lung function after resection to have an acceptable quality of life. This is discussed in detail later.

A substantial majority of cancers of the lung are associated with cigarette smoking; the consequent frequent co-existence of obstructive airways disease, bronchitis and coronary artery disease have obvious implications for anaesthesia.

Assessment of coronary artery disease should be particularly thorough. Factors that may contribute to peri-operative myocardial infarction include hypoxia (intra-operatively on one-lung anaesthesia, post-operatively with atelectasis, sputum retention or the development of pulmonary oedema), arrhythmias, haemodynamic changes (with intra-operative manipulations, peri-operative blood loss and fluid shifts), peri-operative hypothermia and inadequate pain control. It may be necessary to improve coronary blood flow by angioplasty or bypass grafting before operating on the lung. A combined operation, with coronary artery bypass grafting followed by pulmonary resection, is feasible. The increased risk of the combined procedure needs to be weighed against the risk of further significant spread of the tumour if pulmonary resection is delayed by about 4 weeks to allow recuperation from the coronary bypass operation.

Other cardiac problems to consider are pericardial effusions and arrhythmias, both of which may be secondary to tumour invasion.

Patients who have received chemotherapy should be assessed for associated organ damage. A wide range of multi-agent regimens exists. Short- or long-term toxicity of some form is almost universal, though not necessarily serious. Toxicity problems pertinent to anaesthesia include cardiotoxicity (e.g. by doxorubicin), pneumonitis culminating in pulmonary fibrosis (e.g. by mitomycin C or bleomycin, particularly exacerbated by exposure to high inspired oxygen concentrations), nephrotoxicity (e.g. by mitomycin C or cisplatinum), hypomagnesaemia and hypocalcaemia (e.g. by cisplatinum or mithramycin), neuropathy (e.g. by vincristine or vinblastine), and reduced cholinesterase activity (e.g. by alkylating agents, especially cylclophosphamide). The above list of drugs associated with each form of toxicity is not comprehensive, and each regimen needs to be individually evaluated for any potential impact of side effects on anaesthesia.

Treatment of any reversible element to airways obstruction should be optimized. This may necessitate the introduction or optimization of steroid therapy, but it must be borne in mind that patients on high doses of steroids may have impaired wound healing and be more prone to post-operative infections. Patients with chest infections should be treated with antibiotics and physiotherapy. It can be difficult to achieve improvement in chronic bronchitic patients, and impossible in patients with infection distal to an occluded bronchus.

Co-existing pulmonary disease is important not only for its direct impact on the conduct of anaesthesia and influence on the post-operative course, but also in determining how much lung can be safely removed and still leave the patient with adequate respiratory function compatible with a reasonable quality of life.

Assessment of lung function

Prediction of adequate respiratory function is an inexact science, but it is a necessary process before lung tissue is resected from any but the fittest patient. Although lung function tests provide useful information for the conduct of anaesthesia, no test should be considered in isolation. The large standard deviation in the 'normal' values of many of these tests highlights the inexactitude of the process. Furthermore, the parameters deemed acceptable as predictors of increased morbidity after lung resection vary between differing published studies, and the criteria applied at different centres as indicative of suitability for operation also differ. Individual patients' lung function results need to be reviewed in the context of their lung disease, general health and the extent of resection contemplated.

Spirometry

Spirometry is simple, cheap and readily available. The goal is a post-operative forced expiratory volume in the first second (FEV_1) of at least 35 per cent predicted (0.8–1.0 l in an average sized male), and a forced vital capacity (FVC) of at least 40 per cent predicted (2 l in an average sized male). Less than this carries an unacceptable risk of intolerable respiratory failure. The pathologic processes in the patient need to be taken into account when extrapolating from pre-operative measurements to the post-operative status. For example, spirometry may show a 50 per cent reduction in lung volume and flow rates, which would indicate inadequate reserve for a pneumonectomy if that 50 per cent reduction were the result of generalized lung disease. However, this would be acceptable if the reduction was the result of a tumour occluding the left or right main bronchus. Indeed, in the latter situation the patient has already declared what his or her post-pneumonectomy functional status would be; removal of the diseased lung may even improve the condition by removing a source of shunt and by allowing compensatory expansion of the remaining lung. Any patient showing an FEV_1/FVC ratio of less than 60 per cent, or a 30 per cent or more reduction in the maximum expiratory flow rate (MEFR), should be re-tested after administration of a bronchodilator in order to detect any reversibility to the airways obstruction. Nebulized bronchodilator is more effective than that administered via an inhaler, particularly in subjects unfamiliar with inhaler technique and those with significant lung pathology. Salbutamol (e.g. 2.5 mg nebulized) is the usual agent used. The post-bronchodilator results are those to be used if it is anticipated that reasonable medical control of the airways obstruction can be achieved. Significant reversibility is also an indication of the need to optimize peri-operative bronchodilatation and avoid agents likely to exacerbate broncho-constriction.

The maximum voluntary ventilation (MVV), also known as the maximum breathing capacity (MBC), is the volume in litres that can be breathed by an individual over 1 minute. This is an impractical measurement in many people, and is usually extrapolated from the volume breathed in 10 or 15 seconds. Even this can be too volition dependent, so its value can be estimated by multiplying the FEV_1 by 35, to give the so called MVV_i (i for

Table 5.1 Widely accepted lung function criteria for assessing suitability for resection

Pre-op. per cent predicted value	Pneumonectomy	Lobectomy	Wedge/segmental resection
MVV	> 55 per cent	> 40 per cent	> 35 per cent
FEV₁	> 55 per cent (> 2 l)	> 40 per cent (> 1 l)	> 35 per cent (> 0.6 l)

indirect). Alternatively, the FEV over 0.75 seconds can be multiplied by 40. However calculated, the lower acceptable limit for the MVV is a predicted post-resection figure of 20 l per minute per square metre of body surface area.

Table 5.1 summarizes widely accepted criteria for suitability for lung resection.

Diffusion capacity

The diffusion capacity, or transfer factor, of the lungs for carbon monoxide (DLCO or TLCO) is often used as an independent predictor of adequate post-operative respiratory function, with a post-resection minimum of 40 per cent normal being considered acceptable. The DLCO will be reduced if there is either a reduction in available alveolar area, as in emphysema, or a defect in diffusion at alveolar-capillary level, as in interstitial lung diseases. The diffusion at alveolar-capillary level (KCO) is quantified by dividing the DLCO by the available alveolar volume (VA). The VA is determined by a single breath helium dilution test.

Calculation of post-operative lung function

Prediction of post-operative lung function values from pre-operative measurements is attained by calculating how many of the 19 segments of the lungs will remain after resection and multiplying the pre-operative measurement by the resulting fraction. The distribution of the 19 segments is as follows:

right upper lobe – 3
right middle lobe – 2
right lower lobe – 5
left upper lobe   – 5
left lower lobe   – 4.

Ventilation and perfusion scans

These enable the prediction of post-operative lung function from pre-resection measurements if non-uniform lung function is suspected. Radio-active xenon, krypton or DTPA-technetium labelled aerosol tracer is inhaled, and the lungs scanned to observe the distribution of ventilation. Similarly, injected radioactive tracer (e.g. technetium labelled albumin microspheres) demonstrates the distribution of blood flow through the lungs. These results can be quantified into percentages of ventilation and perfusion to each area of the lungs and, by simple arithmetic, the theoretical residual function post-resection calculated.

Blood gas analysis

A P_{CO_2} of greater than 6.0 kPa (45 mmHg) is associated with a greater than average risk of respiratory failure and mortality post-operatively, although this is no longer considered an independent marker. Low P_{O_2} levels may be the result of shunt through non-ventilated lung units destined to be removed at surgery, and are therefore not necessarily a risk factor. Aside from this, an oxyhaemoglobin saturation below 90 per cent with a fall of 5 per cent or more on exercise is associated with a higher risk of complications.

Exercise tests

An old-fashioned but clinically useful test is to see how the patient tolerates a short walk, preferably including two or three flights of stairs, particularly with regard to undue breathlessness and the speed at which it can be accomplished. This has been made more quantifiable in the form of the 'six minute walk test'. The distance covered is measured, enabling the mean speed to be calculated. The pulse rate and arterial oxygen saturation are measured during the test using a portable pulse oximeter. Unacceptable values are a speed of less than 3 km per hour (300 m in 6 minutes), or a fall in oxygen saturation measurements by 5 per cent or more. The test suffers from being dependent on both the motivation of the patient and the encouragement given by the tester. Formal laboratory exercise testing to determine peak oxygen uptake (VO_2 max.) is the most precise way to obtain objective information about the patient's respiratory reserve capacity. A VO_2 max. of less than 15 ml/kg may be associated with an increased risk of post-operative complications.

Pulmonary artery pressure testing

Following lung resection, a small number of patients develop cor pulmonale. This is secondary to the sudden increase in pulmonary vascular resistance caused by removing a proportion of the pulmonary vascular bed. This increase in blood flow to the remaining pulmonary vascular bed is not generally a problem, but can be in patients with already compromised pulmonary vascular compliance, e.g. secondary to obstructive airways disease. Because these patients constitute a relatively small proportion of the total, pulmonary artery pressure (PAP) studies are not routine prior to pulmonary resection. Indirect evidence of raised PAP should, however, be routinely sought. Readily observed signs include a loud pulmonary second sound on auscultation, right atrial or right ventricular hypertrophy on the electrocardiogram and CXR changes. Echocardiography can provide an indirect estimate of pulmonary artery pressure non-invasively, as well as demonstrating right ventricular hypertrophy and dilatation. If raised PAP is suspected, it can then be measured directly; a special type of catheter that permits balloon occlusion of the pulmonary artery on the side to be resected whilst measuring PAP through a lumen proximal to the balloon is positioned transvenously. If the patient then exercises, the post-operative situation can be simulated. A mean PAP higher than 40 mmHg is associated with post-operative development of cor pulmonale. In theory, the bronchus supplying the lung to be resected should also be occluded by a balloon during these measurements in order to eliminate the increase in ventilation–perfusion mismatching that otherwise occurs, but the logistics of this render it imprac-tical. Finally, it is of course possible to measure the PAP at operation after clamping the pulmonary artery on the side to be resected, although by this stage the patient will have undergone an unnecessary thoracotomy should the resection be aborted on the basis of the PAP measurements.

Recommended test protocol

Not every patient needs all of the above tests. If, on simple spirometry, patients achieve their predicted post-resection criteria, no further tests are required. If they do not, or the results are borderline, patients should go on to have full pulmonary function tests including transfer factor estimation and measurement of oxygen saturation at rest and on exercise. If pneumo-nectomy is being considered, a quantitative isotope perfusion scan should be performed. This data should be used to calculate the percentage post-operative predicted FEV_1 and DLCO, using the lung scan for pneumo-nectomy and the anatomical calculation (segments remaining out of nineteen total) for a lobectomy. Patients whose predicted respiratory func-tion from these investigations precludes resection should go on to have formal exercise testing to confirm inoperability. Consideration should be given to a limited wedge resection or non-operative treatment in patients whose respiratory parameters at rest and on exercise predict too limited a reserve for lobectomy or pneumonectomy.

Individual operations

The anaesthetic techniques and post-operative management for specific operations are described below. There is inevitably some overlap between procedures, and repetition has been avoided. This section should therefore be read in its entirety.

Bronchoscopy

Bronchoscopy is the most frequently performed endoscopic examination used for the investigation of intrathoracic disease. Although rigid broncho-scopy has largely been superseded by flexible bronchoscopy in the initial assessment of pulmonary pathology, the rigid bronchoscope is still favoured for surgical assessment prior to mediastinoscopy or thoracotomy. It is also used therapeutically for the removal of foreign bodies, control of massive haemoptysis, placement of stents and endoscopic resection of tracheal or bronchial tumours. Laser resection of tumours may be carried out using fibre-optic bronchoscopy and special metal endotracheal tubes, or more simply by using the rigid metal bronchoscope. Rigid bronchoscopy is a far more stimulating insult to the airway than flexible bronchoscopy, and gives rise to a marked hypertensive response and arrhythmias, most frequently bradycardia as a result of vagal stimulation.

Flexible bronchoscopy

Flexible bronchoscopy is generally performed under sedation with a benzo-diazepine and with topical anaesthesia to the pharynx. Large doses of local anaesthetic may be required, and are best administered by nebulization and by cricothyroid injection. General anaesthesia may occasionally be required. In such cases, the fibre-optic bronchoscope may be passed through a self-sealing cap on the endotracheal tube or laryngeal mask airway to maintain continuity of gas flow to the lungs. The largest endotracheal tube that the patient's airway can accommodate should be used, as passage of the bronchoscope reduces the area of lumen available for ventilation and significantly increases resistance to gas flow. The anaesthetic technique for flexible bronchoscopy under general anaesthesia is essentially the same as that described below for rigid bronchoscopy.

Rigid bronchoscopy

Pre-operative assessment

Patients present for rigid bronchoscopy with a wide variety of pathology. Particular attention needs to be directed to assessment of the upper and lower airways and the lung fields, and the presence of effusions or pneumo-thorax, clinically and from radiographs.

The anaesthetist should be aware of the suspected underlying pathology and co-existent disease, particularly cardiovascular disease. Underlying pulmonary pathologies of note include the following:

- Airway tumours liable to bleed on contact with the bronchoscope or on biopsy
- Emphysematous bullae liable to expand or rupture on application of positive pressure ventilation or administration of nitrous oxide
- Infected lung areas liable to soil healthy lung on loss of the cough reflex following induction
- Foreign bodies lodged in a bronchus acting as a ball valve.

Anaesthetic management

The aims of anaesthesia for bronchoscopy are:

- Provision of anaesthesia of sufficient depth to obtund the extreme car-diovascular responses to passage of the bronchoscope yet, if appropri-ate, allow prompt recovery of laryngeal reflexes and spontaneous respiration at the end of the procedure
- The provision of muscle relaxation for easy passage of the broncho-scope into the trachea and to prevent coughing with the bronchoscope in the airway
- Control of oxygenation in the 'shared' airway.

Premedication is generally omitted, or a benzodiazepine given for anxiolysis rather than sedation. Anticholinergic agents may be useful both for the control of airway secretions (although their use can lead to the formation of dried mucous plugs in the lower airways in patients with asthma, bronchiectasis or chronic obstructive airways disease) and for their protection against bradycardia, which may occur during the procedure.

Following establishment of standard non-invasive monitoring, particularly pulse oximetry, venous access is established, the patient pre-oxygenated and anaesthesia induced with the surgeon at hand to pass the bronchoscope. Short-acting agents are chosen if bronchoscopy is being performed in isolation, rather than immediately prior to a further procedure. A suitable technique is the use of propofol for induction and maintenance (either by infusion or by repeated boluses), alfentanil to obtund the hypertensive reflex response, and repeated doses of suxamethonium for muscle relaxation, bearing in mind the potential for bradycardia. Anaesthesia may be maintained using volatile agents if the type of bronchoscope used permits attachment of an anaesthetic circuit. The use of sevoflurane, isoflurane or halothane with maintenance of spontaneous respiration or with positive pressure ventilation is practised. The flow of gas to the patient is, however, interrupted if the viewing telescope sealing the proximal orifice of the bronchoscope is removed to permit suctioning or biopsy, and may result in awareness.

Oxygenation may be maintained during bronchoscopy by the following methods:

- Maintenance of spontaneous respiration.
- Apnoeic oxygenation; insufflation of oxygen through a catheter placed in the trachea at the carina can satisfactorily maintain oxygenation for prolonged periods, but is limited by progressive hypercapnia and respiratory acidosis. Arterial P_{CO_2} rises by 0.5 kPa per minute.
- Positive pressure ventilation applied via a sideport to the bronchoscope; this is possible if the proximal orifice of the bronchoscope is occluded by the viewing telescope, but is interrupted if this is removed.
- Utilization of a Venturi injector; attachment of an injection needle at the open proximal orifice of the bronchoscope and placed parallel to the long axis of the bronchoscope was first described in 1967 by Sanders. The Sanders injector consists of a pressure-regulating valve connected to an oxygen supply with an on-off valve placed in line between the pressure regulating valve and injector needle (Fig. 5.1). The energy of the compressed oxygen accelerating through the injector needle entrains air at the proximal end of the bronchoscope and generates sufficient pressure at the distal end to ventilate the lungs with a variable FiO_2. The tidal volume generated in an individual patient depends on lung compliance, size of the leak around the bronchoscope and the pressure produced at the distal end. The latter depends on the driving pressure from the pressure-regulating valve, size of the injector needle and dimensions of the bronchoscope. In order to avoid barotrauma, the proximal orifice of the bronchoscope must not be completely occluded during use of the injector, unless there is sufficient gap around the bronchoscope and glottis, and the

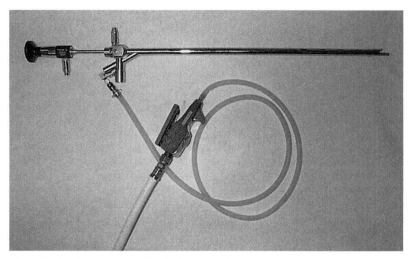

Figure 5.1 Modern version of Sanders' injector showing oxygen pipeline supply and on/
off trigger valve connected to injector needle at proximal end of Storz bronchoscope.

pressure produced at the distal end should be appropriate for the size
of patient. As driving pressure is generally maintained constant, control of flow is achieved by varying the size of the injector needle. At
the standard oxygen pipeline pressure of 410 kPa and using the
correct sized Negus bronchoscope, a 14 standard wire gauge (SWG)
needle is used in adults with poor lung compliance, a 16 SWG needle
for adults with average lungs, an 18 SWG needle for adolescents and
a 19 SWG needle for paediatric cases.

Post-operative care and complications

At the end of the procedure, the airway is suctioned clear of debris, ventilation continued with 100 per cent oxygen by face mask, muscle relaxation
reversed if non-depolarizing agents have been used and the patient placed
in the lateral position with the diseased lung down to prevent soiling of
the 'good' side. Recovery of laryngeal reflexes and spontaneous respiration
should be rapid; if not, insertion of an endotracheal tube or laryngeal mask
may be required.

Common complications include damage to teeth during passage of the
bronchoscope, trauma to the oropharynx or airway resulting in haemorrhage or swelling and airway obstruction, laryngospasm on removal of
the bronchoscope, perforation of the airway or barotrauma during the procedure, leading to pneumothorax or surgical emphysema, and arrhythmias
compounded by hypercapnia.

Open lung biopsy

Biopsy of the lung via a thoracotomy is generally only required when less
invasive approaches such as transbronchial biopsy, transcutaneous needle

biopsy (CT guided in the case of discrete lesions) or video-assisted thoraco-scopic surgery (VATS) have failed to obtain suitable tissue. Diagnostic biopsy of a lesion seen on CXR but of unknown aetiology is the most common indication, the question being whether the lesion is inflammatory scarring from an old insult (e.g. tuberculosis) or tumour. Another common indication is diffuse interstitial disease, although improvements in non-invasive techniques such as high-resolution CT scanning and sero-logical markers in the diagnosis of these diseases have meant that lung biopsy is undertaken less commonly than previously.

There are rarer indications for which open lung biopsy may be carried out, the frequency of which will depend on local factors. One group of note is that of patients who are human immunodeficiency virus (HIV) posi-tive and present with respiratory symptoms and positive CXR findings that elude conventional methods of diagnosis. *Pneumocystis carinii* or cytomega-lovirus infections, tuberculosis and Kaposi's sarcoma may all only be able to be diagnosed with the help of a lung biopsy in these patients. Meticulous attention to aseptic technique in these immunocompromised individuals, as well as protective measures against infection of medical personnel, should be instituted.

Surgical procedure

Only a small thoracotomy incision is required, usually in the axilla. This minimizes both pain and muscle damage, thus reducing impairment of post-operative respiratory function. Localized lesions are identified by pal-pation and biopsied, either by excision and oversewing of the cut edges of the lung or, more commonly, by wedge excision using stapling devices with in-built blades for cutting accurately alongside the staple line. Stapling is faster and generally provides a good result free of air leak from the cut edge. Care must be taken when inflating the lung to avoid over-distension, otherwise the staples may tear out, with ensuing lung air leak. In diffuse lung disease the process is the same, except that the area of lung biopsied is less critical and is usually determined by which area looks most affected on the CXR or CT scan. A chest drain is inserted on closing the wound, to be removed as soon as it has been established that the lung is fully re-inflated and there is no air leak. Haemorrhage is rarely a problem.

Anaesthetic management

Pre-operative assessment

This is of particular importance in patients with diffuse lung disease. Whilst some patients may be virtually asymptomatic, most are at the other end of the spectrum and are short of breath at rest and hypoxic. Auscultation reveals widespread fine crackles. Spirometry reveals a restrictive picture, with a reduced FVC but a preserved or increased FEV_1/FVC ratio. Thus, excessively high ventilation pressures may be generated if care is not taken during positive pressure ventilation. The ability to cough effectively may be impaired, predisposing to post-operative lung infection. Blood gases may show hypoxia, but the $P\text{CO}_2$ is usually normal or low. The patient may have been given a trial of steroids in the recent past in an attempt to control the disease process, or they may still be on steroids. Less commonly, the patient may have received cytotoxic drugs or immunosuppressants.

Anaesthetic techniques and monitoring

Premedication is best minimized or omitted in those whose respiratory reserve is severely compromised.

The procedure is usually short, taking under half an hour, so short-acting anaesthetic agents should be chosen. Although single-lumen endotracheal intubation usually suffices, a double-lumen tube may facilitate surgery and is also an advantage should surgery become more extensive – for example, proceeding to lobectomy if frozen section histology of the biopsied mass shows carcinoma and the patient is considered operable. As in all surgery where lung is resected, the airway should be sucked clear of spilled blood and accumulated secretions before re-expansion and ventilation of the collapsed lung takes place. Gentle and progressive re-expansion of the collapsed lung may help to prevent pulmonary oedema, which may develop at any time in the first few hours after re-expansion.

Monitoring of blood pressure, electrocardiogram (ECG), pulse oximetry, capnography, airway pressure, ventilatory volumes and inspired oxygen concentration should be the routine minimum for thoracic anaesthesia. In those with severe interstitial disease, arterial access is especially useful for monitoring blood gases. A nerve stimulator to monitor adequate reversal of neuromuscular blockade in these patients, who may have very little respiratory reserve, is recommended.

Post-operative care

Patients with severe interstitial disease require particular attention, with a mortality rate of over 4 per cent following open biopsy having been reported. Death is usually in the post-operative period, mainly due to the disease process itself, but inadequate analgesia, over-sedation and a weak cough are all avoidable contributory factors. It may prove necessary to ventilate the most compromised patients post-operatively, although the potential for the patient to become ventilator-dependent is real and the only hope is for the biopsy to reveal a diagnosis amenable to treatment. Air leak from biopsied lung in ventilated patients is a potential problem.

Segmental, limited and wedge resection

These resections are carried out either for excision of localized, discrete lesions of a benign nature, or for malignant lesions in patients with such poor respiratory reserve that lobectomy is foregone in favour of resecting as little functioning lung as possible. The consequence in terms of a reduced chance of having effected a curative resection of a malignant lesion is a reduction in 5-year survival of at least 10 per cent when compared with lobectomy.

Surgical procedure

Access is generally via a lateral thoracotomy; occasionally, an anterior approach may be used. With segmentectomy, the branches of the pulmonary artery, the venous drainage and bronchus supplying the diseased segment are identified and ligated or stapled. Prior to bronchial division the lung is gently re-inflated and the bronchus to be divided is clamped and unclamped to ensure that the correct segmental anatomy has been identified. It should be remembered that a significant degree of small airway communication can exist between adjacent segments, thus bypassing segmental bronchial air supply. After removal of the segment, any intersegmental blood vessels are ligated. Minor air leaks from the raw surface can be tolerated, and usually seal within a few days. Intercostal tube drainage is required until air leakage resolves. More severe leaks can be sealed, as described later under *Lobectomy*. Segmentectomy can be technically demanding and take some time.

Wedge resection involves resection of the lesion and a rim of normal lung, usually using stapling devices, but foregoing dissection of segmental anatomy. It is generally carried out thoracoscopically, but technical difficulties with that approach may result in operation via thoracotomy. The procedure is usually quick and relatively easily accomplished.

Some lesions (for example, hamartomas) can be shelled out with very little dissection, and any blood vessels or air leaks individually ligated, oversewn or stapled. Hydatid cysts can also usually be removed by local excision, though sometimes segmentectomy or lobectomy is required. The cysts may be single or multiple and therefore possibly bilateral, in which case access may be by either midline sternotomy or bilateral thoracotomy. Cysts may be removed from both the lung and liver at the same operation. There are two important considerations relating to their removal. First, the cyst may burst and absorption of the released fluid into the systemic circulation result in an acute anaphylactic reaction with severe vasodilatation and hypotension, necessitating treatment with vasoconstrictors. Second, release of the cyst contents can result in dissemination of the scolices, with subsequent recurrence of hydatid cysts. The risk of this is diminished by pre-operative treatment with albendazole.

Anaesthetic management

The aim of anaesthesia for these procedures is the prompt recovery of spontaneous respiration with extubation at the end of the procedure. Discussion with the surgeon will determine whether one-lung ventilation will be required. Inhalation anaesthesia, or total intravenous anaesthesia with propofol, combined with a short-acting opiate (e.g. alfentanil or remifentanil), will provide an unsedated patient post-operatively with little opiate-induced respiratory depression, particularly if a local anaesthetic block is used to supplement analgesia. Short-acting muscle relaxants, monitored by a nerve stimulator, help to ensure adequate recovery of respiratory muscle function post-operatively. Permissive hypercapnia is preferable to overzealous attempts at normocapnic ventilation in patients with poor lung compliance rendering them at risk of barotrauma. Invasive arterial monitoring is useful for both haemodynamic surveillance and peri-operative blood gas analysis.

Post-operative care

Those with poor lung function demand special care. Pain relief should depress respiration as little as possible, and yet be adequate to prevent inhibition of coughing or breathing, allowing co-operation with physiotherapy. Thus epidural or paravertebral analgesia are usually chosen; alternatively, intercostal blocks may be performed under direct vision prior to chest closure. If an epidural is placed before surgery, then its use intra-operatively can further reduce, or eliminate, the need for respiratory depressant intra-venous opiates during surgery.

(a)

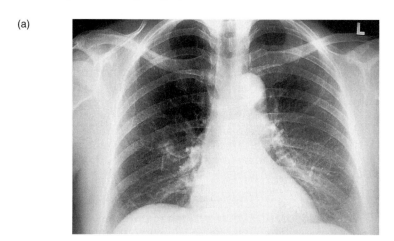

(b)

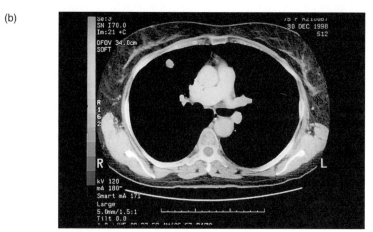

Figure 5.2

(a) Chest X-ray showing lesion in right lung.
(b) CT scan of the same patient showing peripheral location of the lesion in the right lung.

Lobectomy

The main indication for lobectomy is resection of lung cancer (Fig. 5.2). Other indications include bronchiectasis, benign tumours where more limited resection is not feasible, mycetomata and, increasingly, tuberculosis that is resistant to available treatment regimens (Fig. 5.3).

Surgery is indicated in bronchiectasis if there is localized disease, haemoptysis not amenable to treatment by embolization of the responsible artery, a failure of medical therapy (antibiotics, bronchodilators, physiotherapy) with an infectious complication such as lung abscess, empyema or brain abscess or, rarely, secondary amyloidosis. Resection in other circumstances should be avoided, as complete resection is difficult and infection spreads to involve more lung with, subsequently, the ultimate development of respiratory failure. The retention of as much functioning lung as possible is thus desirable. The degree of resection ranges from segmentectomy to pneumonectomy, but lobectomy is most common. The aetiology is only known in about a third of cases of bronchiectasis. Possible causes include pneumonia, measles, pertussis, bronchopulmonary aspergillosis, tuberculosis, alpha-1 antitrypsin deficiency, cystic fibrosis, Kartegener's syndrome (*situs inversus*, bronchiectasis, sinusitis and congenital cardiac lesions) and Swyer–James–MacLeod syndrome (viral lung infection in childhood resulting in unilateral obstruction of distal bronchi, with subsequent non-development of the lung and a unilateral 'translucent lung' on CXR). Bronchiectasis may also be congenital. With appropriate case selection, 60–80 per cent of patients will be symptomatically cured by surgery and most of the rest significantly improved. Patients with bronchiectasis and respiratory failure are best treated by bilateral lung transplantation, particularly those with cystic fibrosis or alpha-1 antitrypsin deficiency.

(a)
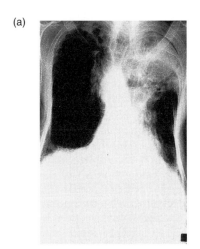

(b)
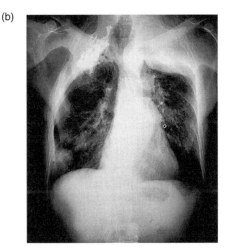

Figure 5.3

(a) Chest X-ray showing mycetoma in upper zone of left lung.
(b) Chest X-ray showing fibrosis and calcification of upper lobes in a patient with tuberculosis.

Mycetomas are fungal balls, usually aspergillus, which have grown in a lung cavity and are frequently of tuberculous origin. They may cause haemoptysis, and the cavity may be secondarily infected by bacteria and thus contain pus. They are difficult to treat with anti-fungal agents and so come to resection, although irradiation is an alternative treatment to be considered if operation is contraindicated. They have a characteristic appearance on CXR of a halo surrounding the fungal ball within the cavity.

Surgery for tuberculosis is becoming increasingly common as a result of the emergence of multi-resistant strains and the increased number of patients who comply poorly with treatment regimens. Prevention of spread of infection to other patients and medical personnel is paramount. In some populations, a significant proportion of these patients may be HIV positive. Surgery varies in extent from segmentectomy or lobectomy to pneumonectomy, and effects a cure in up to 90 per cent of patients. For patients with lung function too poor to tolerate lung resection, interest is reviving in techniques involving partial lung collapse manoeuvres, such as thoracoplasty and plombage.

Superior sulcus (Pancoast) tumours are lung carcinomas situated at the apex of the lung that have extended into the thoracic inlet. They progressively invade local structures, including the brachial plexus, intercostal nerves, the sympathetic chain and stellate ganglion, ribs, vertebrae and the subclavian vessels. They are frequently associated with considerable pain and Horner's syndrome (meiosis, ptosis, anhydrosis of the face and arm and vasodilatation of the arm vessels) as a result of neural involvement. Surgery for superior sulcus tumours is traditionally preceded by radiotherapy 2–4 weeks prior to surgery. Either a segmentectomy or, more commonly, an upper lobectomy is performed, along with resection of the tumour extension into the thoracic inlet, including upper ribs, upper thoracic vertebrae, lower brachial plexus, stellate ganglion, sympathetic chain and subclavian vessels as dictated by the tumour. The approach may either be from above with a cervical incision, or from below via a thoracotomy.

Surgical procedure

Access for lobectomy is usually by lateral thoracotomy, though in the rare instances where bilateral procedures are being carried out a transverse 'clamshell' incision is an alternative to bilateral sequential lateral thoracotomies or midline sternotomy. The lobe is isolated from its neighbouring lobe(s). This can entail delicate dissection if there is incomplete interlobar fissure formation. Care is taken to minimize air leak as a result of damage to the adjacent lung surfaces. The vessels are clamped, ligated or sutured, and divided. The bronchus is identified and clamped. At this point it is prudent to ventilate the lung gently (after endobronchial suction by the anaesthetist) to ensure that the correct bronchus has been identified. It is then divided and oversewn, or alternatively stapled and divided. The lobe can then be removed from the thorax. Sometimes, extensive pleural adhesions or tumour growth into the chest wall require dissection. This can be associated with considerable blood loss and prolongation of the procedure.

If upper lobe tumours involve the upper lobe bronchus, a 'sleeve resection' can be performed as an alternative to pneumonectomy. Sleeve resection entails division of the main bronchus on either side of its junction with the upper lobe bronchus and removal of this sleeve of main bronchus, together with the upper lobe bronchus and upper lung lobe. Re-anastomosis of the cut ends of the main bronchus restores the continuity of the airway. Sleeve resection is of particular benefit in patients who are poor candidates for pneumonectomy.

The bronchial stump is tested for air leaks by progressively inflating the lung to a pressure of 40 cmH$_2$O, having suctioned the bronchus clear of blood and secretions. This manoeuvre also demonstrates any leak of air from the adjacent remaining lung surface. Small leaks usually seal on their own within a few days of surgery, but large leaks can persist and are a source of significant morbidity and prolonged hospitalization. The leaking lung area can be oversewn or stapled. Alternatively, either biological or polymer sealants (such as fibrin glue or polyethylene glycol) can be applied to the lung surface.

If the lobectomy has been performed for malignant disease, the hilar lymph nodes draining the affected lobe are removed.

An intercostal chest drain is placed and the remaining lobe(s) reinflated prior to chest closure.

Anaesthetic management

Pre-operative assessment

Careful evaluation of pre-operative respiratory status and estimation of post-resection lung function are essential. This has already been emphasized in the context of lung cancer, but applies equally to those with bronchiectasis and tuberculosis.

The airway should be assessed clinically and with regard to radiological and bronchoscopic findings. This information is essential to the anaesthetist's choice of technique (type and size of endobronchial tube, bronchus blocker or high frequency jet ventilation), for controlling ventilation and, if necessary, protecting healthy areas of lung intra-operatively.

Patients with tuberculosis may have extensive and widespread damage to their lungs, not just localized infection with cavity formation. Bronchiectasis may be present. Assessment of nutritional status, the possible consequences of co-existing alcoholism and, in HIV positive patients, a search for associated pathologies should be made. Renal function may be affected.

In patients with bronchiectasis, physiotherapy and antibiotic treatment reduce sputum production and bronchodilator therapy may promote the clearance of sputum. CT scanning has almost entirely replaced bronchography in the assessment of the extent and distribution of bronchiectasis.

Patients with malignant disease may have non-pulmonary complications and these should be sought, although they are rare in patients who are operable and are mainly associated with small cell carcinomas. They include the Eaton–Lambert myasthenic syndrome (see Chapter 8), ectopic production of a number of hormones (including ACTH, ADH and parathyroid hormone) and hypertrophic pulmonary osteoarthropathy.

Superior vena caval obstruction can be produced by tumour or, more commonly, associated lymphadenopathy. Considerable swelling of the face and arms can result. The implications for anaesthesia are discussed in Chapter 8.

Premedication

Premedication is satisfactorily and most safely achieved using a benzo-diazepine; opiates may further compromise patients with poor respiratory function and inhibit coughing, resulting in the accumulation of secretions. Anti-sialogogues may cause inspissation of secretions, and are generally best avoided except in patients with discrete lung lesions.

Anaesthetic technique

The principal aims of anaesthesia for lobectomy are as follows:

- Prevention of soiling of undiseased areas of the ipsilateral and contra-lateral lung
- Facilitation of surgical access
- Use of a technique that allows extubation at the end of the procedure
- Provision of sufficient analgesia post-operatively to obtund discomfort on taking deep breaths or expectorating sputum, but without impairment of respiration.

The choice of anaesthetic agents for induction and maintenance is a matter for individual preference, bearing in mind the need for the rapid recovery of spontaneous respiration at the end of the procedure in order to avoid the perpetuation of air leaks from the lung on application of prolonged inter-mittent positive pressure ventilation, and the development of ventilator dependence in patients with diffuse disease. In patients with poor respiratory reserve, tolerance of one-lung ventilation may be improved by the use of total intravenous anaesthesia with propofol, rather than maintenance with volatile anaesthetic agents, because of lesser effects on hypoxic pulmonary vasoconstriction; this is debated in depth in Chapter 19. Planning for post-operative analgesia should form an integral part of the anaesthetic technique. Consideration should be given to the use of regional anaesthetic blocks and non-steroidal anti-inflammatory agents to supplement general anaesthesia, as discussed in Chapter 17.

A widely used anaesthetic technique is the establishment of thoracic epi-dural analgesia with a combination of bupivacaine and fentanyl, induction and maintenance with propofol, and muscle relaxation with atracurium, vecuronium or rocuronium.

The prevention of soiling of undiseased lung and facilitation of surgical access are achieved by lung isolation and one-lung ventilation. This is most commonly and readily attained by the use of a double-lumen tube. Airway distortion as a result of the underlying pathology or previous surgery may preclude the placement of a double-lumen, or even a single-lumen, endobronchial tube. In such cases, provided that there is no gross risk of spillage of infected material from the diseased lobe, endotracheal intubation with surgical retraction of the lung or the use of high frequency jet ventilation, which leaves the lungs partially collapsed, suffices to provide surgical access. If there is a high risk of spillage of contaminated material, then the bronchus to the lobe to be resected may be occluded using a bronchus blocker. The management of one-lung ventilation, the equipment available and specialized modes of ventilation are discussed further in the relevant chapters.

Following excision of the diseased lobe, the lungs, the trachea and bronchi should be thoroughly suctioned and the remaining lobe(s) on the operative side fully re-expanded by gentle manual inflation. Pulmonary oedema on re-expansion of the collapsed lung has frequently been reported, and may occur even at low cardiac filling pressures. Fluid infusion should be judiciously titrated prior to and during one-lung ventilation, although the association between higher volumes of fluid administration and re-expansion pulmonary oedema is debatable as this phenomenon may occur even with rigorous control of intra-operative fluid balance. Should pulmonary oedema occur, treatment is by the application of positive end-expiratory pressure (PEEP), administration of diuretics and limitation of further intravenous fluid administration. Post-operative ventilatory support may be required until resolution of the oedema occurs.

Monitoring

Monitoring for lobectomy should include ECG, blood pressure, temperature, pulse oximetry, capnography, airway spirometry and airway pressure display. Invasive arterial pressure monitoring is particularly useful if there is pre-existing cardiac dysfunction, or if dissection close to the heart or great vessels is anticipated. Pre-induction invasive arterial monitoring is advisable in patients liable to become significantly haemodynamically unstable on application of positive pressure ventilation, e.g. patients with emphysema who may develop a pneumothorax as a result of rupturing a bullous, or develop dynamic hyperinflation as a result of gas trapping. Blood gas analysis is essential peri-operatively in those with poor respiratory reserve or widespread pulmonary disease. In patients with isolated lesions and otherwise healthy lungs undergoing lobectomy, a case can be made for relying on non-invasive blood pressure monitoring, pulse oximetry and capnography as an alternative to invasive arterial monitoring. Central venous pressure monitoring in the lateral position with the chest open may not provide accurate absolute values for right heart filling pressures, but the trend of the observed values does serve as a guide for fluid infusion and is useful post-operatively.

Pulmonary artery (PA) catheterization tends to produce spurious results, as the balloon tends to float towards the upper, operative lung. If this is collapsed, measurements of wedge pressure are an unreliable indicator of filling pressure or ischaemia. Transoesophageal echocardiography provides an alternative means of monitoring cardiac filling and performance that may be more reliable during thoracotomy than PA catheterization.

Post-operative management

Provided that the remaining lung parenchyma is fairly normal, it expands with some degree of hyperinflation and this, along with elevation of the diaphragm on that side, eliminates the space left by the removed lobe. Intercostal tube drainage of lung air leak, effusions and blood post-operatively, along with adequate pain relief, physiotherapy and antibiotics, all play their part in keeping the residual lung expanded and free from accumulation of infected secretions. Lung air leak usually resolves in a few days but, if persistent, may ultimately need surgical exploration and repair. If severe, air leak can result in respiratory failure, necessitating early surgical intervention. The detailed management of persistent air leak, including bronchopleural fistulae, is described in Chapters 16 and 18.

Operative mortality following lobectomy for carcinoma of the lung is about 1 per cent.

Pneumonectomy

The main indication for pneumonectomy is carcinoma of the lung for which lesser resection would not effect a cure. Less frequently, pneumonectomy may have to be performed for severe persistent haemorrhage, chronic infection or as a completion procedure following previous lobectomy with extension of underlying disease to the remaining lobe(s). Extensive tuberculous destruction of a lung, requiring resection, is usually associated with extensive pleural adhesions and may need an extrapleural pneumonectomy, an operation with the potential for considerable blood loss.

Surgical procedure

Access is via a lateral thoracotomy. The pulmonary artery and veins are ligated, divided and oversewn or stapled. If the tumour is very central, the pulmonary veins may be divided within the pericardium. On the right, the azygous veins may be divided to provide better hilar exposure. The main bronchus is exposed up to the carina, divided and stapled or oversewn as close to the carina as possible, leaving as short a stump as feasible. Any bronchial arteries are ligated; these can be a source of significant blood loss post-operatively if not properly secured. The stump may be wrapped over with adjacent tissue. A strip of intercostal muscle with its vascular pedicle may be used for this purpose, but this is rare at primary closure. After suctioning the tracheal lumen of the double-lumen tube, the integrity of the bronchial stump is tested by application of positive pressure up to 40 cmH$_2$O to the airway.

An intercostal chest drain is usually placed prior to closure of the thoracotomy. This enables haemorrhage to be detected and the position of the mediastinum to be controlled. During gentle inflation of the remaining lung, the drain is clamped and is left clamped. This usually leaves the mediastinum in a central position, or slightly towards the pneumonectomized side. The position is checked by CXR immediately post-operatively, and adjusted as required by further suction on, or insufflation of air through, the drain. In cases where no chest drain has been inserted, these manoeuvres are performed percutaneously.

Anaesthetic management

The anaesthetic management for pneumonectomy is essentially similar to that for lobectomy, as described above.

Pre-operative evaluation of lung function should be rigorous, bearing in mind that following a right pneumonectomy lung function may be reduced by roughly 55 per cent, and after a left pneumonectomy by 45 per cent. Careful consideration should also be given to the state of the non-operative lung, ensuring that it is free from infection, oedema and effusions pre-operatively. A more detailed discussion of pre-operative assessment can be found in the above section, *Assessing fitness for surgery*.

The operative lung is ideally isolated by endobronchial intubation of the contralateral lung using a double- or single-lumen endobronchial tube. If this cannot be achieved, then an endobronchial tube may be passed into the operative lung and withdrawn just prior to bronchial resection; alternatively, but less satisfactorily from the point of view of protection of the non-operative lung from soiling, endotracheal intubation and early clamping of the main bronchus of the operative lung suffices.

Hypoxia prior to excision of the operative lung can sometimes be improved by early clamping of the pulmonary artery supplying the operative side, thereby diverting blood to the ventilated lung and reducing the shunt fraction. Other measures to manage hypoxia during one-lung ventilation are discussed in Chapter 4.

Haemodynamic instability may be a particular problem during pneumonectomy; arrhythmias are common during surgical manipulation near the heart, compression of the vena cavae may impair cardiac filling and, finally, clamping of the pulmonary artery to the operative lung may, as discussed earlier in this chapter, increase pulmonary vascular resistance substantially. Anti-arrhythmic agents, inotropes or pulmonary vasodilators may be required to restore haemodynamic stability.

Infusion of fluids should be carefully controlled and monitored because of the risk of post-pneumonectomy pulmonary oedema. This occurs at low filling pressures, with disastrous consequences. Infusion of crystalloid should be limited, and colloid and blood used if required. There is evidence to suggest that both re-expansion and post-pneumonectomy pulmonary oedema may occur even with minimal fluid administration and rigorous control of fluid balance; crystalloid restriction may, however, reduce the severity of the lung injury. As discussed earlier, the value of central venous pressure measurement is debatable during thoracotomy, but it is certainly useful post-operatively. PA catheter measurements are liable to error because the balloon tends to float to the upper, operative side and, even if positioned correctly, should not be wedged following clamping of the pulmonary artery to the operative lung, as inflation of the balloon may occlude a significant proportion of the blood flow to the left side of the heart. Transoesophageal echocardiography is indicated in patients with pre-existing cardiac dysfunction, or if haemodynamic instability arises intra-operatively.

Post-operative management

The patient can usually be extubated at the end of surgery, provided that care has been taken in the choice of anaesthetic technique, temperature control, fluid balance and analgesia, and that the patient's lung function has been correctly assessed. Continued mechanical ventilation, if necessary, should be with the lowest inspiratory pressures feasible and for as short a time as possible. The risk of development of a bronchial air leak and the formation of a bronchopleural fistula is higher after pneumonectomy than lobectomy.

If a chest drain has been left *in situ*, it is unclamped for a minute every hour to alleviate the rise in intrathoracic pressure caused by air, fluid or blood accumulation within the hemithorax, and also to monitor bleeding. The drain is usually removed after 24 hours and the pneumonectomy space left to fill with serosanguinous fluid, which it does substantially within about a further 48 hours. Over a further period the space fills completely and, in the long term, fibroses, with subsequent contraction. The diaphragm rises and the mediastinum shifts with compensatory expansion of the remaining lung (Fig. 5.4).

The patient should be sat up as soon as possible to encourage basal lung expansion and oxygen given as necessary. If the patient lies on one side, the lung should be uppermost in order to prevent its compression by mediastinal structures. Haemodynamic parameters should be closely monitored to manage fluid requirements optimally and to detect haemorrhage, which can be dramatic if a ligature slips off a major vessel. Evidence of myocardial ischaemia or infarction should be sought in those with ischaemic heart disease. If pneumonectomy has involved pulmonary ligation within the pericardium, post-operative pericarditis may occur and the resulting ECG changes should not be confused with myocardial ischaemia.

Arrhythmias, especially atrial fibrillation, are quite common after pulmonary resection. Pre-operative digitalization probably does not reduce the incidence of atrial fibrillation, although it may reduce the ventricular rate should it occur. It is general practice to wait for atrial fibrillation to occur before instituting treatment.

Herniation of the heart into the pleural cavity through an open pericardium produces dramatic cardiac effects, especially on the right side, as the whole heart twists on its pedicle. Recognition of the condition and prompt thoracotomy and correction are needed to save life. Compression of a coronary artery by partial herniation of the heart through the pericardial hole can also occur.

Deep vein thrombosis prophylaxis should be rigorous. Pulmonary embolism in a pneumonectomized patient is a disaster.

Post-pneumonectomy pulmonary oedema is of poorly understood aetiology, presenting as an adult respiratory distress syndrome, complicating about 4 per cent of patients and with an 80 per cent mortality. Excessive

(a)

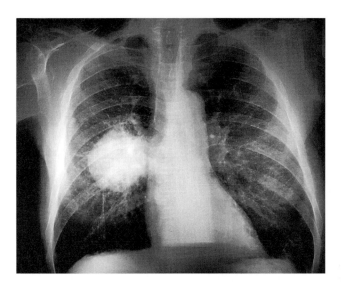

(b)

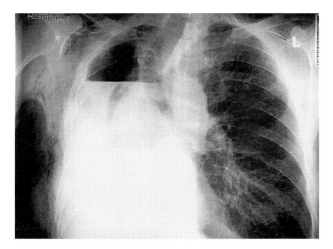

Figure 5.4

(a) Chest X-ray showing a large mass in the right lung pre-
    pneumonectomy.
(b) Chest X-ray of the same patient post-pneumonectomy, showing
    fluid partially filling the right hemithorax and mediastinal shift
    with expansion of the left lung.

peri-operative fluid administration and the relative hyperperfusion of the remaining lung post-operatively may exacerbate the condition if it arises, but these may not in themselves be causative. Treatment is as for the adult respiratory distress syndrome.

Damage to the thoracic duct at operation can result in a chylothorax. Treatment is usually conservative for small leaks, with chest drainage and a low fat diet supplemented with medium-chain triglycerides until resolution of the leak occurs. Larger leaks require surgical correction. Thoracoscopic ligation of leaks has been described.

Operative mortality of pneumonectomy is about 5 per cent.

Bullous lung disease

A bulla is generally a thin walled air-containing cavity within the lung. Some are thicker walled, contain fluid or blood, or may be infected and contain pus. Patients with bullous lung disease present for surgery either when the bulla or bullae are large enough to compress the surrounding lung, thus worsening respiratory impairment, or when they rupture, with resulting pneumothorax. Bullae may be very large, occupying most of a hemithorax, or they may be very small and only reveal their presence by rupturing and causing an air leak. Small bullae are often visible on CT scan, but are sometimes only found on inspection of the lung during pleurodesis for recurrent pneumothoraces. Although bullae are occasionally single, they are usually multiple and bilateral. Thus, although the largest may be targeted for surgery, the possibility of expansion or rupture of a bulla on the contralateral side during surgery is always a danger and can be difficult to diagnose. Many of the signs of pneumothorax from a ruptured bulla (quiet breath sounds, wheeze, poor chest wall movement, hyper-resonance, hypotension with positive pressure ventilation) are those often found with bullous lung disease itself. A chest drain inserted to alleviate a suspected pneumothorax may drain air, even if there is no pneumothorax, by in fact draining a bulla.

A single lung cyst or bulla is often congenital, whereas multiple cysts are usually acquired – for example, in emphysema or post-staphylococcal infection. Congenital lobar emphysema is rare, confined to one lobe (left upper, in over half of all cases), and usually presents in infancy. The cause may related to diminished or absent cartilage in the lobar bronchus, resulting in a dynamic valve-like effect with respiration and distal air trapping, or to lobar bronchial stenosis, again with distal air trapping, but is unknown in 40 per cent of cases.

Surgical procedure

Video-assisted thoracoscopic surgery (VATS) with stapling of the lung tissue around the bulla is the technique of choice. Thoracotomy is resorted to if VATS fails due to adhesions between lung and pleura, or because of technical difficulties in positioning the staple lines in the correct places.

If there are multiple bullae, careful judgement of which to resect needs to be exercised. Only the largest and those that it is possible to remove with minimal loss of adjacent functioning lung should be removed. It is tempting to remove too many, and too much relatively normal lung tissue is sacrificed in the process. This can have serious consequences in patients whose underlying lung function is impaired.

A pleurodesis may be performed, if deemed appropriate, and intercostal tube drains inserted prior to closure of the chest.

Pre-operative assessment

The spectrum of patients varies from the fit young person with a history of recurrent pneumothoraces to an elderly individual in respiratory failure, unable to speak full sentences and with the cardiovascular consequences of a long history of smoking.

Bullae are well demonstrated by CT scans. The presence of any bullae on the contralateral side is important, warning of the potential for enlargement or rupture under positive pressure ventilation. The CT scan, in conjunction with ventilation and perfusion scans, helps to target surgery for multiple bullae on the worst affected areas. A current CXR may reveal the presence of pneumothorax. The functioning of intercostal drains, if present, should be checked. Spirometry reveals any underlying obstructive airways disease. In more severe cases, diffusion studies help to quantify the extent of the disease, and blood gas analysis may show chronic hypercapnia with hypoxic respiratory drive.

Anaesthetic technique and monitoring

Induction can be an extremely hazardous time. Positive pressure ventilation can induce severe hypotension as a result of air trapping. The rise in intrathoracic pressure inhibits venous return and causes so called 'pulmonary tamponade' of the heart. Use of long expiratory times and intermittently discontinuing ventilation to allow air to escape and the blood pressure to recover is necessary. Permissive hypercapnia is safer than vigorous attempts at ventilation to normocapnia with standard tidal volumes in these circumstances. Hypotension may also occur as a result of tension pneumothorax from a ruptured bulla, and ventilation should be pressure limited to avoid barotrauma.

Insertion of a double-lumen tube allows isolation of the affected lung in unilateral disease. Spontaneous ventilation has its theoretical attractions, but the resistance to breathing of a double-lumen tube and the depression of respiration under anaesthesia mitigate in favour of gentle, controlled ventilation, with permissive hypercapnia if necessary. Nitrous oxide is avoided, as it may cause expansion of bullae or pneumothoraces. A combined regional and general anaesthetic technique is optimal, to minimize post-operative respiratory depression. Use of a total intravenous anaesthetic technique may be advantageous, as delivery of inhalational agents may be unpredictable as a result of gas leakage from the lung.

Post-operative care

Chest drains are kept on suction if this does not exacerbate any residual air leakage, and removed once it is apparent there is no further air leak.

Post-operative ventilation is to be avoided because of the possibility of prolonging air leak, rupturing remaining bullae and of air trapping, with adverse haemodynamic consequences.

KEY POINTS

- Cancer is the commonest indication for lung resection.

- Prior to lung resection, assessment of lung function must be performed with appropriate tests to predict adequate post-resection respiratory function.

- One-lung ventilation is usually required for lung resection. It facilitates surgical access and provides protection of the non-operative lung from soiling.

- With bullous emphysema, positive pressure ventilation can cause severe hypotension due to air trapping or development of a tension pneumothorax.

- For those with impaired respiratory reserve, epidural or paravertebral analgesia is optimal.

- Post-operative ventilation is generally to be avoided following lung resection because of the risk of perpetuation of air leak from the lung or airways, and the potential for the development of ventilator dependence in patients with chronic respiratory dysfunction.

- Surgical management for tuberculosis is becoming increasingly common.

- In some populations, lung biopsy is increasingly being used to diagnose lung diseases in HIV positive patients.

Bibliography

American College of Cardiology/American Heart Association (1996). Guidelines for peri-operative evaluation for non-cardiac surgery. *Circulation*, **93**, 1278–1317.

Arcasoy, S.M. and Jett, J.R. (1997). Superior pulmonary sulcus tumours and Pancoast's syndrome. *N. Engl. J. Med.*, **337(19)**, 1370–6.

Barker, S.J., Clarke, C., Trivedi, N. *et al.* (1993). Anaesthesia for thoracoscopic laser ablation of bullous emphysema. *Anesthesiology*, **78**, 44–50.

Conacher, I. (1997). Anaesthesia for the surgery of emphysema. *Br. J. Anaesth.*, **79**, 530–8.

Crapo, R.O. (1994). Pulmonary function testing. Current concepts. *N. Engl. J. Med.*, **331**, 25–30.

Lennon, P.F., Hartigan, P.M. and Friedberg, J.S. (1998). Clinical management of patients undergoing concurrent cardiac surgery and pulmonary resection. *J. Cardiothorac. Vasc. Anesth.*, **12(5)**, 587–90.

Mountain, C.F. (1997). Revisions in the international system for staging lung cancer. *Chest*, **111(6)**, 1710–17.

Olsen, G.N. (ed.) (1993). Peri-operative respiratory care. *Clin. Chest Med.*, **14**, 205–357.

Plummer, S., Hartley, M. and Vaughan, R.S. (1998). Anaesthesia for telescopic procedures in the thorax. *Br. J. Anaesth.*, **80**, 223–34.

Slinger, P.D. (1995). Peri-operative fluid management for thoracic surgery: the puzzle of post-pneumonectomy pulmonary oedema. *J. Cardiothorac. Vasc. Anesth.*, **9**, 442–51.

Thomas, S.D., Berry, P.D. and Russell, G.N. (1995). Is this patient fit for thoracotomy and resection of lung tissue? *Postgrad. Med. J.*, **71**, 331–5.

Williams, E.A., Evans, T.W. and Goldstraw, P. (1996). Acute lung injury following lung resection: is one-lung anaesthesia to blame? *Thorax*, **51(2)**, 114–16.

6

Operations on the pleura, diaphragm and chest wall

D. Smith

Pleura

Pleurectomy

Pleurectomy, removal of the parietal pleural layer from the chest wall, is usually performed for recurrent pneumothorax. Following re-expansion, the lung adheres to the chest wall, obliterating the pleural space. During the procedure, bullae on the lung surface may be obliterated by stapling or suture to prevent the recurrence of air leaks.

Surgical procedure

Pleurectomy may be performed as an open procedure through a thoracotomy, or as a thoracoscopic procedure with or without video assistance. For the open operation, access is gained to the pleural space through a lateral thoracotomy. Irrespective of the means of surgical access, as much parietal pleura as possible is stripped off all but the diaphragmatic surface by blunt dissection. Any remaining parietal pleura and the visceral pleura may then be abraded until capillary bleeding occurs, using either a stiff brush or dry gauze swabs. This abrasion causes inflammation of the pleural surfaces and promotes adhesion. A chest drain is placed at the end of surgery, with low-pressure suction to aid expansion of the lung.

Anaesthetic management

Patients presenting for pleurectomy often have associated lung disease such as asthma or cystic fibrosis, and appropriate measures should be taken to optimize their condition pre-operatively. The patient may come to theatre with an established pneumothorax and a chest drain in place; this should be left unclamped until the chest is opened to prevent the development of a tension pneumothorax when intermittent positive pressure ventilation is commenced. Nitrous oxide should be avoided unless a functional chest drain is in place. Anaesthetic management is as for a standard lateral thoracotomy, with adequate venous access, intra-arterial monitoring and a double-lumen tube. Extubation is usual at the end of surgery. The management of thoracoscopic surgery is dealt with in Chapter 10.

Post-operative care

This operation is extremely painful, and good quality analgesia is vital to post-operative comfort and respiratory function. Thoracic epidural analgesia or paravertebral block should be considered, and the patient should be nursed initially in a high-dependency area. The chest drain remains in place, on suction, until blood and air have stopped draining. The drain tube will limit the mobility of the patient, and also causes additional chest wall discomfort.

KEY POINTS

- Pleurectomy is the removal of parietal pleura from the chest wall, usually for recurrent pneumothorax.

- The chest tube should not be clamped before induction of anaesthesia.

- Single lung ventilation is required.

- Post-operative pain is severe.

Pleurodesis

Pleurodesis is usually carried out for recurrent pneumothorax, generally in patients unfit for the more invasive procedure of pleurectomy. Pleurodesis is preferable to pleurectomy in patients who may require lung transplantation at a future date (for example, cystic fibrotics). Pleurodesis may also be used to prevent the accumulation of pleural effusions, particularly in malignant disease. Although pleurodesis is less invasive than pleurectomy, it is still extremely painful for the patient. An irritant, usually iodized talc or 50 per cent dextrose, is used to produce inflammation of the visceral and parietal pleural surfaces. The resultant scarring and adhesion formation obliterate the pleural space. Alternatively, the pleura can be physically abraded using dry swabs or a stiff brush.

Surgical procedure

The patient is usually laid supine on the operating table, although some surgeons prefer the patient in the lateral position. A short incision is made between two ribs on the antero-lateral chest wall. As the underlying lung collapses, sterile iodized talc is insufflated into the pleural space or the pleura physically abraded. A chest drain tube is then inserted through the same incision, and the collapsed lung should be gently re-expanded once the seal on the drain is established and placed on suction. Pleurodesis may be performed thoracoscopically, and this approach is particularly suited to insufflation of an irritant substance.

Anaesthetic management

The procedure is short. Although a well-collapsed lung allows the cloud of talc to cover most of the pleural surfaces, a double-lumen tube is not normally necessary. However, an appropriate double-lumen tube may occasionally be useful in severe emphysema or in asthmatic patients, when the lung is less likely to collapse adequately if not isolated from the breathing circuit, or when one lung needs isolating from the other to prevent the spread of infection, as in cystic fibrosis.

Post-operative care

For such a simple procedure, the amount of post-operative pain is severe, as the pleural surfaces become inflamed and rub against each other. Good quality analgesia is therefore mandatory. Continuous thoracic epidural infusion of local anaesthetic, with or without opioid, is the method of choice, even though the incision itself may be small.

The chest drain remains in place until blood, serous fluid and air have stopped draining.

KEY POINTS

- Pleurodesis is performed for chronic pneumothorax or pleural effusions.
- An inflammatory agent or physical abrasion is used to produce adhesions between the pleural layers.
- Post-operative pain is severe.

Pleuro-peritoneal shunt

There are occasions when pleurodesis or pleurectomy for malignant pleural effusions fails to provide complete resolution of the effusion. This is usually because of inadequate intercostal tube drainage, allowing large volumes of fluid to maintain separation of the visceral and parietal pleural surfaces. In these circumstances, a pleuro-peritoneal shunt may allow patients with a terminal intrathoracic malignancy to manage their pleural effusion themselves at home. The shunt is a small, valved chamber, connected at each end to a short tube. Repeatedly pressing and releasing the valve with a finger compresses the valve chamber against an underlying rib and pumps fluid along the shunt from the pleural space to the peritoneum. However, the shunt valve often blocks with proteinaceous material, and there is a risk of seeding of an intrathoracic tumour into the abdominal cavity.

Surgical procedure

A short incision is made between the eighth and ninth ribs, and the proximal tube is inserted through this into the pleural space. The distal tube is tunnelled subcutaneously to the abdominal wall, leaving the valved chamber overlying a rib, and inserted into the peritoneum via a second short incision.

Anaesthetic management

Insertion of a pleuro-peritoneal shunt is a usually quick procedure, although patients can be quite sick with advanced malignancy. The patient will often have a chest drain in place, and will have an intrathoracic primary or secondary tumour, which may impair ventilation of the lung on the operative side. Tracheal intubation with a single-lumen tube and intermittent positive pressure ventilation is the technique of choice, in combination with a short duration competitive neuromuscular blocking drug.

Post-operative care

Post-operative pain is not severe, although the patient may find it uncomfortable to operate the shunt valve in the first few post-operative days. The patient needs to be taught how to operate the valve in the shunt to drain fluid from the pleural cavity, increasing dyspnoea being the usual trigger for a further episode of drainage.

KEY POINTS

- Pleuro-peritoneal shunts are used to drain malignant effusions when other measures have failed.
- The shunt enables the terminally ill patient to be nursed at home.
- The shunt valve may become occluded with protein deposits.

Decortication

Decortication is the removal of thickened pleura from either the lung or the chest wall, but often from both. Thickening of the pleural layers to the extent of reducing respiratory excursion of the lung, chest wall and diaphragm sufficient to interfere with the patient's normal activity is the indication for surgery. Pleural thickening may occur as a result of persistent pleural effusion, haemothorax, infection or inflammation, and may be widespread or patchy. Patients presenting for decortication following empyema may have a bronchopleural fistula, and this is discussed in Chapter 16. Decortication is a major procedure, and should not be performed in frail, elderly or sick patients unless there is a real prospect of significant improvement in their quality of life.

Surgical procedure

Access is via a standard lateral thoracotomy, although resection of one of the ribs above or below the incision may be necessary to gain adequate surgical exposure. The thickened pleural layers are stripped first from the chest wall, then from the lung, using blunt dissection. This is a slow process. Planes of dissection can be difficult to identify and the underlying lung may be damaged, resulting in air leaks from open airways.

Anaesthetic management

Pre-operatively, the nature of the underlying disease should be ascertained. If infective, the appropriate antibiotic treatment should be commenced. If significant fluid is present within the hemithorax, this may require drainage pre-operatively. Standard anaesthesia for lateral thoracotomy is used. One-lung ventilation is not essential for this procedure and, as the lung may be difficult to collapse because of fibrous adhesions, a single-lumen tube is satisfactory unless a bronchopleural fistula is present. Bleeding may be considerable, and a central venous catheter is helpful for monitoring and replacing intravascular volume. Adequate cross-matched blood should be available.

Post-operative care

The patient should be nursed in an intensive care unit post-operatively. Post-operative pain is considerable, so good quality analgesia is essential. Continuous thoracic epidural infusion of local anaesthetic, with or without opioid, or patient controlled opiate analgesia combined with a non-steroidal anti-inflammatory drug, are the methods of choice. Significant air leak through the chest drains is common post-operatively. If the leak is small, the patient may be woken up and extubated in the normal way. Application of suction to the drains may exacerbate the leak. It may be necessary to accept that the lung does not completely expand in the first few post-operative days. Larger air leaks may require positive pressure ventilation to prevent respiratory failure if the patient cannot tolerate a partially collapsed lung. The management of ventilation in these patients is complex and demands attention to detail, as discussed in Chapter 18. Positive pressure ventilation may exacerbate the air leak and delay closure of open airways. If ventilation is required, peak airway pressure should be limited and PEEP avoided. High frequency jet ventilation should be considered.

KEY POINTS

- Decortication is the removal of the thickened pleural layers, usually following empyema.

- This is a major procedure, and should be avoided unless the patient will clearly benefit from it.

- A bronchopleural fistula may be present.

- Blood loss may be considerable.

- Air leak intra- and post-operatively is common.

- The patients should be managed in an intensive care unit post-operatively.

Thoracic sympathectomy

Thoracic sympathectomy is carried out for hyperhydrosis of the upper limbs, vasospastic conditions of the upper limbs (for example Raynaud's) or for severe reflex sympathetic dystrophy. It has also been used successfully to treat angina pectoris. The first description of cervical sympathectomy was by Alexander in 1889, although the early procedures were for dubious indications such as exophthalmos, epilepsy and glaucoma. It was not until the 1920s that the true indications for cervical sympathectomy became clear, but at this time it was realized that the upper thoracic ganglia must also be removed for successful sympathetic denervation of the upper limbs.

Surgical procedure

The surgery may be by an open or thoracoscopic approach. Open surgery may be performed via many different routes, the most popular being the extrapleural approach via a supraclavicular incision through the bed of the resected first rib as described by Roos in 1971. Access may also be gained through the dorsal midline approach described by Cloward, which is popular with neurosurgeons; this approach is useful for bilateral sympathectomy, but has not achieved popularity with thoracic surgeons. The thoracoscopic approach is now the most common, since it is less complex than open surgery and leaves less scarring.

The first thoracoscopic sympathectomy was performed by Hughes in 1942, but this approach only became popular with the advent in the 1980s of improved surgical instruments and the development of video-assisted thoracoscopy. The patient is positioned supine on the operating table with the ipsilateral arm abducted to 90°; the operating table is adjusted to a 20–30° head-up position. After isolation of the lung on the operative side, the thoracoscope is then inserted into the chest through a short incision and the thoracic sympathetic chain destroyed by electrocautery. Insufflation of carbon dioxide to induce a pneumothorax is unnecessary and may be dangerous, particularly in the prescence of adhesions.

Anaesthetic management

A left-sided double-lumen tube is employed, with competitive neuro-muscular blockade and mechanical ventilation of the lungs. The procedure is of short duration, and appropriate anaesthetic agents should be chosen. One-lung ventilation should be established before the surgeon introduces the thoracoscope into the chest. At the end of the procedure, the collapsed lung on the operated side should be manually re-inflated under direct vision; a chest drain tube is usually not inserted, provided that full inflation of the lung is achieved.

Post-operative care

Pain is not severe, and opiate analgesics will not usually be required.

A chest X-ray should be taken in the recovery room to ensure that there is no residual pneumothorax before the patient returns to the ward.

The patient should be warned about the possibility of a Horner's syndrome, and also of possible compensatory hyperhidrosis in other parts of the body.

> **KEY POINTS**
>
> - Thoracic sympathectomy is performed for hyperhidrosis, to promote vasodilatation, or for reflex sympathetic dystrophy of the arms.
> - The operation is usually performed thoracoscopically, and there is little post-operative pain.
> - Provided the lungs are fully inflated during chest closure, chest drains are not required.
> - A chest X-ray should be performed post-operatively to exclude residual pneumothorax.

Diaphragm

Plication

Eventration of the diaphragm, where one or both leaflets of the diaphragm are situated in an abnormally high position, most frequently occurs as a result of iatrogenic phrenic nerve palsy following cardiac or thoracic surgery. However, congenital hypoplasia or acquired atrophy of the muscle fibres may also cause elevation of the diaphragm on one or both sides. Diaphragmatic eventration is usually tolerated by adults, but not by neonates and infants. Plication of the hemidiaphragm flattens it, fixing it in the inspiratory position, thereby increasing lung volume on that side of the chest and aiding ventilation by minimizing paradoxical movement of the diaphragm and mediastinum.

Surgical procedure

Plication of the diaphragm is usually performed via a lateral thoracotomy because it is easier to visualize the branches of the phrenic nerve from above than via the abdominal approach. An upper abdominal incision may be used for the plication of bilateral eventrations. Four or five rows of non-absorbable suture material are inserted in an antero-lateral to postero-medial direction across the diaphragm to form five to six pleats across the diaphragm at 90° to the sutures. Alternatively, a continuous nylon running suture is placed in a repeating 's' or 'z' shaped pattern from the medial edge of the hemidiaphragm to the chest wall. The sutures should not pass through the full thickness of the diaphragm, as there is a risk of damaging the underlying viscera. Pulling the suture tight then puckers the central portion of the hemidiaphragm, flattening the dome shape. A chest drain is usually placed at the end of the intrathoracic procedure.

Anaesthetic management

Patients are often on intensive care pre-operatively, unable to be weaned from mechanical ventilation. Respiratory function may be severely compromised in patients who are not already ventilated. Standard anaesthesia for lateral thoracotomy should be used, with neuromuscular blockade of sufficient degree to prevent movement of the diaphragm. A double-lumen tube should be used in adult patients to allow deflation of the lung on the affected side. In infants, the lung is retracted away. Hand ventilation may improve surgical access and permit better control of blood gas tensions in small children and neonates.

Post-operative care

Patients who were already on the intensive care unit will probably be returned there for respiratory management after the operation. Other patients can be extubated at the end of surgery and observed in the recovery room. Adequate post-operative analgesia, consistent with lateral thoracotomy, will improve respiratory function and compliance with physiotherapy in the post-operative period.

KEY POINTS

- Plication of the diaphragm is carried out for restoration of lung volume when the paralysed hemidiaphragm occupies a high position in the chest.

- The procedure is rarely necessary in adults, but children may be severely compromised by a paralysed hemidiaphragm.

Repair of hiatus hernia

Tightening of the diaphragmatic hiatus is usually carried out as part of other operations for hiatus hernia with associated gastro-oesophageal reflux, such as Nissen fundoplication, Collis gastroplasty or insertion of an Angelchick Ring. However, tightening of the diaphragmatic hiatus may be performed in isolation for uncomplicated hernias. The management of hiatus hernia is discussed further in Chapter 9, but a brief description is included in this chapter for completeness.

Surgical procedure

The surgical approach may be via an abdominal incision or a left lateral thoracotomy, although the procedure may also be performed through the thoracoscope. Occasionally, if the herniated gastric fundus is adherent to mediastinal structures or is difficult to reduce, a thoraco-abdominal approach may be required. Irrespective of the surgical approach, the oesophagus is first mobilized from its bed, along with the left vagus nerve, and the hernia is reduced into the abdomen. A gastric fundoplication may be carried out at this time. Three or four linen sutures are used to appose the crurae of the diaphragm, such that the remaining hiatus admits a single finger.

Anaesthetic management

Standard anaesthesia for lateral thoracotomy is used, with a double-lumen tube to facilitate access into the left chest. Rapid sequence induction of anaesthesia may be required if there is severe gastro-oesophageal reflux.

Post-operative care

Post-operative management is as for any other lateral thoracotomy, with the same consideration for post-operative analgesia. It is important to check that the patient has no obstruction to swallowing as a result of the repair constricting the lower oesophagus.

KEY POINTS

- Tightening of the diaphragmatic hiatus is performed for uncomplicated hiatus hernia.
- The operation may be performed via the thoracoscope.
- The ability of the patient to swallow must be confirmed post-operatively.

Chronic diaphragmatic rupture

Traumatic rupture of the diaphragm is rare in isolation, but is approximately three times more common on the left than the right side because of the protection afforded by the liver on the right side. Rupture of the diaphragm usually presents early, associated with abdominal injuries, after major trauma. However, a lacerated diaphragm is often overlooked at laparotomy. The signs of respiratory distress and the presence of bowel sounds in the chest may be masked by positive pressure ventilation, which may also reduce the herniated gut back into the abdomen. The presentation of a diaphragmatic rupture may therefore be delayed (sometimes for years) until the complications of the herniated abdominal contents, notably intestinal obstruction, occur. The diaphragmatic defect tends to enlarge steadily over time if not closed.

Surgical procedure

Ideally, the diaphragm should be repaired via a lateral thoracotomy, particularly on the right side, but a thoraco-abdominal incision may be required to deal with any adhesions that prevent complete reduction of the herniated gut. For this approach, the patient is rotated approximately 30° so the affected side is uppermost, supported on sandbags or a vacuum cushion, and an upper quadrant laparotomy incision is extended into the eighth intercostal space. When the herniated gut has been mobilized and returned to the abdominal cavity, the diaphragmatic tear is repaired in two layers with non-absorbable sutures.

Anaesthetic management

The repair of a chronic diaphragmatic rupture is usually performed electively. However, the herniated gut may become incarcerated, in which case an emergency procedure may be required to relieve obstruction. In such cases, careful attention to pre-operative fluid and electrolyte status will be required and induction of anaesthesia should be by a rapid sequence technique.

Post-operative care

Patients with chronic diaphragmatic ruptures can be managed in the same way as a standard lateral thoracotomy or thoraco-laparotomy, paying attention to post-operative analgesia.

KEY POINTS

- A ruptured diaphragm may be missed on initial trauma assessment or during laparotomy.

- The defect in the diaphragm should be closed as soon as possible.

- Chronic diaphragmatic rupture may present late as bowel obstruction.

Chest wall

Thoracoplasty

Rarely performed nowadays, thoracoplasty was common in the early part of the twentieth century for treatment of pulmonary tuberculosis with cavitation. The aim was to collapse the affected lung by producing multiple fractures of the ribs overlying the affected lung lobe(s), and so deprive the tubercle bacilli of oxygen. Thoracoplasty was often performed under local anaesthesia in an era when general anaesthesia was unsafe for patients with respiratory disease. The main indication currently for thoracoplasty is to obliterate or reduce the size of the residual space in patients with chronic empyema or bronchopleural fistula, usually following pneumonectomy. Thoracoplasty may be performed following lobectomy if it is felt that the lung will fail to expand to fill the thoracic cavity.

Surgical procedure

The operation is performed in two or possibly three stages, depending on the extent of the disease process. The first stage is an extrafascial apicolysis, in which the first three ribs are removed (while leaving the periosteum and pleura intact) and the parietal pleura is freed from Sibson's fascia, any fibres of scalenus anterior and from the mediastinum. The pleural cavity is not breached, and the first three intercostal bundles are divided posteriorly, leaving the apex of the lung free to collapse. Thoracoplasty for the management of pleural spaces does not usually require this first stage, and the second stage procedure is performed in isolation.

The second stage is performed about 10–14 days after the first operation, when the wound has healed. A sufficient number of ribs are removed to allow the scapula to embed itself in the chest wall without riding over any remaining ribs. The pleural space is again left intact, and the neurovascular bundles are divided in the same way as described above.

Anaesthetic management

The patients may be quite unwell as a result of their underlying disease. A standard thoracic anaesthetic with an appropriate double-lumen endo-bronchial tube allows isolation of the diseased lung and can improve surgical access, although a single-lumen tube will obviously suffice for thoracoplasty over a pneumonectomy space.

Post-operative care

Post-operative pain is not severe, partly because the neurovascular bundles are obliterated at the level of the rib resections. Although the chest wall is not rigid on the operated side, this does not usually embarrass respiratory function.

KEY POINTS

- Thoracoplasty is performed infrequently, although it used to be a common treatment for tuberculosis of the lung.

- The procedure is often performed in several stages, requiring two or three operations.

Rib resection and thoracostomy

These procedures are used to aid drainage of stubborn empyemas, but they should only be used as a last resort when intercostal tube drainage has failed. Tube drainage may fail due to antibiotic resistance in the infecting organism, the nature of the organism itself (actinomyces, aspergillus), the presence of a bronchopleural or oesophago-pleural fistula (especially in the presence of residual tumour), the presence of a foreign body, or locu-lation of the empyema contents. Further details of the management of empyema and bronchopleural fistula are covered in Chapter 16.

Surgical procedure

A 5-cm section of rib over the most dependent part of the empyema cavity is removed completely. The cavity is debrided and loculations broken down. A large-bore drainage tube is then inserted a short distance only into the cavity, allowing the contents of the empyema to drain.

Thoracostomy is a variant of rib resection in which short lengths of two adjacent ribs are removed via an H-shaped incision straddling the intercostal space. After resection of the ribs, the skin flaps formed by the H-shaped incision are sewn to the parietal pleura, allowing the contents of the empyema to drain directly through the chest wall.

Anaesthetic management

The anaesthetic technique needs to be chosen carefully, since there is the possibility of an undiagnosed bronchopleural fistula. Good pre-operative preparation, with adequate intercostal tube drainage or physiotherapy and postural drainage, is important to prevent soiling of the respiratory tract if there is a known bronchopleural fistula. If a bronchopleural fistula is present or suspected, the surgeon may elect to perform the rib resection under local anaesthesia with the patient sitting up. If the rib resection is being carried out under a general anaesthetic, serious consideration should be given to managing the patient as described for bronchopleural fistula.

Post-operative care

Post-operative pain is not severe unless ribs have been resected, and a standard regimen of intramuscular opiates and oral non-steroidal analgesics usually suffices. Instillation of antibiotics into the empyema cavity via a small tube (i.e. size 10 nasogastric tube) passed through the chest wall at the time of surgery may be required to sterilize the cavity.

KEY POINTS

- Thoracostomy is used for the drainage of stubborn empyemas.
- There is a risk of an undiagnosed bronchopleural fistula.
- Antibiotics may be instilled into the empyema cavity post-operatively.

Pectus repair

Pectus excavatum (funnel chest) and pectus carinatum (pigeon chest) deformities of the sternum are not usually a danger to life or physical health, but are often a cause of psychological distress in adolescents and their parents. Pectus excavatum may displace the heart to the left, and may also cause respiratory difficulty if the depression is deep, especially during episodes of chest infections.

Pectus excavatum

A vertical skin incision is made along the length of the sternum. The lower costal cartilages are detached from the sternum on both sides, and a transverse osteotomy is performed at one or two points across the sternum to enable it to be flattened. The deformed costal cartilages are often removed completely, leaving the perichondrium intact. The new sternal shape is maintained by supporting the underside of the sternum on a metal bar that rests on the rib cage on either side. The costal cartilages are then reattached to the sternum, if they are being retained. The bar is removed at a later date, once the sternum has healed, to prevent later complications due to its migration.

Pectus carinatum

This is treated by a similar procedure to pectus excavatum, with resection of the excessive lengths of the lower costal cartilages. The ends of the costal cartilages, or the remaining perichondrium, are reattached to the sternum.

Anaesthetic management

These patients are usually fit, and no special anaesthetic precautions are needed. Anaesthesia follows standard practice, with tracheal intubation and positive pressure ventilation. Bleeding may be profuse, and large bore venous access is recommended. It is important to bear in mind that the pleura may be breached on either or both sides of the chest during surgery.

Consideration should be given to use of a mid-thoracic epidural for post-operative analgesia.

Post-operative care

There is no particular post-operative concern apart from the maintenance of adequate analgesia. Some surgeons prefer the patient to be nursed supine for 24–48 hours after repair of pectus carinatum, often with a large sandbag over the sternum to apply corrective pressure to the chest wall.

KEY POINTS

- Pectus repair attempts to restore the shape of the anterior chest wall.
- The repairs are entirely elective, usually performed for psychological indications.
- Bleeding may be profuse, and the surgeon may unintentionally enter one or both pleural cavities.

Chest wall resection

Tumours of the chest wall are uncommon, but may be primary or secondary. Neurofibromata and Schwannomas may extend through intervertebral foraminae, and a collaborative neurosurgical and thoracic surgical approach may be necessary.

Surgical procedure

Usually, surgery involves removal of part of the bony structure of the chest wall along with the tumour. When the defect in the chest wall is not covered by the scapula, a patch of Marlex mesh may be required to support the chest wall. Larger defects may need the added rigidity of a Marlex and methyl methacrylate sandwich, or titanium mesh.

Anaesthetic management

There are no specific anaesthetic issues related to the removal of chest wall tumours. Although a double-lumen tube may be useful to allow the lung to be deflated to improve surgical access to the tumour, it may not be possible to collapse the lung completely if it is anchored to the chest wall by adhesions to the tumour.

Post-operative care

Resection of part of the chest wall is often very painful, and good quality post-operative analgesia is essential. Thoracic epidural analgesia or patient controlled opiate analgesia is effective, and the patient is best nursed in a high dependency area post-operatively. There may be an air leak post-operatively if the underlying lung was adherent to the chest wall. Most post-operative complications are due to sputum retention and atelectasis of the underlying lung, which can be minimized by good physiotherapy.

KEY POINTS

- Removal of chest wall tumours leaves a defect which may need prosthetic support.

- Nervous system tumours may need a combined thoracic and neurosurgical approach.

- Post-operative pain is severe, and post-operative care is best provided on a high dependency ward.

Chest drainage

Intercostal drainage tubes may be used to drain air or liquid (blood, pus or effusions) from the pleural cavity (Figs 6.1 and 6.2). Pneumothorax may be spontaneous, secondary to interventions close to the pleura (e.g. subclavian cannulation, cervical sympathectomy, brachial plexus or intercostal nerve block), or due to trauma. Pneumothorax may be suspected if there is dyspnoea or unequal movement of the two sides of the chest during respiration, and confirmed by absence of breath sounds on the affected side. However, clinical signs are not completely reliable, and the exact location of the pneumothorax should be confirmed by chest X-ray before insertion of a drain tube, unless the patient is in danger of respiratory or CVS collapse. Tension pneumothorax may occur when the tear in the lung forms a one-way valve, allowing air into the pleural space but not back out. Intrathoracic pressure increases as air accumulates in the affected side, causing shift of the mediastinum to the opposite side and haemodynamic compromise as the great vessels in the chest are distorted and compressed.

Pleural effusions may be transudative or exudative, depending on their cause, and may be infected or sterile. Most commonly, effusions are associated with cardiac failure, pneumonia or tumours. Blood or chyle may accumulate in the pleural space after trauma or surgery. If left undrained, even small accumulations of fluid may cause respiratory embarrassment in patients with impaired lung function. Undrained fluid may also lead to empyema formation.

Surgical procedure

A short incision is made over a suitable rib space, most commonly the fourth or fifth space in the mid-axillary line. Anterior drains penetrating

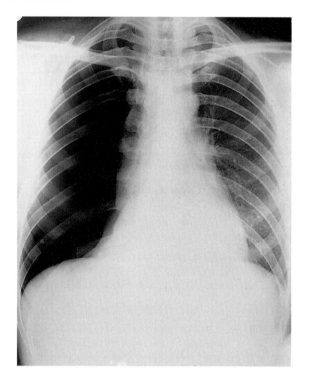

Figure 6.1 PA chest X-ray showing right-sided pneumothorax.

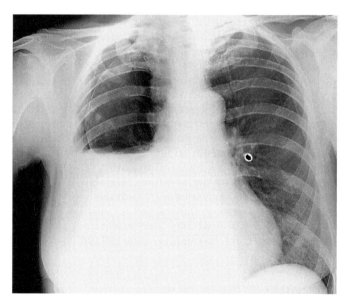

Figure 6.2 PA chest X-ray showing right-sided haemo-pneumothorax.

the pectoral muscles should be avoided, as they cause more pain than those in the lateral chest wall. A horizontal mattress suture should then be inserted across the centre of the incision, but not tied down, the ends being left long to allow airtight closure of the incision when the tube is removed later. Purse-string sutures should be avoided, because puckering of the skin when they are tied produces an ugly scar. Blunt dissection with a Spencer Wells forceps is used to open a track down to and through the pleura, and the drain is advanced into position through the track without a trocar; forceful penetration of the chest wall with sharp trocars is dangerous as the lungs, heart, oesophagus, great vessels or liver can be damaged when the trocar suddenly advances after the pleura has been breached. The drain tube is held in place by an anchoring suture in the skin tied round the tube at the point of entry. The tube is attached to an underwater seal drainage bottle. Low-pressure suction (5–15 kPa) may aid re-expansion of the lung. A chest X-ray should be taken to confirm the intrathoracic position of the drain.

Anaesthetic management

Insertion of a tube drain can normally be accomplished under local anaesthesia in adults. A general anaesthetic will usually be necessary in small children. Nitrous oxide should be used with care in pneumothoraces; because it is less soluble in blood than nitrogen, there will be an increase in gas volume (or pressure) over the first 20–25 minutes of administration as the nitrous oxide diffuses into the pneumothorax faster than nitrogen can diffuse out. Vigorous positive pressure ventilation should be avoided as it may worsen the air leak; spontaneous ventilation is ideal if the patient is well enough to tolerate this.

Post-operative care

Re-expansion pulmonary oedema may occur in the affected lung (Fig. 6.3), even after a short period of lung collapse, and staff caring for the patient should be warned of this possibility. A regimen of intermittent clamping of the drain prior to removal to confirm that pneumothorax does not recur is unnecessary. The drain tube can usually be safely removed when air or fluid is no longer draining and the absence of air or fluid within the pleura is confirmed radiologically. Entonox administered through a demand apparatus provides good analgesia for this procedure. The retaining suture is cut and a single throw is taken on the mattress skin suture and gently tensioned by an assistant. The operator pulls the drain tube out smoothly while the patient holds his or her breath at maximal inhalation or exhalation; the assistant simultaneously tightens the mattress skin suture around the emerging drain and knots it upon complete removal. A chest X-ray should be taken post-drain removal to confirm the absence of pneumothorax.

KEY POINTS

- Intercostal tubes are used to drain air or fluid from the pleural space.

- The drain should be inserted using blunt dissection to avoid damage to intrathoracic organs or liver.

- Avoid the anterior approach as this is more painful than insertion in the lateral chest.

- Low-pressure suction may aid drainage of the pleural space and expansion of the lung.

- Re-expansion pulmonary oedema is a significant risk, even after lung collapse of short duration.

- Mattress sutures rather than purse-string sutures should be used to close the incision after removal of the drain tube.

- The absence of residual pneumothorax should be confirmed by chest X-ray after the drain has been removed.

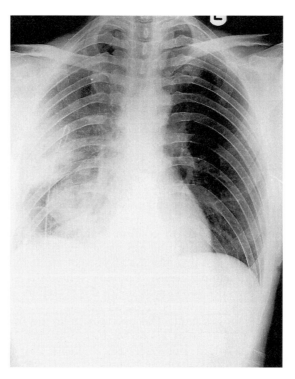

Figure 6.3 PA chest X-ray showing pulmonary oedema of right lung after re-expansion following insertion of a chest drain for pneumothorax.

Bibliography

Hartrey, R., Poskitt, K.R., Heather, B.P. and Durkin, M.A. (1994). Anaesthetic implications for transthoracic endoscopic sympathectomy. *Eur. J. Surg.*, **572**, 33–6.

Kam, A.C., O'Brien, M. and Kam, P.C.A. (1993). Pleural drainage systems. *Anaesthesia*, **48**, 154–61.

Kraenzler, E.J. and Hearn, C.J. (1993). Anaesthetic considerations for video-assisted thoracic surgery. *Sem. Thorac. Cardiovasc. Surg.*, **15**, 321–6.

Robinson, D.A. and Branthwaite, M.A. (1984). Pleural surgery in patients with cystic fibrosis. A review of anaesthetic management. *Anaesthesia*, **39**, 655–9.

Roos, D.B. (1980). Transaxillary extrapleural thoracic sympathectomy. In *Operative Techniques in Vascular Surgery* (J.J. Bergan and J.S.T. Yao, eds). Grune and Stratton.

Waldschmidt, M.L. and Laws, H.L. (1980). Injuries of the diaphragm. *J. Trauma*, **20**, 587.

Walsh, T.S. and Young, C.H. (1995). Anaesthesia and cystic fibrosis. *Anaesthesia*, **50**, 614–22.

7

Tracheal and bronchial surgery

I. D. Conacher

Introduction

Early bronchial surgery goes back to the era of tuberculosis, with the operation of sleeve resection. In this, the right main bronchus was sectioned, this sleeve with the bronchus for the upper lobe was removed, and the bronchus intermedius was re-anastomosed to the trachea. The need for this kind of surgery, in which the anaesthetist may potentially be cut off from the means to oxygenate a patient, has always been rare, and few centres have much experience of its management. What experience there is, is largely case report and anecdote.

The principal indications for surgery on the major airways are stenotic or malacic segments that have resulted in stridor and respiratory obstruction. Primary causes are:

- Congenital, where resection of trachea and bronchi may be required for paediatric cases.
- Post-traumatic, notably after prolonged tracheal intubation or complications of tracheostomy.
- Slow growing tumours, characteristically benign, or of low grade malignancy.

The vascular supply to the trachea and the main bronchi is precarious and this, together with the difficulty of splinting a new anastomosis, has led to a very cautious attitude to the use of surgical options. The potential for dehiscence, mediastinal sepsis and erosion of major blood vessels is significant. Developments in less irritant plastic materials for tracheal intubation, lasers and other methods of debulking intraluminal obstructions, and of stents (Fig. 7.1), has meant that the need for resection and reconstruction is unusual except in paediatric practice.

Techniques such as the laser debulking of tumours or tracheal or bronchial stenting are largely dependent on bronchoscopy for implementation.

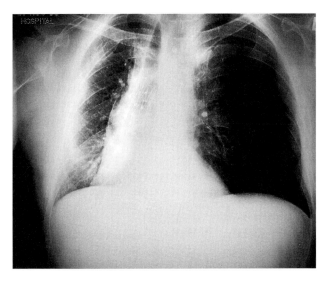

Figure 7.1 Chest X-ray showing stents placed bronchoscopically in the right main bronchus.

Surgery

Surgical management

Access to the middle and lower third of the trachea, and to isolated stenoses of the main bronchi, can be gained from a standard antero-lateral thoracotomy. Lesions involving the carina and both bronchi are approached through a sternotomy. Partial cardiopulmonary bypass may be instituted for paediatric cases and those requiring extensive central airways and bilateral bronchial surgery. Femoro-femoral bypass is suitable, as the need is to secure gas exchange rather than to replace the function of the heart. Long segments of airway may be replaced with prostheses. Cartilage substitutes, such as pieces of rib, may also be inserted. Pieces of pericardium, or intercostal muscle on vascular pedicles, may have to be interposed. Some surgeons routinely protect against dehiscence and encourage healing by wrapping anastomoses in omentum or intercostal muscle on a vascular pedicle. Some plastic repair techniques conducted to widen and lengthen the trachea may involve the larynx. Plastic surgical techniques occasionally require stabilization of the chin and/or head in the flexed position for a period post-operatively.

Anaesthetic management

Pre-operative assessment

Presenting symptoms range from a persistent dry cough to wheeze or stridor. Severity of symptoms may be dependent on posture and rate and depth of respiration. Symptomatic relief may be obtained by the use of steroids and breathing of low-density gas, such as a helium–air mixture. It is important to get as much information as possible about the site, type and limits of the narrowing or obstruction. By studying chest radiographs and CT scans it is possible to build up a three-dimensional image of most stenoses, and to put this into the context of the sizing of tracheal tubes and the optimum positioning of the tip of the tube. In adults in whom the airway is not too compromised, useful information can be obtained from fibre-optic bronchoscopy under local anaesthesia. Small fibre-optic broncho-scopes are now available for infants, which can be threaded through a laryngeal mask airway, maintaining spontaneous respiration using a volatile agent. Sevoflurane would appear to have many of the properties that are regarded as ideal for this type of procedure. A plan of airway management needs to be established with the surgeon prior to the pro-cedure. The possibilities that the artificial airway may have to be adjusted, removed, displaced or altered, or may be lost, should be taken into account. This calls for considerable flexibility and ingenuity on the part of the anaesthetist.

Anaesthetic technique and monitoring

Establishment of monitoring, commensurate with a major procedure, is best conducted in the awake patient, who may be most comfortable sitting up. Before induction of anaesthesia, a rigid bronchoscope and a choice of sterile tracheal tubes (cuffed, uncuffed and uncut), as well as alternative methods of ventilation, should be to hand. A Sanders jet injector connected to an oxygen supply is particularly useful.

In considering the induction of anaesthesia, the events most likely to pro-duce a catastrophic obstruction of the central airways are coughing and the loss of upper airway muscle tone. Coughing is a risk of both local anaes-thetic techniques and of volatile agents. The latter also have a propensity to affect muscle tone. Sevoflurane will undoubtedly have an impact on these considerations, particularly in paediatric practice. Although it is possible to use sevoflurane to produce rapid induction of anaesthesia with a reduced risk of coughing, it still has the genre's effects on muscle tone. A volatile induction is useful for those in whom a tracheostomy is present. Because of the vicious circle of airway irritation, coughing and loss of muscle tone leading to respiratory obstruction and further irritation and hypoxia, rapid induction of anaesthesia and intubation of the upper trachea following muscle relaxation with suxamethonium is often regarded as being indicated. Muscle relaxation should, however, only be used after balancing the relative risks of loss of spontaneous respiration and inability to artificially ventilate the patient against the feasibility of safely and rapidly securing the airway without paralysis. Maintenance of anaesthesia should be by a total intravenous technique because of the risk of awareness if ventilation is interrupted resulting in unpredictable delivery of volatile agents.

Apart from airway management at induction of anaesthesia, separate planning and action may be necessary during the resection and reconstruction and post-operatively. Much tracheal surgery can be conducted without displacement of the tracheal tube. For central airway lesions, in which tracheo-bronchial separation is required, long flexible catheters sited by the surgeon through the surgical field have proved successful. The use of two catheters, or a bifurcated one, is reported for carinal lesions. The onus is on the surgeon to ensure the stability of the catheters and to prevent aspiration of blood, as the protection of the lower airway is minimal. High frequency ventilation techniques have proved popular, but the usual risks of barotrauma and consequences of dynamic hyperinflation particularly pertain, as the presence of the narrow conduits employed may interfere with expiration and encourage air trapping.

For the insertion of stents and other endoscopic procedures, such as the use of lasers, the airway may need to be maintained with a rigid bronchoscope. In this case, the standard anaesthetic techniques discussed in Chapter 5, with total intravenous anaesthesia, are suitable.

Post-operative care

Patients should be advised in advance about their post-operative care as, in some cases, it can mean a period on a ventilator, a period with a tracheal tube *in situ* and the possibility of a prolonged period in which the head will be maintained flexed, either by fixation of the chin or with plaster casts.

Optimally, spontaneous respiration and extubation is achieved as soon as possible post-operatively, as this provides the best chance for successful healing of the newly fashioned airway anastomosis. Early extubation has to be carefully conducted, and is best managed with the patient conscious and co-operative. Suitable equipment must be available by the bedside in case respiratory obstruction should occur.

KEY POINTS

- Resection and reconstruction techniques are associated with significant surgical morbidity and are major undertakings.

- Tracheal surgery is the most challenging for techniques of airway management, and requires careful planning and co-operation with the surgeon and flexibility on the part of the anaesthetist.

- Lasers are commonly employed. The risk of fire is minimized by using metal instrumentation.

- The most commonly employed techniques for lasers and stents are based on requirements for rigid bronchoscopy.

- To reduce traction on tracheo-broncheal anastomoses, the patient may have to maintain a position of neck flexion for 2 or more weeks.

- Early extubation is required to minimize trauma to the airways.

Bibliography

Conacher, I.D., Paes, M.L., McMahon, C.C. and Morrit, G.N. (1998). Anaesthetic management for central airways obstruction. *J. Cardiothorac. Vasc. Anaesth.*, **12,** 153–6.

Grillo, H.C., Mathisen, D.J. and Wain, J.C. (1992). Laryngotracheal resection and reconstruction for subglottic stenosis. *Ann. Thorac. Surg.*, **53,** 54–63.

Pollard, J. and Harrison, M.J. (1985). Subtotal tracheal resection. *Eur. J. Anaesthiol.*, **2,** 387–94.

Rowe, R.W., Betts, J. and Free, E. (1991). Peri-operative management for laryngotracheal reconstruction. *Anesth. Analg.*, **73,** 483–6.

Sonnet, J.R., Keenan, R.J., Ferson, P.F. *et al.* (1995). Endobronchial management of benign, malignant and lung transplantation airway stenoses. *Ann. Thorac. Surg.*, **59,** 1417–22.

Young-Beyer, P. and Wilson, R.S. (1988). Anaesthetic management for tracheal resection and reconstruction. *J. Cardiothorac. Anesth.*, **2,** 821–35.

8

Mediastinal surgery (including thymectomy, myasthenia gravis and retrosternal goitre)

R. O. Feneck

Introduction

Previously, surgery of the mediastinum was considered to be of relatively minor importance to the thoracic surgeon. In the pre-antibiotic era, surgery for the complications of pulmonary infection, particularly tuberculosis, was pre-eminent. In the era immediately following the introduction of antibiotics, pulmonary resection for the treatment of pulmonary neoplasm and its complications has achieved greater prominence.

The advent of chemotherapy/radiotherapy for mediastinal tumours, including lymphoma, has meant that many of these tumours, previously considered fatal, now have a relatively good prognosis. There is, however, an absolute need for a tissue diagnosis and, in a proportion of cases, successful biopsy will only be achieved by mediastinoscopy or anterior mediastinotomy. These procedures have thus become important as part of the diagnostic and staging process, and there has been an increase in mediastinal surgery in recent years. Tumours of the thymus and retrosternal thyroid have long been managed surgically, but these are relatively rare. They are, nonetheless, an important group, and their anaesthetic management may be both theoretically and practically demanding, particularly in patients with myasthenia gravis.

In order better to understand the anaesthetic implications and potential complications of mediastinal surgery, it is necessary to have an understanding of the anatomy of the mediastinum.

Normal anatomy and pathology

The mediastinum is a wide, organ filled space between the two pleural sacs. It is divided into two parts (Fig. 8.1): the upper part, or superior mediastinum, and the lower part, which is divided into three sections – the anterior mediastinum in front of the pericardium, the middle mediastinum containing the heart and pericardium, and the posterior mediastinum behind the pericardium. The anatomy of and surgical access to these areas is discussed below.

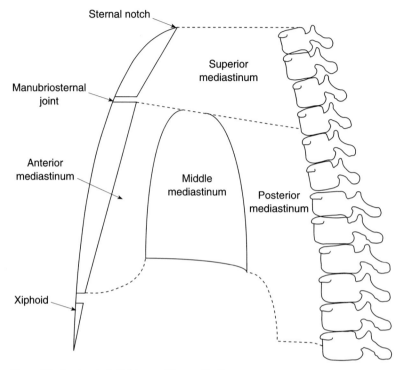

Figure 8.1 Anatomical divisions of the mediastinum.

The superior mediastinum

- *Boundaries*: the thoracic inlet superiorly, the mediastinal pleura of the lungs laterally, the manubrium of the sternum anteriorly and the thoracic verterbrae posteriorly. Inferiorly, its lower extent is the plane from the sternal angle to the 4th thoracic vertebra.
- *Contents*: the aortic arch, the innominate artery, the intrathoracic portion of the left common carotid and subclavian arteries, the innominate veins, the upper halves of the superior vena cava, trachea and oesophagus, the thoracic duct, the thymus, the recurrent laryngeal and phrenic nerves and lymph nodes. A retrosternal thyroid is usually contained mostly within the superior mediastinum.
- *Surgical access*: mediastinoscopy, anterior mediastinotomy or median sternotomy.

The anterior mediastinum

- *Boundaries*: the body of the sternum anteriorly, the parietal pericardium posteriorly and the diaphragm inferiorly.
- *Contents*: lymph nodes, thymic remnant, thyroid remnant (occasionally).
- *Surgical access*: anterior mediastinotomy or median sternotomy.

The middle mediastinum

- *Boundaries*: the upper border of the pericardium superiorly, the dia-phragmatic pericardium inferiorly and the pericardial edge antero-laterally.
- *Contents*: the heart, ascending aorta, lower half of the superior vena cava, the main pulmonary artery with its left and right branches, left and right pulmonary veins and the phrenic nerves.
- *Surgical access*: median sternotomy.

The posterior mediastinum

- *Boundaries*: the posterior pericardium and lower diaphragm anteriorly, the 4th to 12th thoracic vertebrae posteriorly, the mediastinal pleura laterally on both sides.
- *Contents*: the thoracic part of the descending aorta, the azygos veins, the bifurcation of the trachea and main bronchi, the oesophagus, the thoracic duct and lymph nodes.
- *Surgical access*: thoracoscopy, lateral or postero-lateral thoracotomy.

Incidence and anatomical location of tumours and cysts

The relative incidence of different types of mediastinal tumours is given in Table 8.1a. Neurogenic tumours are usually confined to the posterior mediastinum, and pericardial and bronchogenic cysts to the middle medias-tinum. The common locations of mediastinal tumours and other mediastinal pathology are shown in Table 8.1b.

Table 8.1a Incidence of primary mediastinal tumours

Type of tumour	Incidence (per cent)
Neurogenic tumour	20
Thymoma	19
Lymphoma	13
Germ-cell neoplasm	10
Primary carcinoma	5
Mesenchymal tumour	6
Endocrine tumour	6
Other	3
Cysts	
Pericardial	6
Bronchogenic	6
Enteric	2
Other	4

Table 8.1b Incidence of anatomic location of primary tumours and cysts of mediastinum

Type	Percentage
Anterosuperior mediastinum	
Thymic neoplasms	31
Lymphomas	23
Germ cell	17
Carcinoma	13
Cysts	6
Mesenchymal	4
Endocrine	5
Other	1
Middle mediastinum	
Cysts	61
Lymphomas	20
Mesenchymal	8
Carcinoma	6
Other	5
Posterior mediastinum	
Neurogenic	50
Cysts	32
Mesenchymal	10
Endocrine	3
Other	4

Table 8.1c Presenting symptoms in patients with a mediastinal mass

Symptoms	Patients (per cent)
Chest pain	29
Dyspnoea	22
Cough	18
Fever	13
Weight loss	9
Superior vena caval syndrome	8
Myasthenia gravis	7
Fatigue	6
Dysphagia	4
Night sweats	3

Clinical presentation and investigation of mediastinal disease

Signs and symptoms

The signs and symptoms of mediastinal disease can range from relatively trivial to life threatening. The most serious complications include superior vena caval (SVC) obstruction, pulmonary artery obstruction, right heart compression and compression of the major conducting airways. SVC obstruction may present as dyspnoea, orthopnoea, cough, headache and acute facial swelling. Later, superficial veins in the neck and chest wall may become prominent as these collateral vessels open up. Pulmonary artery obstruction may present as acute right ventricular strain or failure, and postural hypotension. Right heart compression presents in a similar manner. Compression of the carina or major conducting airways may produce respiratory distress.

Lesser complications include oesophageal compression, with dysphagia, and neural or other compressive symptoms manifesting as pain, which may be severe. If the spinal cord is involved in neurogenic tumours, a range of neurological symptoms (including paralysis) may occur.

Recurrent laryngeal nerve entrapment may cause vocal cord palsy. Horner's syndrome may result from posterior mediastinal tumour involvement of the sympathetic chain. The incidence of presenting symptoms is given in Table 8.1c.

Investigations

In general, patients presenting with the symptoms and signs described above will have a plain film chest X-ray as part of their initial work-up (Fig. 8.2a). However, once mediastinal disease is suspected, CT is clearly the best and most effective single investigation for localizing a mediastinal mass (Fig. 8.2b). Furthermore, CT is effective in differentiating between mainly fatty, cystic, vascular or soft tissue masses. Although CT cannot primarily differentiate between benign and malignant conditions, it may demonstrate invasive disease affecting the airways, heart and great vessels, pleura and lung parenchyma, thereby helping to differentiate between benign and malignant conditions.

In order to establish a conclusive diagnosis, a tissue biopsy must be obtained. This is particularly important with mediastinal pathology, as a high proportion of mediastinal masses are malignant and the optimum treatment varies between chemotherapy, radiotherapy, combined chemotherapy and radiotherapy, combined chemotherapy and radiotherapy followed by surgery, or surgery alone. The mass of biopsy tissue required to make a definitive diagnosis also varies. Needle biopsy under fluoroscopic, ultrasound or, most effectively, CT control may be sufficient for most diagnostic purposes, but if tissue is required for immunophenotyping, an open surgical biopsy is usually necessary.

If there are significant respiratory symptoms, or signs of respiratory impairment, pulmonary function tests should be carried out before initial biopsy. Simple spirometry (FEV_1 and FVC) and peak expiratory flow

(a)

(b)

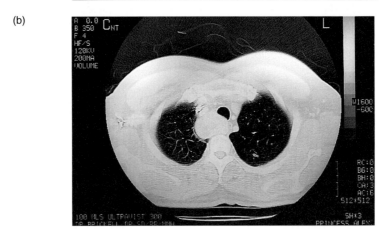

Figure 8.2

(a) Chest X-ray showing mediastinal mass causing tracheal
    deviation.
(b) CT scan of superior mediastinum showing mass located behind
    and to the right of the trachea.

measurements may be valuable. Where the patient has a background of pulmonary disease such as pulmonary fibrosis, chronic bronchitis or emphysema in addition to the mediastinal pathology, tests of total lung capacity, residual volume and gas transfer factor are appropriate. Flow volume loops in the erect and supine posture may be useful in determining whether an obstructive lesion is intra- or extrathoracic.

If there is evidence of right ventricular outflow tract compression, or obstruction of right ventricular function, transthoracic echocardiographic examination is warranted.

The primary focus of the thoracic surgery team will be on the patient's mediastinal pathology, but it is essential to consider the general health of the patient and that the patient may be suffering from unrelated, but significant, disease that compromises the safe delivery of anaesthesia. Hypertension, ischaemic heart disease and cerebrovascular disease are obvious examples that require further investigation pre-operatively.

Some patients, particularly those with severe compressive symptoms, may undergo radiotherapy to reduce both the tumour size and surrounding oedema before any further treatment takes place. This initial reduction in tumour size reduces the immediate life-threatening risk of surgical intervention. Furthermore, it is now possible to shield a portion of the tumour from radiotherapy, thereby protecting it as a source of 'clean' tumour tissue for histological diagnosis.

Invasive diagnostic surgical techniques and their anaesthetic implications

The surgical procedures commonly undertaken include needle biopsy, fibre-optic or rigid bronchoscopy, mediastinoscopy, anterior mediastinotomy and thoracoscopy. The preferred route of surgical access will be determined by the location of the mass within the mediastinum.

Needle biopsy

Needle biopsies are usually taken under radiographic guidance, without general anaesthesia. It may occasionally be necessary to perform a needle biopsy through a surgical incision; the anaesthetic considerations are similar to those for mediastinoscopy/mediastinotomy.

Diagnostic bronchoscopy and tissue biopsy

Patients with severe symptoms require a fibre-optic bronchoscopy to evaluate the integrity of the airway. This fibre-optic examination is usually carried out by the initial team evaluating the patient before surgical referral, invariably under topical anaesthesia. There may be tumour invading the trachea or main bronchi, but if disease is restricted to the mediastinum, external compression of the trachea and/or main bronchi is usually the only feature.

This initial evaluation may be of considerable use to the anaesthetist, since it provides the first assessment of the patient's airway. However, further bronchoscopic examination may be required at the time of surgery, particularly if endobronchial intubation is required. Although rigid bronchoscopy is not usually considered to be a particularly useful investigation of mediastinal disease, many thoracic surgeons will take the opportunity to assess the patient's respiratory tract immediately before or after carrying out other surgical procedures (e.g. mediastinoscopy, mediastinotomy). In particular, the degree of extrinsic compression of the airway, invasion of the airway by tumour, mobility of the carina and alteration of the carinal angle is of interest.

The detailed considerations for anaesthesia for diagnostic rigid bronchoscopy are described in Chapter 5.

Mediastinoscopy and anterior mediastinotomy

These procedures are indicated for examination of, and biopsy from, the anterior and superior mediastinum. They are most frequently carried out under general anaesthesia.

The usual technique for mediastinoscopy is more accurately described as cervical mediastinoscopy, and consists of making a small incision at the suprasternal notch, carrying out blunt dissection of the pretracheal fascia into the mediastinum, and then inserting the mediastinoscope under the manubrium sternae. When positioned behind the thoracic aorta but anterior to the trachea, the mediastinoscope may be used to gain access to superior mediastinal lymph nodes and masses. Some lesions are more easily approached via a left anterior mediastinotomy. This is performed by dissection through the second rib interspace via a small incision just lateral to the sternum. This approach gives useful access to centrally located and left-sided pathology, as well as to the thymus and structures of the anterior mediastinum. The relative indications and contraindications to these procedures vary between different authorities. They are certainly more hazardous in the presence of tumour causing SVC obstruction, compression of the heart or great vessels or severe tracheal deviation or narrowing; the anaesthetic implications of these conditions are discussed in detail under *Resection of large anterior mediastinal masses*.

Particular attention should be paid to evaluation of the airway prior to surgery. Chest X-ray, chest CT and bronchoscopy will reveal the extent and level of any tracheal deviation and external compression of the trachea or main bronchi. This is usually distal to the tip of an appropriately sized single-lumen endotracheal tube, which is usually sufficient for securing the airway. Endobronchial intubation should only be undertaken after specific discussion with the surgeon, since it may be of little value and is rarely required for mediastinal procedures. Use of an armoured or non-kinking endotracheal tube may be advisable. The procedure is usually carried out with the patient's head placed on a head ring and fully extended, with the patient tilted slightly head-up to minimize venous engorgement, although this may slightly increase the risk of venous air embolism. The endotracheal tube should be firmly secured so that it does not interfere with the surgical field.

Anterior mediastinotomy is largely extrapleural. However, a small tear in the pleura may occur, and an early post-operative chest X-ray is advisable.

The surgery is not usually prolonged, and the anaesthetic and muscle relaxants chosen should reflect both the duration of the procedure and the patient's general condition. Inhalational induction of anaesthesia has theoretical advantages in patients in whom there is any doubt about the ease of securing the airway. With the advent of sevoflurane there is now a volatile anaesthetic agent whose odour is easily tolerated by most patients. A total intravenous anaesthetic (TIVA) technique, supplementing a propofol induction and maintenance infusion with alfentanil (20–30 mg/kg) and

Table 8.2 Complications of mediastinoscopy

- Haemorrhage
- Pneumothorax
- Recurrent laryngeal nerve injury
- Air embolism
- Arterial compression:
  aorta
  right carotid
  right subclavian
- Tracheal compression
- Infection
- Others:
  tumour implantation
  phrenic nerve injury
  oesophageal injury
  chylothorax
  air embolism
  transient hemiparesis

atracurium (5–7 mg/kg), is satisfactory. Ventilation is with either oxygen and nitrous oxide or oxygen enriched air, as appropriate. The aim should be to awaken and extubate the patient at the end of the procedure.

The usual minimum monitoring standards should be observed, but it may be best to place the blood pressure cuff on the left arm and gain access to palpate the right radial artery in order to exclude mediastinoscopic compression of the major vessels during the procedure. Compression of the innominate, right subclavian or carotid arteries may theoretically occur. If an indwelling arterial cannula is placed, it may be most suitably sited in the right arm for the same reason. Large bore venous access should be established using lower limb veins if there is evidence of SVC obstruction.

Neither mediastinoscopy nor anterior mediastinotomy are without complications, and these are shown in Table 8.2. Although the overall mortality from the procedure is low (0.1 per cent), major complications occur frequently (1.5–3 per cent), and many need rapid and urgent attention. Clearly haemorrhage is a recognized complication, and blood should be available, particularly for higher risk cases. Catastrophic haemorrhage is rare, but emergency sternotomy or thoracotomy may be necessary to locate and stem the source. The usual resuscitative measures include massive volume replacement, pharmacologic support of the circulation as appropriate, and maintenance of oxygenation. Cardiopulmonary bypass has been used in an attempt to provide haemodynamic support and a route for massive transfusion; in this patient group, in these emergency circumstances, the outcome is usually poor. Nonetheless, cardiopulmonary bypass standby is frequently recommended in patients undergoing high risk mediastinoscopy or resection of mediastinal masses.

Pneumothorax is a not infrequent finding post-operatively, especially after mediastinotomy, but rarely requires chest tube drainage. Recurrent laryngeal nerve damage may also occur, and may be permanent in approximately 50 per cent of patients. If injury is suspected, then vocal cord movement under direct laryngoscopy should be checked at the end of the procedure immediately after extubation.

Venous air embolism is rare (less than 0.1 per cent), particularly if the patient is being ventilated with intermittent positive pressure ventilation rather than breathing spontaneously.

Pressure on, or compression of, vascular structures can cause arrhythmias, hypotension and impaired cerebral perfusion. This latter complication, though rare, may be catastrophic in outcome, and invasive monitoring of the arterial pressure in the right arm should therefore be considered, as mentioned earlier.

Thoracoscopy

The technique of thoracoscopy is not used *per se* in the surgical management of masses arising from the anterior or superior mediastinum. However, it is still relevant because it may form part of the surgical procedures necessary to establish a diagnosis in patients with thoracic neoplasm – in particular, bronchogenic carcinoma. A detailed discussion of anaesthesia for thoracoscopy can be found in Chapter 10.

Resection of large anterior mediastinal masses

The anaesthetic significance of large masses in or near the anterior mediastinum can be divided into factors associated with compression, resulting from the physical size of the tumour, and disorders of the thyroid and thymus. Thyroid goitre may extend retrosternally and, apart from the physical size of the tumour (which may be considerable), it is important to ensure that the patient is euthyroid before the procedure. Tumours of the thymus may also be of significant size. However, most important is the presence of myasthenia gravis, and the effect that this has on the perioperative management of patients undergoing surgery. This is discussed in detail below.

Compression

Symptoms and signs of compression most frequently affect the airway (trachea and main bronchi), the heart (right ventricle and pulmonary artery) and the SVC. In some patients, very large tumours will produce symptoms and signs of compression affecting all three.

Compression of the tracheobronchial tree

A variety of tumours may cause major airway compression, including cystic hygroma, teratoma, thymoma, retrosternal thyroid tumour and lymphoma. Since the therapeutic management of these conditions differs, patients will require a biopsy procedure, either a needle or open biopsy. Patients who have symptoms of airway compression are more likely to suffer from serious respiratory complications peri-operatively, but a proportion of patients who are relatively asymptomatic will also suffer a stormy peri-operative course. Anaesthesia in these patients must therefore be recognized as hazardous at all times, and steps taken accordingly.

In a proportion of patients there may be some doubt as to whether the respiratory symptoms result from intrathoracic or extrathoracic airway obstruction. In these patients, a flow–volume loop, preferably in the erect and supine positions, may help to make the distinction.

The majority of patients will have undergone a needle biopsy with CT guidance under local anaesthesia, and initial radiotherapy or chemotherapy (or both) to produce shrinkage of the tumour. This latter point is important, since the tumour size and effects of compression may be profoundly reduced. If the patient is to be anaesthetized, the tracheobronchial tree should be inspected before any attempt is made to intubate the patient. In practice, this will usually have been carried out before surgery, but the anaesthetist must be satisfied that an appropriately sized endotracheal tube can be safely placed. It may be necessary to change the patient's position during and after induction if symptoms of respiratory obstruction develop. Although inhalational induction has theoretical advantages, an intravenous induction with a short-acting agent is usually well tolerated. In severe cases it is necessary to be able to place the tip of the endotracheal tube distal to the tumour, and a range of endotracheal tube sizes should therefore be at hand. It should be noted that complete airway obstruction has been reported both with an inhalational induction and after positioning the tip of the tube distal to the tumour. Availability of a rigid bronchoscope is thus of value, since this will not become obstructed as a result of kinking, and has been used frequently as a way of establishing and maintaining a patent airway in an emergency.

In addition to the kinking of an endotracheal tube in a deformed trachea, obstruction of the tube may occur if the orifice impinges on a deformed tracheal wall. Other causes include bleeding and haematoma formation after tumour manipulation and tracheomalacia. Post-operatively, respiratory distress may occur as a result of recurrent laryngeal nerve damage or collapse of malacic tracheal cartilages after removal of adherent tumours.

The details of anaesthetic technique are less important than the guiding principles, which in summary are as follows:

- Pre-operative evaluation of the state of the airway, including simple spirometry, flow–volume loop assessment, fibre-optic bronchoscopy, and other lung function tests as appropriate.
- Needle biopsy under local anaesthesia if possible.
- Chemotherapy or radiotherapy to shrink the tumour and reduce the immediate life-threatening aspects of the procedure.
- Induction of anaesthesia in whatever position the patient will tolerate best, preferably supine with mild head-up tilt. However, be prepared to move the patient quickly if respiratory obstruction should occur.
- A wide range of endotracheal tube sizes and lengths should be available, as well as a rigid bronchoscope.

- The patient should be fully pre-oxygenated to allow for maximum time if problems in securing the airway do occur.
- An intravenous induction of anaesthesia is usually acceptable, but an inhalational induction or the use of helium/oxygen mixture may be necessary.
- Muscle relaxants should only be administered after checking that the patient's lungs can be adequately ventilated artificially. Adequate ventilation of the lungs should be rechecked after the endotracheal tube has been passed. It may be necessary to change the patient's posture, remove the endotracheal tube and start again.
- Airway management problems may become apparent in the post-extubation period. Removal of the tumour may not relieve the symptoms of obstruction, particularly if resection leads to partial collapse of the tracheal wall.

Compression of the pulmonary artery and right ventricle

Compression of the pulmonary artery and right ventricle is fortunately rare because these structures lie underneath the aortic arch and tracheobronchial tree and are thus partially protected by them. However, in patients with evidence of severe tracheobronchial compression, compression of the pulmonary outflow tract may also occur.

The consequences of pulmonary outflow tract compression are worsening right ventricular function, right ventricular dilatation, functional tricuspid regurgitation and raised central venous pressure, shift of the intraventricular septum leading to a reduced left ventricular end diastolic volume, and reduced cardiac output. As pulmonary blood flow is reduced, pulmonary gas exchange is worsened and hypoxia may ensue.

Patients with lymphoma and pulmonary outflow tract compression may benefit from a pre-operative course of radiotherapy to reduce the tumour bulk, which may relieve respiratory and vascular obstruction.

All the factors relating to the anaesthetic management of tracheobronchial compression as described earlier apply.

It may be important to vary the patient's posture in order to reduce the effects of the obstruction, and steps should be taken to ensure that this is possible quickly at any time during surgery. The anaesthetic technique should take into account both airway considerations and the preservation of right ventricular filling and contractile function. In this regard, ketamine may be a useful agent for induction of anaesthesia and analgesia. Volume loading may be required, although care must be taken not to overload the right ventricle, particularly in the presence of poor contractile function.

Compression and obstruction of the superior vena cava

SVC obstruction is a particularly sinister sign in patients with mediastinal pathology. Lesions responsible for SVC obstruction are frequently malignant, and include bronchial carcinoma and lymphoma. The SVC syndrome is characterized by obstruction and therefore engorgement of veins that drain into the SVC, most obviously from the head and neck and upper limbs. The venous pressure in these veins may be markedly raised, and flow from the veins to the right atrium will be sluggish at best. There may be an increased incidence of venous thrombosis as a result.

Respiratory symptoms are usual, although they may be associated with other abnormalities, including partial airway obstruction. Dyspnoea and cough are frequent, and orthopnoea may be marked due to further postural venous engorgement. If the central venous pressure is markedly raised, cerebral venous engorgement may occur, leading to headache, cerebral oedema and altered mental state. These problems are more likely to occur in patients in whom SVC obstruction develops rapidly. A slower onset is more likely if an adequate collateral circulation, characterized by prominent veins on the upper chest wall, develops.

SVC obstruction should always be investigated, and the investigative work-up will be similar to that of other mediastinal masses. CT should identify the location of the mass. Initial radiotherapy to reduce the tumour size is particularly useful simply because the symptoms are so distressing to the patient. Although many consider needle biopsy to be contraindicated, each patient is best assessed individually.

The anaesthetic implications of a patient with SVC obstruction may be variable, ranging from of little concern in patients with very mild symptoms to extremely hazardous. The main points of management are summarized below:

- Pre-operative radiotherapy should be undertaken in all but the mildest of cases. Every attempt should be made to reduce upper airway and head and neck oedema, and the patient's airway should be carefully evaluated because the haemorrhagic consequences of even the mildest trauma may be severe. The use of an anticholinergic drying agent is recommended.
- The patient may be at risk from postural exacerbation of the compression, similar to patients with tracheobronchial compression.
- Radial arterial monitoring and lower limb venous access is preferable in all but the mildest cases. Cannulation of central veins that drain into the SVC should be avoided.
- Induction of anaesthesia may be associated with a reduction in venous pressure and, thus, a substantial fall in cardiac output. Consider an agent that preserves venous tone, such as ketamine. Vasopressors should be available.
- Blood should be cross-matched and, in severe cases, available in the operating theatre at the time of surgery.
- Great care should be taken during induction and emergence to avoid coughing, straining, etc., which may further increase venous pressure.

Exacerbation of the obstruction leading to a profound reduction in cardiac output, respiratory obstruction and massive haemorrhage may occur during the procedure. In the post-operative period, haemorrhage and respiratory dysfunction may occur, possibly necessitating re-intubation and a period of IPPV as well as other supportive measures. In view of the overall perioperative risks, patients with SVC obstruction are best managed in an intensive care unit during the immediate post-operative period.

Thyroid goitre

The resection of a thyroid goitre that is invading the mediastinum can, on occasion, be a fairly remarkable sight, as these tumours may grow to a considerable size. However, the vast majority of thyroid goitres with retrosternal extension have clearly identifiable connections in the neck, and indeed most of them are resectable through the neck without having to extend the incision. In the remainder, excision from the superior and anterior mediastinum will warrant a median sternotomy.

It is important to ensure that patients are euthyroid before surgery. However, significant abnormality in thyroid function is uncommon in the majority of patients, and toxic symptoms are very rare. The usual symptoms are those of dyspnoea and dysphagia, representing either tracheobronchial or oesophageal compression. Symptoms of vascular compression are very rare but, if they do occur, may be particularly troublesome, as thyroid goitres are not as amenable to radiotherapy as other mediastinal tumours. In fact, retrosternal thyroid goitres are very rarely malignant, but they may be relatively vascular, and difficult resection may be complicated by significant blood loss.

The general condition of the patient presenting for surgery will be variable, but the general points of management are summarized below:

- Significant weight loss and cachexia are rarely a problem, unless symptoms of dysphagia have been severe and prolonged.
- Abnormalities of thyroid function are rare. Patients are no more prone to cardiovascular and other endocrine disease than the general population.
- The main problem is airway management, and details of postural control, airway assessment and intubation are described earlier.
- The surgery may be complex, prolonged and complicated by haemorrhage. Full patient monitoring, blood cross-matching and vascular access for both monitoring and volume replacement are advisable.

Thymectomy and myasthenia gravis

Myasthenia gravis was first described by Thomas Willis in 1672, although the electrophysiological diagnosis was described much later by Freidrich Jolly. The condition was named myasthenia gravis by Campbell in 1900. It is a disease of neuromuscular transmission resulting in early fatigue of muscle, and the exact signs and symptoms will depend on which groups of muscles are affected.

The incidence of myasthenia is approximately 1 in 30 000. Without treatment, the 10-year mortality was about 40 per cent; however, with modern pharmacological and surgical therapy, death from myasthenia is now rare.

Pathology

In normal tissues, acetylcholine is released from vesicles in the nerve terminal and combines with acetylcholine receptors at the post-synaptic receptor on the motor end plate. Acetylcholine is hydrolysed by choline-sterase, and choline is taken up into the nerve terminal to aid further synthesis of acetylcholine. The receptors on the postsynaptic terminal are constantly being formed and sequestrated; the lifespan of an acetylcholine receptor is normally about 7 days.

In myasthenia, the post-synaptic receptors are attacked by immuno-globulin G auto-antibodies, which bind to the receptor and consequently substantially reduce the number of functional receptors at the motor end plate, hence reducing neuromuscular function. Not only is the number of receptors reduced, but the average life span of a post-synaptic acetylcholine receptor is reduced to approximately 1 day once auto-antibody is bound to it. A thymoma is commonly, but not invariably, present.

Clinical presentation

The clinical status of the myasthenic patient may be classified as shown in Table 8.3. Ocular symptoms include diplopia, which is the most common early symptom, followed by ptosis, which may be unilateral or bilateral, fleeting, and is frequently missed if mild.

Dysarthria is a sign of bulbar involvement. If difficulties in chewing or swallowing are prolonged, progressive weight loss may ensue. In more advanced cases, facial weakness or weakness of the extremities in either limb may be noted. The hallmark of the disease is weakness and rapid fatiguability of skeletal muscles with repetitive use, followed by partial recovery on resting.

Myasthenia and other auto-immune diseases are frequently associated, and commonly co-existing conditions are listed in Table 8.4.

Tests

Anti-acetylcholine receptor antibody is specific for myasthenia. The anti-body titre is raised in over 90 per cent of patients with generalized myasthenia, and in 75 per cent of patients with the ocular form of the disease only. Anti-striated muscle antibody is raised in 90 per cent of myasthenic patients with thymoma, but in less than a third of non-thymoma myasthenics.

Table 8.3 Patient clinical status in myasthenia gravis

● Group I	● Ocular myasthenia gravis (ocular symptoms only)
● Group II (A & B)	● Mild/moderate generalized myasthenia gravis (bulbar and skeletal)
● Group III	● Acute severe myasthenia gravis with respiratory muscle involvement
● Group IV	● Chronic severe disease
● Group V	● Myasthenia gravis with muscle atrophy

Table 8.4 Autoimmune disorders linked to myasthenia gravis

- Hyper/hypothyroidism
- Rheumatoid arthritis
- Polymyositis
- Systemic lupus erythematosus
- Pernicious anaemia
- Pemphigus
- Sjögren's syndrome

Electromyography shows a characteristic decremental response to repetitive stimulation, which is reversed by administration of an anti-cholinesterase. Edrophonium, an anticholinesterase of very short duration, is usually used for diagnostic purposes.

Studies of oesophageal manometry may be useful, and abnormalities have been found in many patients, not only those with dysphagia or bulbar symptoms. Radiological investigations, in particular CT, may identify a thymoma. Approximately one-third of patients with thymomas have myasthenia gravis, although of all myasthenic patients only approximately one in eight has a thymoma.

Pharmacological treatment

The pathological processes involved in myasthenia indicate that there are three broad therapeutic strategies available: first, to increase the amount of acetylcholine available in order to maximize occupancy of a reduced mass of receptors; second, to modify the auto-immune process by pharmacological means; and third, thymectomy to remove the source of the auto-antibody.

The amount of acetylcholine available for receptor occupancy is increased by oral anticholinesterase therapy, thereby inhibiting the enzymatic breakdown of acetylcholine. Pyridostigmine is usually preferred to neostigmine, since it has a longer duration of action and fewer muscarinic side effects – particularly sweating, salivation, abdominal pain, diarrhoea and bradycardia. Successful anticholinesterase therapy requires some receptor availability, and the greater the proportion of receptor destruction, the more difficult the pharmacological management will be. Furthermore, prolonged use of high doses of anticholinesterase drugs appears to induce a decreased sensitivity to them.

Overdosage with anticholinesterases may be particularly difficult to differentiate from a myasthenic crisis. A myasthenic crisis may be provoked by physical and psychological stress, drug interactions and other factors, but the symptoms of overdosage with anticholinesterases are similar, including muscle weakness, which may affect the respiratory muscles and necessitate ventilatory support. Although a small dose of anticholinesterase may prove diagnostic, the need for a period of ventilatory support should be recognized.

Corticosteroid therapy may be particularly successful in achieving remission of myasthenia in a high proportion of cases, and is frequently valuable in patients with ocular myasthenia. In more generalized cases, high doses of prednisolone may be necessary to achieve initial remission, but the dose can then frequently be reduced to a maintenance dose of 10 mg on alternate days. Remission may be achieved in 2–3 weeks.

When the dosage of prednisolone cannot be reduced to an appropriately low level, aziothiaprine may be added. The onset of action of azothiaprine is slow (8–12 weeks), with a peak effect not seen for as many months.

Plasmaphoresis has also been used successfully, although this is best reserved for short-term benefit such as management of a myasthenic crisis or optimization of the patient peri-operatively. There is no evidence that repeated plasmaphoresis improves long-term outcome.

Surgery

Surgery is generally very effective in myasthenia. Thymectomy should be considered in all patients other than those who have minimal symptoms; however, surgery is not uniformly successful in all groups. For example, thymectomy is less successful in older patients with thymoma and severe disease, but more successful in patients less than 40 years old with less severe myasthenia, clear evidence of other auto-immune involvement and thymitis rather than thymoma. In this latter group, substantial improvement can be expected to occur in 90 per cent of patients, although the full benefit may take years to become evident. In thymoma patients, excision is still recommended because thymomas may grow to a size that produces compressive symptoms and may become malignant. Surgery involves radical resection of tumour, thymic remnant, nodes and surrounding fatty tissues, and is usually carried out through a median sternotomy, although lateral sternotomy and even lateral thoracotomy have been used.

Anaesthetic considerations

Thymectomy is a major surgical procedure, and requires full haematological and biochemical investigations and cross-matched blood available. The following features are worthy of special attention.

Airway

Patients with thymoma may have symptoms of tracheobronchial compression. In these patients, the airway should be fully assessed by plain film radiography, CT scan and fibre-optic bronchoscopy as appropriate. The most appropriate action will be determined by the findings, but the anaesthetist must be prepared to have all the necessary airway apparatus to hand as described previously.

Respiratory function

It is essential to have baseline tests of respiratory function, as a guide to the likely post-operative course and as a means of assessing early post-operative progress. Spirometry (FEV_1 and FVC) and blood gases will be of most benefit.

In cases with bulbar involvement, the cough reflex may be impaired and soiling of the lungs may result. Care must be taken to ensure that patients are free from chest infection at the time of surgery.

Cardiovascular function

Myasthenic patients may suffer from associated myocardial degenerative changes, and cardiovascular investigation is essential. However, the extent of the investigation will be dictated by the age and general condition of the patient and degree of cardiovascular co-morbidity, rather than by any cardiovascular changes specific to myasthenia. In most patients an ECG should suffice; in patients with suspected myocardial dysfunction, a transthoracic or transoesophageal echocardiogram may be appropriate.

It should be borne in mind that patients in the older age group may have cerebrovascular disease.

Other

There may be associated thyroid abnormalities, and thyroid function should be checked pre-operatively. In addition to lung soiling, patients with chronic bulbar symptoms may suffer from chronic dehydration and nutritional deficiency. Where this is evident, fluid and electrolyte replacement therapy may be necessary.

Medical management before surgery

Plasmaphoresis may be of value in the immediate pre-operative period in order to optimize the patient's condition before surgery. Anticholinesterase therapy should be continued pre-operatively and, in all but the mildest cases, a full dose of anticholinesterase should be given on the morning of surgery. In patients with mild myasthenia, a reduced dose should be given or the anticholinesterase omitted completely. Steroid therapy should also be continued, and care should be taken to continue steroid replacement therapy throughout the early peri-operative period.

Some consideration should be given to the psychological preparation of the patient, particularly since emotional stress may act as a trigger factor for a myasthenic crisis.

Anaesthetic management

The surgical procedure is usually carried out through a median sternotomy, for which an endotracheal tube will be required. In rare circumstances the thymoma may not be situated in the midline, necessitating an endobronchial tube to facilitate surgical access to the thoracic cavity.

The relative merits of different anaesthetic techniques have been debated. Of more importance is the recognition of the nature of the problems involved in delivering safe anaesthesia.

The following should therefore be noted:

- Intravenous or inhalational induction of anaesthesia is perfectly acceptable, using carefully titrated doses of anaesthetic agents. Once the patient is anaesthetized, however, ventilation may need to be assisted immediately.
- Endotracheal intubation may be carried out following intravenous or inhalational induction of anaesthesia only, avoiding the use of muscle relaxants. However, the use of muscle relaxants is not contraindicated providing they are used appropriately.
- Patients with myasthenia are resistant to the effects of suxamethonium, and an increased dosage should be used (2 mg/kg). This may be followed by a prolonged phase II block.
- Patients with myasthenia are sensitive to the effects of non-depolarizing relaxants, and these should be used in markedly reduced dosage. Between one-quarter and one-half of the normal dose may be appropriate. Atracurium has the advantage of Hofmann degradation and elimination, and may be considered to be the relaxant of choice.
- The myorelaxant properties of volatile anaesthetics are enhanced in myasthenia.
- The time course of small doses of neuromuscular blocking drugs in myasthenic patients is similar to larger doses given to normals. However, the extent of neuromuscular blockade and the effectiveness of reversal should be monitored by a nerve stimulator.
- Thoracic epidural anaesthesia has been used as a means of providing intra- and post-operative analgesia. Ester-type local anaesthetics (procaine, chloroprocaine, amethocaine) are best avoided because they are metabolized by plasma pseudocholinesterase, whose activity may be inhibited by anticholinesterase therapy, thereby increasing the possibility of local anaesthetic toxicity.
- Although a median sternotomy is one of the least painful thoracic incisions, post-operative analgesia will be necessary. There is no contraindication to the use of opioids and, indeed, good analgesia will potentiate post-operative chest physiotherapy. Although the concerns about opioid-induced respiratory depression combined with weak muscular power are understandable, they should not be allowed to result in inadequate post-operative analgesia.

Without doubt, the greatest concern is the use and reversal of neuromuscular blocking drugs. The resistance to suxamethonium is easily explained by the reduced number of effective acetylcholine receptors, but this is usually followed by a prolonged phase II block. Once intubation has been achieved, non-depolarizing agents should only be used if clinically indicated. Atracurium in 2.5–5 mg doses as required is sufficient. The use of a nerve stimulator to check neuromuscular conduction and adequate reversal of neuromuscular blockade is essential.

The decision to extubate the patient at the end of surgery should be individually based, but some indication of likely success may be given by the patient's pre-operative history, anticholinesterase dosage and respiratory status (see Table 8.5).

Table 8.5 Scoring system used to predict post-operative ventilatory requirements in patients undergoing thymectomy via median sternotomy under specified anaesthetic conditions

• History > 6 years	•	12 points
• Other respiratory disease	•	10 points
• High anticholinesterase requirement (> 750 mg/day pyridostigmine)	•	8 points
• Vital capacity < 2.91	•	4 points

Ten points or more predicts the need for post-operative ventilatory support (predictive accuracy 80 per cent)

Anticholinesterase therapy is likely to be required in the post-operative period, and some thought should be given to this aspect of management, particularly if the patient cannot tolerate oral medications. Despite an initial and often dramatic improvement in the early post-operative period, the full benefit of thymectomy can take weeks or even years to become apparent, and the patient must be psychologically prepared for this delay. Of more obvious relevance is the variable need for post-operative anticholinesterase therapy for some considerable time.

Myasthenic (Eaton–Lambert) syndrome

Myasthenia gravis differs from the myasthenic syndrome in a number of important ways, and although patients with myasthenic syndrome (Eaton–Lambert syndrome) are not candidates for thymectomy, they may, nonetheless, present a problem for the thoracic anaesthetist. The main differences between myasthenia gravis and myasthenic syndrome are as follows:

- Myasthenic syndrome occurs more commonly in males, in contrast to myasthenia gravis.
- Myasthenic syndrome occurs due to a pre-synaptic defect in neuro-muscular transmission, similar in effect to that produced by magnesium, neomycin or botulinus toxin. There is a decrease in the number of quanta of acetylcholine released from the nerve terminal in response to a nerve impulse. This occurs following destruction of the acetylcholine release zones in the nerve terminal. The aetiology is auto-immune.
- Although weakness and fatiguability are features, initial activity produces a transient increase in strength followed by weakness, primarily in the proximal muscles of the extremities (e.g. thighs). Muscle pain is common.
- Myasthenic syndrome is frequently associated with bronchial neoplasm, especially small cell lung cancer, although evidence of tumour is not invariably found.
- Myasthenic syndrome patients respond poorly to anticholinesterases; effective drugs are those that aid release of acetylcholine from motor

nerve terminals by blocking potassium channels. 4-aminopyridine and its derivatives have been used.

- Patients are sensitive to both depolarizing and non-depolarizing muscle relaxants.

Patients with myasthenic syndrome may present for thoracotomy and lung resection or for diagnostic thoracic surgery, and the above features should be borne closely in mind when dealing with them.

Bibliography

Akhtar, T.M., Ridley, S. and Best, C.J. (1991). Unusual presentation of acute upper airway obstruction caused by an anterior mediastinal mass. *Br. J. Anaesth.*, **67**, 632–4.

Baraka, A. (1992). Anaesthesia and myasthenia gravis. *Can. J. Anaesth.*, **39**, 476–86.

Eaton, L.M. and Lambert, E.H. (1957). Electromyography and electrical stimulation of nerves in disease with motor units. Observations on myasthenic syndrome associated with malignant tumours. *JAMA*, **163**, 1117–24.

Ferrari, L.R. and Bedford, R.F. (1990). General anaesthesia prior to treatment of mediastinal masses in paediatric cancer patients. *Anesthesiology*, **72**, 991–5.

Mackie, A.M. and Watson, C.B. (1984). Anaesthesia and mediastinal masses. *Anaesthesia*, **39**, 899–903.

Morton, J.R. and Guinn, G.A. (1971). Mediastinoscopy using local anaesthesia. *Am. J. Surg.*, **122**, 696–8.

Plummer, S., Hartley, M. and Vaughan, R.S. (1998). Anaesthesia for telescopic procedures in the thorax. *Br. J. Anaesth.*, **80**, 223–34.

Robertson, R. and Muers, M. (1995). Mediastinal masses. *Medicine*, **23**, 369–71.

Sabiston, D.C. and Spencer, F.C. (1990). *Surgery of the Chest*. WB Saunders.

Telford, R.J. and Holloway, T.E. (1990). The myasthenic syndrome: anaesthesia in a patient treated with 4-diaminopyridine. *Br. J. Anaesth.*, **64**, 363–6.

9

Oesophageal surgery

K. J. Benson and R. P. Mahajan

Introduction

Anaesthetic techniques that were originally developed to facilitate lung surgery are frequently employed to permit intrathoracic oesophageal surgery. These techniques include use of a double-lumen tube and maintenance of one-lung anaesthesia. The anaesthetic considerations are broadly similar to those for any major surgical intervention. However, the nutritional state of the patient and the potential for soiling of the bronchial tree with oesophageal contents require special care. In order to safely anaesthetize patients presenting for oesophageal surgery, a background understanding of the relevant anatomy and physiology of the oesophagus is essential.

Anatomy and physiology of the oesophagus

It was once thought that the oesophagus was a passive drainage tube from the mouth to the stomach. Following the introduction of manometry in the 1950s, the function and physiology of the oesophagus was defined as a highly complex integration of muscular activity and sphincter control.

Gross anatomy

The oesophagus is a tubular structure, 23–25 cm in length, extending from the pharynx at the lower border of the cricoid cartilage to the stomach. It is basically a midline structure, though it lies more to the left in the neck, lower thorax and abdomen. In the neck, the oesophagus is posterior to the trachea and projects slightly beyond the tracheal border on the left, providing a more accessible surgical approach on this side.

In the thorax, the posterior relations of the oesophagus are the first to seventh thoracic vertebrae, the azygos and hemi-azygos veins, the intercostal arteries, thoracic duct and left recurrent laryngeal nerve. Anteriorly, the left main bronchus and pericardium separate the oesophagus from the left atrium. Below this level, the aorta gradually takes a posterior position and the oesophagus lies more to the left. The lateral margin on the left relates to the common carotid artery, subclavian artery, arch of aorta and descending aorta, which separate it from the mediastinal pleura and lung. On the right, the oesophagus lies next to the pleura and lung.

The oesophagus is innervated by both sympathetic and parasympathetic trunks together with local plexuses (pharyngeal, cervical splanchnic and coeliac), which create co-ordinated muscular activity.

Arterial blood supply to the oesophagus comes from the inferior thyroid artery in the neck, the descending aorta and bronchial and intercostal arteries in the thorax and the left gastric artery in the abdomen. Venous drainage is complex, though ultimately the inferior thyroid, azygos and gastric vessels anastomose and drain into the portal and systemic circulations.

Microscopic anatomy

The muscular wall of the oesophagus is composed of two layers, the outer longitudinal and the inner circular. Both the layers have striated and/or smooth muscle. The upper third of the oesophagus is predominantly striated muscle, the middle third is mixed and the lower portion becomes smooth muscle. The lining of the oesophagus is of stratified squamous non-keratinizing epithelium, with mucous glands scattered throughout.

Physiology

Both ends of the oesophagus form sphincters that protect against regurgitation of the stomach contents. The upper sphincter, which is normally closed except during swallowing, is formed by the cricopharyngeus muscle. The lower sphincter is of prime importance to the anaesthetist, since its major function is as a barrier to reflux and regurgitation of acidic gastric contents, which may cause aspiration pneumonitis.

Although the lower sphincter is not anatomically identifiable, it exists functionally as a 2.5–5 cm long zone, extending both above and below the diaphragm, that exerts an increased pressure of 30 cmH$_2$O. In a normal person, any increase of intra-abdominal pressure results in an adaptive increase in the lower oesophageal pressure, maintaining a constant barrier.

Peristalsis is initiated in the pharynx as alternating waves of contraction and relaxation. This is predominantly under vagal control. The lower oesophageal sphincter maintains its tone by the circular muscle fibres in the oesophageal wall. Nervous control is derived principally from parasympathetic fibres, with additional input from the sympathetic trunk. A number of factors can affect the lower oesophageal sphincter tone, and these are summarized in Table 9.1.

Abnormalities of the oesophagus such as hiatus hernia can be associated with an inability to adapt to changes in intra-abdominal pressure, with an increased risk of regurgitation and reflux of gastric acid. Patients with motility disorders may have poorly digested remnants of food within a dilated portion of the oesophagus. Positioning such patients supine increases the risk of regurgitation and aspiration of products that have not been exposed to the acidic pH of the stomach, and thus may contain bacterial over-growth, leading to pulmonary complications. The anaesthetist must

Table 9.1 Factors affecting lower oesophageal sphincter (LOS) tone

---

Factors that increase LOS tone

Hormones
- gastrin
- acetylcholine

Drugs
- antiemetics – metoclopramide, cyclizine, prochlorperazine
- antacids
- β-blockers – metoprolol
- α-adrenergic stimulators
- anticholinesterases – edrophonium, neostigmine
- muscle relaxants – suxamethonium, pancuronium

Miscellaneous
- increased intra-abdominal pressure – maintains barrier pressure constant

Factors that decrease LOS tone

Hormones
- prostaglandins E and A
- secretin
- gastric inhibitory peptide (GIP)
- vasoactive intestinal peptide (VIP)
- glucagon

Drugs
- opioids
- inhalational anaesthetics – halothane, enflurane, isoflurane
- β-stimulants
- ganglion blockers
- anticholinergics – atropine, glycopyrrolate
- dopamine
- thiopentone

Miscellaneous
- stimulation of pharynx – LMA insertion, cricoid pressure
- oesophageal disease
- persistent swallowing – usually at emergence from anaesthesia

---

assume that all patients with symptoms of heartburn and other abnormalities of the oesophagus are at risk of regurgitation and aspiration of gastric contents.

Oesophageal disease

The most commonly encountered lesions of the oesophagus are as follows:

- Tumours – usually squamous cell and adenocarcinoma
- Hiatus hernia
- Benign strictures caused by reflux oesophagitis in the lower third of the oesophagus, or by ingestion of caustic fluid affecting the upper oesophagus

- Motility disorders – achalasia and collagen diseases (e.g. scleroderma)
- Tracheo-oesophageal fistula – congenital, malignant or traumatic
- Oesophageal perforation and rupture.

The operative procedures undertaken for the diagnosis and surgical management of oesophageal disease include endoscopy, laparotomy, thoracotomy and, more recently, laparoscopic or thoracoscopic techniques.

Anaesthesia for oesophageal surgery

This section presents an overview of the conduct of anaesthesia for oesophageal surgery. Considerations that are specific to a particular type of oesophageal disease or surgical procedure are included in the relevant part of the next section.

Pre-operative management

Patients presenting with oesophageal disease may be of any age, from infant to the elderly, and complain of a wide range of symptoms and signs. Risk factors associated with benign oesophageal disease have been identified as excessive tobacco and alcohol consumption. The aetiology of malignant oesophageal disease is more complex, and there is no single environmental factor that accounts for the disease. Due to the multifactorial nature of the disease process, it is imperative that all patients undergo a thorough pre-operative evaluation, including a detailed history, to elicit the presence of symptoms of heartburn and regurgitation and also of unrelated disease.

Examination must include primarily the pulmonary and cardiovascular systems, along with an assessment of the overall nutritional status of the patient.

Respiratory system

Anaesthesia for surgical procedures may induce many physiological changes affecting the pulmonary system and its defence mechanisms. The presence of risk factors – for example, smoking, chronic obstructive pulmonary disease (COPD) and severe obesity – can contribute to the development of pulmonary complications. Patients with a history of oesophageal obstruction and increasing dysphagia may have been affected by chronic aspiration. They may have symptoms and signs of pneumonitis and recurrent infections, with associated reduction in respiratory reserve and bronchospasm.

Pulmonary complications are the commonest cause of increased post-operative morbidity and mortality during oesophageal surgery. General anaesthesia alone reduces functional residual capacity. Reductions of up to 50 per cent of pre-operative values have been seen in upper abdominal and thoracic surgery. There are also large reductions in peak expiratory flow rate (PEFR) and the FEV_1/FVC (forced expiratory volume in 1 second/forced vital capacity) ratio. Such reductions in respiratory reserve, in combination with surgical trauma and post-operative pain, can provoke complications including retention of bronchial secretions, atelectasis and inadequate gaseous exchange, which lead to increased morbidity. The pulmonary consequences of obesity are the exaggerated reductions in lung and chest wall compliance, further loss of functional residual capacity, increased work of breathing and increased ventilation–perfusion mismatch resulting in systemic arterial hypoxaemia and risk of respiratory insufficiency.

Following clinical assessment, all patients should have a pre-operative chest radiograph in order to determine changes due to COPD or aspiration pneumonitis. Hiatus hernia may be seen, along with consequent reduced lung volumes, on the affected side. Lung function tests are justified in patients undergoing upper abdominal or thoracic surgery, and should probably be extended to include obese patients, smokers and patients with COPD. Since no single test has been identified as being consistently predictive of pulmonary complications, it is appropriate to combine various techniques of assessing respiratory reserve. Baseline spirometry, both before and after a nebulized bronchodilator, and the maximal voluntary ventilation (MVV) can be measured. Arterial blood gas analysis provides further information regarding baseline gaseous exchange, and identifies patients with chronic hypoxaemia and hypercarbia. Additional studies, including measurement of lung volumes and diffusing capacity, may further define abnormal pulmonary physiology, but these are not performed routinely.

If the vital capacity is less than 70 per cent of the predicted value, FEV_1 is less than 2 l, or MVV is less than 50 per cent of that predicted, then thoracotomy is likely to be poorly tolerated, with the increased risk of respiratory failure and increased mortality. Blood gas analysis alone may be a poor index of post-operative recovery, but ventilatory problems should be anticipated post-operatively in patients identified as hypoxaemic and hypercarbic at pre-operative testing.

Having identified those patients at risk of respiratory complications, a suitable prophylactic regimen should be employed pre-operatively in order to minimize these risks. Instructions to patients should include the cessation of smoking and deep breathing exercises. Medical interventions may include the use of bronchodilator therapy, antibiotic treatment for infection as appropriate and intensive physiotherapy as required. In those patients presenting the greatest risk, facilities for post-operative respiratory support should be confirmed prior to anaesthesia and surgery.

Cardiovascular system

There is no direct correlation between oesophageal and cardiovascular disease. However, this group of patients may have a history of exposure to risk factors such as cigarette smoking, and they are also often elderly. Widespread atherosclerosis and ischaemic heart disease should therefore be anticipated.

All elderly patients and those with risk factors or signs of cardiovascular disease should have a pre-operative electrocardiogram (ECG) in order to determine the presence of arrhythmias, previous infarction, signs of ischaemia and changes associated with hypertension. If further investigations are necessary, an echocardiogram can be obtained to assess valvular and left ventricular function. A more accurate assessment of cardiac performance is derived from the radionucleotide ejection fraction (EF). This has been found to be a useful predictor of cardiac complications in patients undergoing non-cardiac surgery.

More recent advances in cardiac assessment include the use of an ambulatory (Holter) ECG to detect silent ischaemia, and stress echocardiography to identify regional wall abnormalities, which are associated with ischaemic damage to the myocardium. Where there is doubt regarding cardiac status, pre-operative referral to a cardiologist is wise. Cardiac function should be optimized with treatment of arrhythmias, hypertension and cardiac failure.

Invasive monitoring is indicated in most patients undergoing major surgery, and is imperative in patients with poor cardiac performance. Intra-operative invasive monitoring and post-operative intensive care have been shown to reduce the incidence of myocardial re-infarction after elective surgery.

Nutritional status

Nutritional impairment may occur with benign oesophageal disease, i.e. motility disorders, but occurs most commonly in patients with malignancies of the oesophagus. Initially, patients present with increasing dysphagia for solids, but this progresses until ingestion of fluids also becomes difficult. Such disorders of nutrition may have been present for several months prior to surgery, and are compounded by the cachexic effects of the tumour. The ensuing weight loss is thus associated with a number of physiological problems, including the following:

- Dehydration, leading to a reduced extracellular volume, exacerbating hypovolaemic hypotension, and increasing the tendency to develop acute renal failure.
- Electrolyte imbalance, most importantly hypokalaemia, hypocalcaemia and hypomagnesaemia.
- Reduced protein intake, resulting in hypo-albuminaemia. This leads to a fall in colloid osmotic pressure with disruption of Starling forces across capillary beds. Patients are particularly at risk of developing pulmonary oedema. There is an altered volume of distribution for protein bound drugs with a higher proportion of unbound or active drug within the plasma. This may result in more side effects at lower doses.
- Anaemia, occurring due to chronic blood loss from the gastrointestinal tract and also as a result of nutritional deficiency.
- Impaired immune response.

Pre-operative malnutrition is associated with a high risk of post-operative morbidity and mortality. It is therefore important to identify patients at risk, correct simple metabolic deficiencies and consider nutritional supplementation. In patients with severe dysphagia, major surgery will be better tolerated with improved nutritional status.

Total parenteral nutrition (TPN) given to malnourished patients in adequate amounts for 7–15 days pre-operatively significantly improves both the nutritional status and post-operative outcome. Enteral nutrition given pre-operatively is as effective as TPN in improving the post-operative outcome. Enteral feeding, if possible, is preferable to TPN on the basis of several factors – better substrate utilization, prevention of mucosal atrophy, preservation of normal intestinal flora and immune competence. However, where enteral feeding is impossible, TPN is of benefit.

Identifying patients at risk can be difficult. Pre-operative factors, including albumin and serum transferrin concentrations, triceps skinfold thickness and delayed cutaneous hypersensitivity, may predict post-operative morbidity; serum albumin concentration has been found to be the most reliable predictor of mortality.

Patients requiring nutritional support will have a history of progressive weight loss, and show signs of physiological imbalance such as dehydration, anaemia, etc. Nutrition indices are not routinely used, but nutritional support is warranted pre-operatively if moderate hypo-albuminaemia (albumin less than 30 g/l) is present. Where TPN has been instituted pre-operatively, the anaesthetist should be aware of the risk of intra-operative hypoglycaemia, and continue an infusion of dextrose-containing fluid.

All patients undergoing oesophageal resection should have nutritional support post-operatively until oral intake is resumed. Following nutritional intervention, it is important that the patient's metabolic state is monitored. Measurements should include weight, fluid input and output and caloric and protein intake. Serum urea and electrolytes, including phosphate, should be measured at least twice weekly, though more frequent assessments may be indicated.

Further pre-operative evaluation includes a haematological screen, with assessment of liver function and clotting pathways as well as serum urea and electrolytes.

Conduct of anaesthesia

There are no specific rules applying to anaesthesia for oesophageal surgery, but certain general principles can be suggested.

All patients presenting for oesophageal surgery should be assumed to be at risk of regurgitation and aspiration of gastric contents. Pre-operatively, where oesophageal obstruction is present, a large-bore nasogastric tube may be inserted with care to aspirate residual food debris from dilated oesophageal pouches and the stomach.

Patients with an incompetent lower oesophageal sphincter should be given antacid therapy pre-operatively. Drugs including H_2 receptor antagonists, proton pump inhibitors and prokinetics can be used. Non-particulate antacids may be administered immediately prior to theatre, and are useful adjuncts in minimizing morbidity from aspiration.

Selection of the appropriate endotracheal tube depends on the type of oesophageal surgery that will take place. For procedures requiring thoracotomy, a double-lumen tube is normally used in order that the lung on the appropriate side may be deflated. A standard oral endotracheal tube is suitable for abdominal procedures or oesophageal anastomoses that are to be performed in the neck.

Induction

As suggested above, all patients must be considered at risk of regurgitation and aspiration, even when starved pre-operatively. The options for securing a protected and safe airway include an awake fibre-optic intubation of the trachea using local anaesthetic techniques, or a rapid sequence induction. It is essential that the anaesthetist uses the technique appropriate to the level of his or her expertise and, in cases where a difficult intubation is anticipated, the help of an anaesthetist experienced in this field of anaesthesia is imperative. In most centres, the use of the rapid sequence induction is normal practice for oesophageal surgery.

Maintenance

Specific anaesthetic technique is a matter for individual preference, and must take into account the type and duration of surgery and the potential for blood loss and hypotension, together with the overall medical status of the patient.

Acceptable anaesthetic techniques include maintenance with oxygen, nitrous oxide and supplemental volatile agents with adequate opioid analgesia. Alternatively, total intravenous anaesthesia using standard protocols or target-controlled infusions is appropriate. Intrathecal, extradural or paravertebral local anaesthetic with or without opioids are useful adjuncts. Such techniques enable optimal pain management intra-operatively and in the early post-operative period. The presence of bowel within the thorax (e.g. due to hiatus hernia) may be a contraindication to the use of high (50 per cent) inspired concentrations of nitrous oxide; expanded bowel may cause atelectasis both intra- and post-operatively.

The most common intra-operative complications include hypotension secondary to blood loss and manipulation of the great vessels within the chest, arrhythmias (particularly bradycardia following vagal stimulation) and, finally, damage to structures adjacent to the surgical field (e.g. perforation of the trachea and dependent pleura).

In general, the usual considerations for major surgery apply. Care must be taken to avoid injury to pressure areas, using padding and careful positioning. Maintenance of body temperature is important since large areas are exposed, and this may be achieved using warmed fluids and humidified gases, warming blankets and warm air blowers.

Monitoring

Normal standards of monitoring apply for all the surgical procedures outlined below. Depending on the medical condition of the patient, further invasive monitoring should be applied either prior to or following induction. Invasive arterial blood pressure monitoring allows accurate assessment of blood pressure and serial arterial blood gas measurements as deemed necessary by the anaesthetist. Central venous pressure monitoring by means of internal jugular or subclavian lines or peripherally inserted long lines gives an objective measure of fluid balance status. Patients with poor cardiac function may benefit from the insertion of a pulmonary artery catheter for assessment of pulmonary capillary wedge pressure and mixed venous oxygen content (SvO_2), though the readings may be affected by one-lung ventilation.

Recovery and post-operative care

The immediate recovery phase depends on the procedure performed. Patients undergoing uncomplicated abdominal surgery may be extubated at the termination of anaesthesia. However, it is prudent to ensure full recovery of airway reflexes prior to extubation in those patients in whom the oesophago-gastric junction was impaired.

Most patients will be transferred directly to a high dependency or intensive therapy unit, depending on artificial ventilation requirements and the nature of the surgery.

The most common complications post-thoracotomy include atelectasis, pulmonary oedema, respiratory infection and ventilatory insufficiency. Such complications are exacerbated by poor tidal volumes and by the inability to cough post-extubation in the presence of inadequate pain management. This is discussed further in Chapter 17. Additional complications include fluid depletion, which may be masked in the cold, vasoconstricted patient. On warming, hypovolaemia may be manifest as hypotension. During this phase, patients often require large volumes of fluids to replace excessive third space losses and maintain peripheral perfusion as vasodilatation occurs.

Post-thoracotomy haemorrhage can be profound, and should be investigated and managed immediately.

Oesophageal disease and surgery

Oesophagoscopy

Oesophagoscopy, the visual inspection of the oesophagus using a flexible or rigid scope, may be performed for diagnostic or therapeutic purposes. The principal indications are dysphagia, oesophagitis and haematemesis. Conditions that most frequently give rise to symptoms requiring oesophagoscopy are hiatus hernia, achalasia, oesophageal tumours or varices. Occasionally, oesophagoscopy may be required for confirmation of an oesophageal tear, fistula or congenital anomaly. Conditions pertinent to thoracic surgery and their management are discussed later in this chapter.

Inspection, biopsy and dilatation of the oesophagus or injection of varices can be adequately performed via a flexible scope. Rigid oesophagoscopy is required for assessment of oesophageal fixation by tumour, removal of impacted material, or passage of stents through strictures or obstructive tumours. Rigid oesophagoscopy is preferred by some surgeons for dilatation using bougies, and is routinely used by most cardiothoracic surgeons.

Flexible oesophagoscopy is generally performed under sedation with a benzodiazepine and topical anaesthesia to the pharynx. Rigid oesophagoscopy requires general anaesthesia.

Anaesthetic management

The main hazard of anaesthesia for oesophagoscopy is aspiration of gastric or oesophageal contents. The patient should be starved for 6 or more hours beforehand. A barium swallow may have been performed prior to oesophagoscopy, and time should be allowed for residual barium to be expelled prior to anaesthesia.

While oesophagoscopy itself is a relatively minor procedure, the patient may present the anaesthetist with a wide variety of problems relating to the underlying pathology. Patients with strictures, achalasia or tumours are generally emaciated, while those with hiatus hernia tend to be obese. Patients with haematemesis may have associated liver disease. Anaemia is common, either due to malnutrition or chronic bleeding.

Premedication is not required; however, an anti-sialagogue may be useful in limiting the accumulation of secretions in the pharynx peri-operatively.

The aims of anaesthesia are protection of the airway and a rapid return of laryngeal reflexes at the end of the procedure, which is generally of short duration. Induction and maintenance are best achieved using short-acting agents, and a suitable combination is alfentanil, propofol, suxamethonium and isoflurane. Rapid sequence intubation is recommended. If required, muscle relaxation can be maintained with intermittent boluses of low doses (25 mg) of suxamethonium. The potential for bradycardia on repeat administration of suxamethonium should be anticipated, and atropine either given prophylactically or kept to hand. Alternatively, a small dose of atracurium may be used following rapid sequence intubation with suxamethonium.

The oesophagus and pharynx should be thoroughly suctioned, and the patient placed in the lateral position prior to extubation.

Post-operatively, patients are generally maintained nil by mouth for a variable period, depending on underlying pathology and the procedure performed. Some patients may require intravenous fluids, particularly if their presenting symptom was dysphagia.

A post-operative chest X-ray is required to exclude oesophageal perforation following biopsy, dilatation or passage of stents.

Analgesia is generally not required following oesophagoscopy but, if the patient is in discomfort, paracetamol or diclofenac by rectal administration suffice.

Carcinoma of the oesophagus

Surgical resection is the only proven curative treatment for carcinoma of the oesophagus. It remains the 'gold standard' by which all other therapeutic modalities are measured. The aims are:

- To eradicate the tumour and lymph nodes.

- To provide relief from dysphagia and commencement of alimentary tract nutrition.

The best chance of 5-year survival after surgical resection is approximately 20 per cent. Surgery may be combined with chemotherapy, with or without radiotherapy. The choice of operation depends mainly upon the location of the tumour and the preference of the surgeon. Other factors that may influence the decision are body habitus, prior operation, condition of the patient, choice of oesophageal substitute and prior radiation therapy.

For upper oesophageal (in the neck) carcinoma, combined chemotherapy and radiation without surgery may be indicated. Surgery may be in the form of pharyngo-laryngectomy with extra-thoracic oesophagectomy and gastric interposition. For carcinoma at the thoracic inlet, extra-thoracic oesophageal gastrectomy without laryngectomy is possible. For carcinoma at the middle and lower curve of the oesophagus, combined thoracic and abdominal approaches are usually used for oesophagectomy.

Ivor Lewis operation

This is a common technique for middle and lower third carcinoma, including the gastric cardia. It is performed through an abdominal and right thoracic approach. Laparotomy is performed with the patient in the supine position. If there is no evidence of metastatic liver disease, extensive coeliac node involvement or tumour fixation to the aorta, the patient is considered a candidate for surgical resection. The stomach is mobilized with preservation of the right gastro-epiploic artery. Pyloroplasty is usually performed, and the oesophageal hiatus is enlarged and widened. The abdominal incision is then closed and the patient is turned to the left lateral decubitus position. A standard postero-lateral right thoracotomy is performed through the fourth or fifth intercostal space. The oesophagus is totally mobilized, and the tumour lying in the middle third is carefully dissected off the posterior wall of the main stem bronchi and pericardium. The stomach is delivered into the thoracic cavity and the oesophageal tumour is resected. Anastomosis is performed as end-to-side oesophago-gastrostomy. Approximately 7 days later, a gastrographin or barium swallow is performed. If the anastomosis is leak-proof, oral intake is allowed.

Left thoraco-abdominal approach

This approach is indicated for tumours in the lower third and the gastric cardia. The disadvantage is that the heart limits the extent of proximal resection and makes intrathoracic anastomosis more difficult. The patient is positioned in the right lateral decubitus position, with the left thorax and abdomen prepared and draped. A thoracotomy incision is made through the bed of the resected sixth or seventh rib. Once in the thoracic cavity, the diaphragm is incised along its periphery, preserving a 1-cm attachment for reconstruction. The entire thoracic oesophagus and stomach is mobilized, the distal oesophagus and stomach is resected and an oesophago-gastric anastomosis is performed.

Anaesthetic considerations for oesophagectomy

In addition to the general considerations discussed above, specific attention should be given to the following.

Pre-operatively:

- Moderate to severe undernourishment and cachexia.
- Collection of food in the dilated oesophagus above the tumour site. This food usually becomes infected with bacterial growth, as it is not exposed to gastric acid.
- Aspiration pneumonitis.
- Patients may have received bleomycin as part of chemotherapy, and 5–10 per cent of patients who have received bleomycin may develop pulmonary toxicity. This manifests as a cough, restlessness, basal creps, interstitial pneumonia and pulmonary fibrosis. There may be an increased alveolar to arterial oxygen gradient, with impaired diffusion capacity. In patients who have received bleomycin, controlled use of inspired oxygen is indicated. Exposure to higher concentrations of oxygen peri-operatively can lead to adult respiratory distress syndrome (ARDS).
- Patients may have received doxorubicin, an antibiotic derivative, as part of chemotherapy. This can lead to myelosuppression and cardiomyopathy. The acute form of cardiomyopathy shows non-specific ST changes, reduced QRS voltage, tachyarrhythmias, conduction abnormalities and left axis deviation on ECG. A slowly progressive form of cardiomyopathy can lead to heart failure. Pre-operative echocardiography is indicated in patients who have received doxorubicin.

Intra-operatively, management is to some extent dictated by the pre-operative condition of the patient. The following considerations apply:

- Invasive monitoring, including a central venous line, arterial pressure monitoring, urinary catheter.
- Placement of a nasogastric tube to empty debris from the oesophagus and stomach – this should be carefully passed, avoiding excessive force, as oesophageal perforation may occur. The surgeon will usually position the nasogastric tube across the anastomosis when this is completed, and the tube should be firmly secured at this stage.
- Double-lumen endotracheal intubation and one-lung anaesthesia.
- Because of their poor nutritional status, the patients are particularly prone to develop hypothermia; therefore, the use of warming devices is indicated.
- At the time of dissection of tumour near the pericardium, a careful watch should be maintained for surgeon-induced arrhythmias.
- In the presence of an unresectable tumour, the placement of wide-bore tubes such as a Celestin's tube can be used to provide palliation of dysphagia. To insert such tubes, a gastrostomy is performed. A risk of this procedure is oesophageal perforation.

Post-operatively, the patient should be admitted to a high dependency area, where gradual recovery is allowed and extubation is performed only once the following have been achieved:

- Core temperature more than 36° C.
- Adequate haemoglobin.
- Electrolytes within normal limits.
- No evidence of bleeding.
- Adequate pain control.
- Adequate urine output.
- No evidence of arrhythmias, or well controlled arrhythmias.
- Good respiratory effort, as judged by tidal excursion or airway occlusion pressure.
- Normal gas exchange on less than 40 per cent FiO_2.

The methods of pain relief after thoracotomy are discussed in Chapter 17. Mid-thoracic epidural analgesia is the analgesia of choice in patients undergoing oesophageal resection.

Expected complications after oesophagectomy and their incidence are given in Table 9.2.

Hiatus hernia

Heartburn is a symptom of decreased barrier pressure across the lower oesophageal sphincter, and indicates the presence of gastro-oesophageal reflux. Most patients with gastro-oesophageal reflux have a sliding hernia, but every patient with a hiatus hernia does not necessarily have significant reflux. Two types of hiatus hernia have been described:

Table 9.2 Complication rate following oesophagectomy

Complication	Rate (per cent)
• Death	3
Lung complications	
• pneumonia	10
• adult respiratory distress syndrome	4
Cardiovascular complications	
• myocardial infarction	1
• arrhythmias	10
• pulmonary embolus	1
Gastrointestinal complications	
• anastomosis leak	7
• gastric stasis	2
• splenic injuries	3
Miscellaneous	
• vocal cord palsy	4
• chylothorax	1

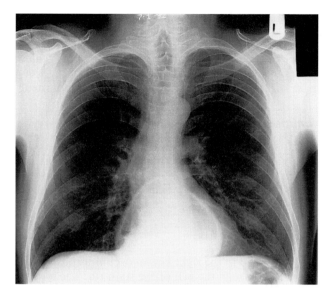

Figure 9.1 PA chest X-ray showing hiatus hernia. The stomach, with a fluid level, can be seen behind the cardiac shadow.

1. Sliding hernia (Type I). These constitute 90 per cent of total hiatus hernias. The lower end of the oesophagus, oesophago-gastric junction and fundus of the stomach herniate axially into the thorax through a hiatus in the crus of the diaphragm (Fig. 9.1). The herniated segment may move cephalad or caudad, depending upon the pressure changes in the chest and abdomen. Since the lower oesophageal sphincter ends up in the thorax, it may not respond appropriately to the raised abdominal pressure. This may be one of the reasons for the increased incidence of reflux in these patients. Oesophagitis and, ultimately, stricture formation is common.

2 Para-oesophageal (rolling) hernia (Type II). In this type of hernia, the fundus and body of the stomach enter the thorax but the oesophago-gastric junction remains within the abdomen. Reflux is less likely, as the lower oesophageal sphincter remains unaffected. However, the stomach is prone to chronic haemorrhage due to venous congestion. Associated features are blood loss and anaemia, acute dilatation of the stomach with respiratory distress, and volvulus of the stomach.

The aims of surgical treatment are:

- To prevent reflux
- To preserve normal swallowing
- To obtain gastro-oesophageal competence.

These aims can be achieved by:

- Restoration of normal anatomy at the hiatus

● Ensuring that an adequate length of oesophagus remains in the abdomen.

In the majority of cases the anatomical correction can be achieved through the abdominal route, but in a few very obese patients or in those with a very large and fixed hernia, the thoracic approach may be indicated.

Trans-abdominal approach

With the patient supine, an upper paramedian incision is made. The lower oesophagus is mobilized and the crus of the diaphragm is sutured to repair the hernia. Patients are usually obese, and a head-up tilt may therefore be requested by the surgeon to help to reduce the hernia with the aid of gravity.

Thoracic approach

The patient is positioned in the right lateral decubitus position. Left thoracotomy is performed through the bed of the sixth rib. The lower oesophagus is mobilized, the hernia reduced and the hiatus repaired.

Nissen's fundoplication

There is growing realization that the anatomical correction of hiatus hernia by itself does not prevent reflux. The 'wrap-around' procedure, fundoplication, with or without anatomical correction, is found to be more successful in preventing reflux.

The fundus of the stomach is mobilized, and a cuff is created around the abdominal oesophagus by passing the fundus behind the oesophagus, pulling it over the anterior aspect and suturing it to the body. This procedure achieves the following objectives:

● It ensures that an adequate length of oesophagus stays in the abdomen.
● It increases the efficiency of the circular muscles of the lower oesophageal sphincter.
● It ensures that the pressure changes from alterations of intraabdominal pressure are reflected equally inside and outside the oesophagus.

Recently, it has been possible to perform Nissen's fundoplication using a laparoscopic approach. From the patient's point of view, this is minimally invasive and has all the associated advantages.

Anaesthetic considerations

The principal anaesthetic problems associated with hiatus hernia repair are as follows:

● The patients are often obese.
● There is potential for aspiration of gastric contents; antacid prophylaxis and rapid sequence induction/intubation should be routine.

- One-lung ventilation may be required.
- If the fundoplication causes excessive compression of the lower oeso-phageal sphincter this can lead to dysphagia, and gastric dilatation as air and fluid accumulating in the stomach cannot be expelled via the oesophagus. The treatment for this is the passage of a nasogastric tube into the stomach intra-operatively, and removal of the tube 3 days after the procedure, once the bowel function has returned to normal.

Oesophageal strictures

Reflux is the most common cause of benign strictures in the lower oeso-phagus (Fig. 9.2). It may or may not be associated with hiatus hernia. Chronic reflux of gastric acid leads to ulceration, inflammation and, eventually, stricture formation. The aim of treatment is to either reduce gastric acidity or prevent the contact of oesophageal mucosa with gastric acid. Major surgery may be necessary if medical treatment and oesophageal dilatation are inadequate in controlling reflux and dysphagia. There are two types of surgical procedures, both of which are usually approached by a left thoraco-abdominal incision.

Gastroplasty

The stricture is dilated and a left thoraco-abdominal incision is made. A part of the stomach fundus is then interposed between the oesophageal mucosa and the acidic milieu of the stomach. The remaining fundus is sewn to the lower oesophagus to create a valve-like effect.

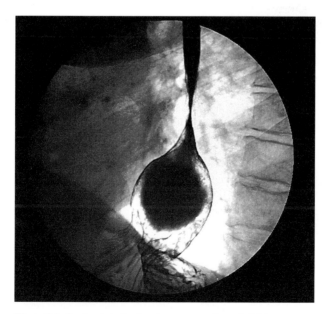

Figure 9.2 Contrast study showing an oesophageal stricture.

Resection of the stricture

This is also performed through a left thoraco-abdominal incision. The stricture is resected in the thorax, and the oesophagus is joined to the stomach in an end-to-side oesophago-gastrostomy. To eliminate stomach acidity, vagotomy and antrectomy are performed. Roux-en-Y gastric drainage procedure is performed to prevent alkaline intestinal reflux.

Anaesthetic considerations

The anaesthetic considerations are essentially the same as those for patients with hiatus hernia. Careful attention needs to be given to fluid and electrolyte balance as well as to physiotherapy and analgesia. Parenteral nutrition should be continued for at least 1 week, when enteral nutrition can be started if the anastomosis is confirmed to be intact radiologically.

Achalasia of the oesophagus

Achalasia is characterized by a lack of peristalsis in the oesophagus. The lower oesophageal sphincter also fails to relax in response to swallowing, resulting in oesophageal distension (Fig. 9.3). The most likely aetiology is neurogenic. Clinically, patients present with chronic regurgitation. Repeated chest infections or a pulmonary abscess may result from aspiration of residual food from the oesophagus.

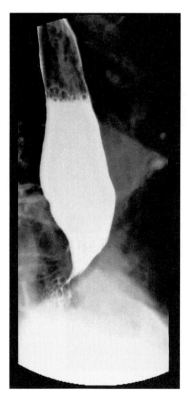

Figure 9.3 Barium swallow in a patient with achalasia. Note the distended, barium filled oesophagus above the lower oesophageal sphincter.

The aim of surgical treatment is to alleviate the obstruction. This can be achieved either by repeated dilatation or by major surgery. Dilatation carries the risk of oesophageal perforation, and is reserved mainly for poor risk patients or for those who refuse surgery. Surgical repair consists of Heller's myotomy, in which circular muscle fibres of the oesophageal gastric junction are divided. The myotomy is often combined with hiatus hernia repair to prevent subsequent reflux. The procedure is usually performed via a thoracic incision, but an abdominal approach is also possible. Recently, a laparoscopic approach for the surgery has been introduced into practice.

Anaesthetic considerations

The anaesthetic considerations are similar to those for patients with hiatus hernia. Due to the presence of residual debris in the dilated oesophagus, there is a risk of aspiration at induction. In addition, some patients with achalasia are prone to chronic aspiration with consequent pneumonitis. In some centres, oesophageal washouts are performed prior to surgery.

Fistula between oesophagus and respiratory tract

In adults, the commonest cause is malignancy. Other causes are summarized in Table 9.3.

If the cause of the fistula is a benign condition, it is usual to perform a full surgical correction. However, in the presence of malignancy only palliative procedures are performed. The aim is to prevent soiling of the lungs and restore continuity of the gut.

If the patient is assessed to be a poor risk with limited life expectancy, an endo-oesophageal intubation is all that can be offered. Occasionally, for healthier patients, a bypass or exclusion procedure can be performed. For this, the oesophagus is divided in the neck as well as at the cardia. The fundus of the stomach is then connected to the proximal part of oesophagus directly or via a jejunal or colonic connection, which is placed in either the pre-sternal or retrosternal space.

Anaesthetic considerations

- Patients with an oesophago-gastric fistula are usually debilitated, and present an extremely high risk of peri-operative mortality. Lung soiling resulting in bronchospasm, pneumonia, abscess formation and systemic sepsis should be anticipated and treated.

Table 9.3 Causes of oesophago-respiratory tract fistulae

- Malignancy
- Congenital tracheo-oesophageal fistula without oesophageal atresia
- Inflammation
- Chest trauma
- Endotracheal tube injury
- Endoscope injury

- Intra-operatively, positive pressure ventilation may result in loss of inspired gas through the fistula, leading to abdominal distension, respiratory insufficiency or even cardiac arrest. Spontaneous breathing should preferably be maintained during induction of anaesthesia, until it has been ascertained that positive pressure ventilation is not likely to cause significant leak through the fistula.
- Inhalational induction with sevoflurane may be particularly advantageous, but experience is limited.
- For high tracheal fistulae, a single-lumen tube might isolate the lungs by blocking the tracheal end of the fistulae.
- For low tracheal or left bronchial fistulae, a right-sided double-lumen tube is indicated. For right bronchial fistulae, a left-sided double-lumen tube is indicated.
- A nasogastric tube should be passed to vent the stomach to prevent distension on application of IPPV.
- High frequency ventilatory methods have a role if ventilation is compromised by excessive loss of airway gas through the fistula.
- Post-operatively, spontaneous ventilation should be allowed to resume as soon as possible, as positive pressure ventilation and the presence of an endotracheal tube can disrupt the surgical repair.

Oesophageal perforation and rupture

The upper oesophageal sphincter is the narrowest point in the oesophagus, and is the region most likely to be perforated by an endoscope. Perforations resulting from the passage of bougies are common at the level of the lesion. Other causes for oesophageal perforation are given in Table 9.4.

A rupture is a bursting injury. The commonest cause is unco-ordinated vomiting. Other causes of oesophageal rupture are given in Table 9.5.

The important difference between perforation and rupture is that, in the latter, the gastric contents enter the mediastinum under high pressure and the patient becomes symptomatic much more abruptly. The rupture is usually located on the left side within 2 cm of the gastro-oesophageal junction. The cause is a sudden increase in abdominal pressure with a relaxed lower oesophageal sphincter and an obstructed oesophageal inlet.

Patients with intrathoracic oesophageal perforation or rupture may develop the following:

Table 9.4 Causes of oesophageal perforation

- Endoscopic procedures
- Foreign bodies
- Bougies
- Oropharyngeal suction
- Accidental traumatic oesophageal intubation
- Oesophageal obturator airways
- Oesophageal balloons
- Nasogastric tubes

Table 9.5 Causes of oesophageal rupture

- Unco-ordinated vomiting

- Strain during:
  weight lifting
  childbirth
  defecation

- Crush injury to chest
- Crush injury to abdomen

- Pain, which is unresponsive to the administration of opioids
- Labile blood pressure, sweating and peripheral cyanosis
- Tachypnoea
- Surgical emphysema (in up to 60 per cent of cases)
- Unilateral or bilateral hydrothorax or hydropneumothorax
- Mediastinitis and sepsis.

Radiological changes may be apparent as:

- Subcutaneous emphysema
- Pneumomediastinum
- Widening of mediastinum
- Pleural effusion
- Pneumoperitoneum.

A barium swallow may localize the injury. Air may be seen in the mediastinum on a CT scan of the chest.

The key principle of surgical treatment for a perforation or rupture of the oesophagus is drainage and prevention of further contamination. Oesophagoscopy may first be required to diagnose and localize the site of perforation or rupture. Definitive surgery for the upper half of the thoracic oesophagus is via a right-sided thoracotomy, while a left-sided thoracotomy is used when the injury is in the lower third of the oesophagus. On exposure, if the oesophageal wall is healthy, a primary closure may be performed. If the perforation is at the lower end of the oesophagus, an attempt is made to patch it with the fundus of the stomach. However, if the perforation has occurred in the presence of an operable carcinoma of the oesophagus, an oesophagectomy may be performed. In poor risk patients, thoracotomy may be avoided by dividing the oesophagus in the neck and performing a cervical oesophagostomy. The distal oesophagus is then divided via an abdominal incision and a feeding gastrostomy is placed.

Anaesthetic considerations

- Surgery is usually urgent. Transfer of patients to a high dependency area may be indicated to optimize their condition pre-operatively. Optimization may require commencement of inotropes in addition to fluid resuscitation, and should be guided by appropriate invasive cardiovascular monitoring. Insertion of intercostal drains may be required to relieve hydropneumothorax prior to induction.

- Post-operatively, pulmonary dysfunction is likely and ventilatory support will usually be required.
- There is at least a 50 per cent chance of repair dehiscence with the formation of an oesophageal-pleural-cutaneous fistula.
- Cardiac arrhythmia, particularly atrial fibrillation, is common due to mediastinitis.
- Gram-negative septicaemia in the early post-operative period should be anticipated.
- Parenteral nutrition, or enteral nutrition if a gastrostomy feeding tube has been inserted, should be commenced early.

KEY POINTS

- Patients may be of any age – for example, young children with congenital pathology or the elderly and infirm with co-existent disease.

- Pre-operative assessment should encompass the 'whole' patient, with particular attention directed to the cardiovascular, respiratory and nutritional status.

- Nutritional support should be considered as early as possible.

- Consider high dependency facilities prior to surgery.

- Consider the risks of aspiration of gastric contents or oesophageal debris, and take appropriate precautions peri-operatively to minimize the hazard.

- Assess the need for one-lung ventilation; for most oesophageal surgery, one-lung ventilation is only required to facilitate surgical access and can be dispensed with if placement of the double-lumen tube proves difficult or hazardous.

Bibliography

Aitkenhead, A.R. (1987). Anaesthesia for oesophageal surgery. *Baillière's Clin. Anaesthesiol.*, **1(1)**, 181–205.

Campos, A.C.L. and Meguid, M.M. (1992). A critical appraisal of the usefulness of perioperative nutritional support. *Am. J. Clin. Nutr.*, **55(1)**, 117–30.

Earlam, R. (1995). The oesophagus. In *Bailey and Love's Short Practice of Surgery*, 22nd edn (C.V. Mann, R.C.G. Russell and N.S. Williams, eds), pp. 641–68. Chapman and Hall.

Forshag, M.S. and Cooper, A.D. Jr (1992). Post-operative care of the thoracotomy patient. *Clin. Chest Med.*, **13(1)**, 33–45.

Heslin, M.J., Latkany, L., Leung, D. *et al.* (1997). A prospective randomized trial of early enteral feeding after resection of upper gastrointestinal malignancy. *Ann. Surg.*, **226(4)**, 567–80.

Kavanagh, B.P. and Sandler, A.N. (1996). Anaesthesia for thoracic surgery. *Baillère's Clin. Anaesthesiol.*, **10(1)**, 77–98.

Mohr, D.N. and Lavender, R.C. (1996). Pre-operative pulmonary evaluation: identifying patients at increased risk for complications. *Postgrad. Med.*, **100(5)**, 241–56.

Sydow, F.W. (1989). The influence of anaesthesia and post-operative analgesic management on lung function. *Acta Chir. Scand.* (suppl.), **155(550)**, 159–68.

Vaughan, R.W. (1983). Anaesthesia for the morbidly obese patient. *Clin. Anaesth.*, **1(2)**, 337–55.

10

Video-assisted thoracoscopic surgery (VATS)

M. Zammit and E. Mackson

Introduction

Thoracoscopy, the passage of a telescopic viewing device through the chest wall, was first described in 1910 by Jacobeus, a Swedish Professor of Medicine. Jacobeus used modified cystoscopy instruments for intrapleural pneumolysis in patients with pulmonary tuberculosis, and this technique was widely adopted in Europe and the United States until 1945, when the introduction of streptomycin resulted in a rapid decline in the incidence of tuberculosis. The use of thoracoscopy then became confined mainly to diagnostic rather than therapeutic interventions.

Major technological advances have led to the development of a wide range of operating instruments and high resolution cameras, which have resulted in renewed interest in thoracoscopy for both diagnostic and therapeutic purposes.

Video-assisted thoracoscopic surgery (VATS) has largely superseded thoracoscopy because of the superior quality of visualization of the operative field that can be obtained, and because it frees the surgeon's hands to manipulate operating instruments rather than holding the scope to maintain a view. The surgical and anaesthetic considerations are essentially the same for VATS and thoracoscopy.

Indications

VATS has revolutionized the management of a wide variety of intrathoracic pathology. The indications for VATS may be described in terms of four main categories:

1. Pleural pathology
2. Pulmonary pathology
3. Mediastinal pathology
4. Oesophageal pathology.

Pleural pathology

VATS is invaluable as a diagnostic intervention for pleural pathology. In tuberculosis and cancer, the reported diagnostic sensitivity of biopsy and brush samples ranges from 93 to 97 per cent. There has been some concern about the possibility of seeding of mesothelioma along the thoracoscope track, although the incidence of this may be decreased by post-operative radiotherapy.

Pleural effusions

VATS permits drainage of effusions, visualization and biopsy of pleura and lung parenchyma and re-expansion of the lung under direct vision.

VATS is the early intervention of choice in the management of empyema, as drainage, adhesiolysis, irrigation and decortication can all be performed thoracoscopically. Delayed intervention results in organization of the collection into a fibrotic peel, which encases the lung and contracts. At this stage the method of choice is a formal thoracotomy and decortication, but this is often complicated by lung laceration and prolonged air leak as discussed in Chapter 16.

Pulmonary pathology

Pneumothorax

The primary aims in management of pneumothorax are re-expansion of the lung and prevention of recurrence. Resection of emphysematous bullae, division of pleural adhesions, decortication and pleurodesis may be carried out via VATS, and lung re-expansion directly visualized. VATS resection of emphysematous blebs is recommended if there is persistent air leak after 72 hours of conservative management by underwater seal drainage. Recurrence of pneumothorax is higher for VATS when compared to formal thoracotomy. VATS, however, is associated with lower post-operative analgesic requirement, earlier mobilization and improved post-operative respiratory function.

Lung parenchymal disease

VATS plays a major role in the diagnosis of lung parenchymal lesions when pleural biopsy and pleural cytology have failed. Peripheral solitary lung lesions and pulmonary metastases may be biopsied and resected. Major lung resection is possible, but the limitations of VATS, such as loss of palpation and incomplete lymph node dissection, render this intervention of uncertain value as a therapeutic procedure in oncological surgery.

Lung volume reduction surgery

This intervention is usually reserved for patients with extensive emphysematous lung disease and poor respiratory reserve. Lung volume reduction surgery (LVRS) is thought to improve outcome by increasing the pulmonary and thoracic elastic recoil and improving diaphragmatic function. This is discussed in detail in Chapter 13. VATS has several advantages over formal thoracotomy in these patients in that it is associated with a decreased incidence of lobar atelectasis, less diaphragmatic disturbance and decreased analgesic requirement post-operatively. The mortality and morbidity in this group of patients remains high, and further studies are in progress to evaluate long-term results.

Mediastinal pathology

The mediastinum is easily visualized using VATS. Discrete lesions and lymph nodes may be biopsied under direct vision, and staging of malignant disease is possible. Radiotherapy may be required post-operatively, and in this circumstance healing is less likely to be impaired in the smaller and more laterally placed incisions required for VATS as compared to median sternotomy.

Thymectomy in patients with myasthenia gravis has been carried out using VATS; however, in the presence of a thymoma, extended resection by an open approach is preferable.

Pericardial disease

VATS allows direct access to the pericardium for biopsy, and a pericardial window may be created for drainage of a pericardial effusion.

Oesophageal pathology

The role of VATS in malignant oesophageal disease is mainly in pre-operative staging. Surgery for oesophageal carcinoma requires wide exposure and mobilization of the oesophagus, as well as extensive lymph node dissection; thus, an open transthoracic approach is the method of choice. Enucleation of benign tumours and treatment of benign motility disorders is possible via VATS.

Miscellaneous

Other indications for VATS include sympathectomy, minimally invasive coronary artery surgery and biopsy of neurogenic tumours.

The list of procedures performed by VATS is constantly lengthening. However, for some procedures, although VATS may be technically feasible, it may not necessarily be the most sensible surgical technique.

Surgical procedure

The patient is generally placed in the lateral decubitus position. The table is maximally flexed, or a support is placed underneath the thorax, in an attempt to maximize the exposure of the thorax and widen the intercostal spaces. For procedures on the apical region of the lung or thorax, or for cervical sympathectomy, access may be improved by placing the patient supine in the semi-upright chair position, with the arm on the appropriate side abducted and the hand placed under the head. This approach is particularly appropriate for bilateral procedures, as it obviates the need for turning the patient. It does, however, have haemodynamic disadvantages in terms of maintenance of venous return to the heart and cerebral blood flow and, most pertinently, in terms of loss of the effect of gravity in diverting blood flow to the ventilated lung during one-lung ventilation. Hence, during one-lung ventilation with the patient in the supine semi-upright position, shunt is greater than in the lateral decubitus position and the risk of hypoxia during one-lung ventilation increased.

The skin is prepared and draped, giving sufficient exposure of the chest if the need for conversion to a formal thoracotomy arises.

One-lung ventilation is established, and the non-dependent lung collapsed. The use of actively insufflated gas (e.g. CO_2) to aid induction of pneumothorax is both unsafe and unnecessary.

The initial intrathoracic access port is usually placed in the sixth intercostal space at the mid- to posterior axillary line, but this is subject to change according to the nature of the procedure and surgical preference. The lung is collapsed before insertion of trocars to prevent iatrogenic trauma to the lung. A wide angle, $0°$ 10-mm operating thoracoscope is passed through an introducer port. Additional access sites are established as necessary to allow the passage of instruments.

Anaesthetic considerations

- Patients presenting for VATS fall within a broad spectrum of disease. Careful patient selection and optimization of pre-operative condition is as essential as for thoracotomy.
- Surgical access requires collapse of the lung within the operative hemithorax. Adequate collapse of the lung may not always be possible to achieve because of adhesions. Under such circumstances, visualization of structures is impaired and the underlying lung may be damaged by insertion of trocars through the chest wall; there should therefore be a low threshold for conversion to open thoracotomy.
- The anaesthetic technique should allow for a variable length of procedure and possibility of conversion to formal thoracotomy. While extubation is usual at the end of VATS procedures, high dependency or intensive care facilities may be required to accommodate patients with poor pre-operative respiratory function.

Pre-operative assessment

The goal of pre-operative consultation is to define the patient's medical problems and optimize the patient's condition, principally to ensure that one-lung ventilation will be tolerated safely during the procedure.

History and physical examination

The history and physical examination are focused on the respiratory and cardiovascular systems, and on any co-existing disease.

- The degree of functional limitation is assessed, as indicated by the severity of symptoms such as dyspnoea, cough and sputum production, poor exercise tolerance and the presence of signs such as cyanosis, clubbing and additional sounds on auscultation of the chest.
- Information about the upper and lower airway should be obtained by clinical examination and review of radiological investigations, to determine if endobronchial intubation can be accomplished.
- The presence of coexistent ischaemic heart disease is associated with increased morbidity, and patients with valvular heart disease may be poor candidates for the haemodynamic changes associated with one-lung ventilation and the lateral position.
- Any co-existent disease should be noted, for example, diabetes or renal impairment.

Investigations

In addition to routine pre-operative tests, blood should be grouped and saved or cross-matched since the procedure is associated with the potential for major haemorrhage. Pulmonary function tests, and arterial blood gases in patients with severe lung disease, are helpful in assessing the patient's suitability for one-lung ventilation and the need for post-operative respiratory support.

Chest X-rays and, if appropriate, computerized axial tomograms (CT scans) should be reviewed, as the nature and extent of adhesions or tumour invasion may preclude collapse of the lung or passage of the endobronchial tubes and thus render VATS impractical.

Premedication

This is tailored to individual requirements; the use of a benzodiazepine for anxiolysis and sedation is satisfactory. Opioids may be associated with excessive respiratory depression in patients with poor respiratory reserve. Anti-sialogogues may lead to inspissated secretions, predisposing to increased post-operative complications.

Monitoring

Basic non-invasive monitoring is instituted in all patients. However, the use of invasive intra-arterial blood pressure monitoring and blood sampling is desirable for various reasons:

- One-lung ventilation may be complicated by hypoxaemia, necessitating more accurate monitoring than can be attained by pulse oximetry. If one-lung ventilation is complicated by high airway pressures, necessitating permissive hypercapnia to reduce the risk of barotrauma, direct measurement of arterial P_{CO_2} is required rather than relying on end-tidal CO_2.

- Haemodynamic instability may arise as a result of surgical manipulation, especially in patients with pre-existing cardiovascular disease.
- There is the ever-present possibility of conversion to thoracotomy, particularly for more complex VATS procedures.

Trans-oesophageal echocardiography may be indicated in procedures on the pericardium.

Induction and maintenance of anaesthesia

Thoracoscopy may be performed under local, regional or general anaesthesia. Local anaesthesia is by infiltration of the incisions and parietal pleura. Regional techniques used are intercostal nerve blocks, paravertebral blocks or thoracic epidural block.

The choice of anaesthetic technique is aimed at optimizing surgical conditions whilst ensuring maximal patient comfort and safety. Local and regional techniques are rarely used in isolation, except in extremely ill patients, but are frequently used together with general anaesthesia.

Anaesthesia may be satisfactorily induced with any of the widely used agents, e.g. propofol, thiopentone or etomidate, and maintained by inhalational or total intravenous techniques with no significant difference in outcome. The use of shorter-acting agents predictably promotes earlier ambulation, and this is desirable for minimally invasive procedures.

The intra-operative use of narcotics should be minimized; 1.5–2 μg/kg of fentanyl given intra-operatively and combined with local infiltration is generally satisfactory in providing post-operative analgesia and early mobilization.

Muscle relaxation facilitates intubation and ventilation, and the application of intermittent positive pressure ventilation prevents mediastinal shift and paradoxical respiration during one-lung ventilation. The muscle relaxant should be of intermediate duration of effect, e.g. vecuronium, atracurium.

One-lung ventilation is attained by the use of a double- or single-lumen endobronchial tube or bronchial blocker, as discussed in Chapters 1 and 4.

Large bore peripheral venous access should be established in view of the potential for significant haemorrhage. Central venous access may be required, depending on the patient's condition and the nature of the procedure.

Post-operative management

The majority of patients undergoing VATS procedures may be extubated in theatre, or early in recovery. Supplemental oxygen is administered and the patient nursed sitting up to optimize lung mechanics. Patients with severe pre-existing lung disease may require prolonged ventilation, and in these cases the endobronchial tube should be replaced by a single-lumen endotracheal tube at the end of the procedure.

A post-operative chest X-ray is taken in recovery to exclude residual pneumothorax, persistent atelectasis or haemothorax, and to check the correct positioning of chest drains.

Early mobilization is encouraged.

Post-operative analgesia

VATS procedures are associated with less analgesic requirement than formal thoracotomy, which has been described as one of the most intensely painful procedures. A multimodal approach to pain management is generally used. Following diagnostic VATS procedures, opioids are generally not required if simple local anaesthetic techniques combined with the use of non-steroidal anti-inflammatory agents are used. Local infiltration of incision sites and single-shot intercostal blocks may be useful in the short term. Intrapleural anaesthetics have been shown to have no significant opioid-sparing effects, and are of doubtful value.

For complicated VATS procedures and for VATS pleurodesis, which is extremely painful post-operatively, regional local anaesthetic blocks are appropriate. Paravertebral blocks are increasingly being used, and offer significant benefits in that they are simple and quick to carry out. Furthermore, the concomitant unilateral sympathetic block is associated with a lower incidence of hypotension than epidural block. Epidural local anaesthetics are associated with excellent pain relief but, on risk–benefit assessment for VATS, are usually deemed unnecessary unless there is a high possibility of conversion to formal thoracotomy (such as for a pneumonectomy) or the procedure is deemed to be particularly painful. More detailed discussion of the techniques of pain relief can be found in Chapter 17.

Complications

Intra-operative complications include:

- Hypoxia on one-lung ventilation: Some degree of hypoxia is inevitable on one-lung ventilation as a result of ventilation–perfusion mismatch and obligatory shunt; this is seen more commonly with right thoracoscopies because the right lung receives 55 per cent of the total pulmonary blood flow. The incidence of hypoxaemia is increased in the presence of pre-existent lung disease, and may also occur as a result of suboptimal positioning of the endobronchial tube.
- Haemorrhage.
- Air embolism.
- Surgical emphysema.
- Cardiac arrhythmias; these are more common in patients older than 70 years, with co-existent heart disease or lung carcinoma, or during mediastinal tumour or lymph node dissection.
- Trauma to liver or para-oesophageal hernia.
- Creation of aorto–pleuro–cutaneous fistula (rare).

Early post-operative complications include:

- Persistent air leak.
- Pulmonary oedema.
- Empyema.
- Chylothorax.
- Wound infection.
- Respiratory insufficiency.

Late post-operative complications include:

- Incisional pain; 7 per cent of patients complain of persistent pain at the incision sites. This may be secondary to direct or indirect trauma to the intercostal nerves by large trocars.
- Malignant spread; the reports of tumour seeding along entry tracts are anecdotal, no clinical trials are available.
- Septicaemia.

Advantages and disadvantages of VATS compared to thoracotomy

Advantages include:

- Decreased incidence of post-operative pain.
- Improved post-operative respiratory function as a result of lesser use of opioids, less interference with diaphragmatic function and improved clearance of secretions.
- Decreased incidence of post-operative lobar atelectasis and pneumonia.
- Faster post-operative recovery and earlier socio-economic re-integration.
- Improved cosmetic result.

Disadvantages include:

- Lack of tactile discrimination.
- Lack of three-dimensional visualization.
- Difficulty in assessing and controlling haemorrhage.
- Limitations of instrumentation.
- Expensive equipment.

Conversion of VATS to formal thoracotomy is often necessary in the following conditions: presence of tight pleural adhesions, failure to establish one-lung ventilation, inability to locate the pulmonary lesion, technical difficulty, and major haemorrhage.

VATS is a considerably less invasive technique than thoracotomy, and can be used as a diagnostic and therapeutic intervention in a wide range of intrathoracic pathology. In general, it allows earlier post-operative mobilization and is better tolerated by sicker patients than thoracotomy.

KEY POINTS

- VATS is a much less invasive alternative to thoracotomy for many diagnostic and therapeutic thoracic procedures.

- VATS is performed by placement of trocars and a thoracoscope through the chest wall. This requires collapse of the lung to prevent iatrogenic injury to the lung and permit visualization of intrathoracic structures.

- Anaesthesia for VATS should be tailored to allow prompt recovery and early mobilization – a multimodal approach to analgesia, minimizing opioid usage, is optimal.

- VATS should not be regarded as a minor operation; the potential need for conversion to open thoracotomy must be borne in mind.

Bibliography

Boutin, C., Viallat, J.R., Cargnino, P. *et al.* (1981). Thoracoscopy in malignant pleural effusions. *Am. Rev. Resp. Dis.*, **124**, 588–92.

Boutin, R., Loddenkemper, R., Astoul, P. *et al.* (1993). Diagnostic and therapeutic thoracoscopy: techniques and indications in pulmonary medicine. *Tubercle Lung Dis.*, **74**, 225–339.

Coosemans, W. and Lerut, T. (1997). Risks and benefits of thoracoscopic surgery. *Curr. Opin. Anaesthesiol.*, **10**, 41–3.

Harris, R.J., Kavuru, M.S., Rice, T.W. *et al.* (1995). The diagnostic and therapeutic utility of thoracoscopy. *Chest*, **108**, 828–41.

Haselrigg, S.R., Landreneau, R.J., Boley, T.M. *et al.* (1991). The effect of muscle sparing versus standard postero-lateral thoracotomy on pulmonary function, muscle strength and post-operative pain. *J. Thorac. Cardiovasc. Surg.*, **46**, 266–70.

Hill, R.C., Jones, D.R., Vance, R.A. *et al.* (1996). Selective lung ventilation during thoracoscopy: effects of insufflation on haemodynamics. *Ann. Thorac. Surg.*, **61**, 945–8.

Horsewell, J. (1993). Anaesthetic techniques for thoracoscopy. *Ann. Thorac. Surg.*, **56**, 624–9.

Janovici, R., Lang-Lazdunski, L., Pons, F. *et al.* (1996). Complications of video-assisted thoracic surgery. A 5-year experience. *Ann. Thorac. Surg.*, **61**, 533–7.

Kavanagh, P.P., Katz, J., Sandler, A.N. *et al.* (1994). Pain control after thoracic surgery. *Anesthesiology*, **81**, 737–59.

Krashna, M.J., Deshmukh, S. and McLaughlin, J.S. (1996). Complications of thoracoscopy. *Ann. Thorac. Surg.*, **61**, 1066–9.

Landreneau, R.J., Hazelrigg, S.R., Mack, M.J. *et al.* (1993). Post-operative pain related morbidity: video-assisted thoracic surgery versus thoracotomy. *Ann. Thorac. Surg.*, **56**, 800–9.

Larbuisson, R. and Lamy, M. (1997). Anaesthesia for thoracoscopic surgery. *Curr. Opin. Anaesthesiol.*, **10**, 44–7.

Plummer, S., Hartley, M. and Vaughan, R.S. (1998). Anaesthesia for telescopic procedures in the thorax. *Br. J. Anaesth.*, **80**, 223–34.

Wakabayashi, A. (1995). Thoracoscopic laser pneumoplasty in the treatment of diffuse bullous emphysema. *Ann. Thorac. Surg.*, **60**, 936–42.

11

Chest trauma

W. T. McBride

Introduction

Throughout all age groups, trauma is the third highest cause of death after cancer and atherosclerosis. If we focus on the first three decades of life, trauma becomes the foremost cause of death; in children of school age it is responsible for 50 per cent of deaths.

Thoracic trauma

In lethal trauma chest injury is particularly important, accounting for 56 per cent of deaths due to trauma every year. Although trauma is the most common cause of death in children, the incidence of chest injury in children (under 15 years old) is rare: approximately 5–10 per cent. The effects of thoracic trauma are mostly immediately life threatening, and yet lend themselves to treatment in the accident and emergency department during the initial survey phase of the advance trauma and life support protocol (ATLS). Furthermore, there is a high probability of serious co-existing injury, of which central nervous system damage is the most frequent. Such a combination is especially lethal.

The role of the anaesthetist

Only a minority (less than 30 per cent) of thoracic trauma patients require anaesthesia for thoracotomy. Nevertheless, the anaesthetist makes an important contribution to the care of these patients throughout the course of their hospital stay. This is seen in the emergency room in the immediate resuscitation phase, in the operating room in provision of anaesthesia for surgical treatment of thoracic and non-thoracic injuries, in the intensive care unit in the management of multiple organ support, and in pain management on the ward.

Anaesthetic management in the emergency room as part of the trauma team

The anaesthetist should be part of a trauma team, composed of the accident and emergency physician, trauma surgeon and support staff.

When called to the acutely distressed patient, the team should pursue the basic principles of the ATLS protocol: airway, breathing and circulation, primary and secondary surveys.

In such a team approach to trauma, a dedicated member of the team (usually the Accident and Emergency physician or surgeon) is involved in diagnosis, decision making and co-ordinating the therapeutic actions of the other team members. However, in some centres this may be the role of the anaesthetist. The team co-ordinator should constantly re-evaluate, in collaboration with the other team members, the success of the resuscitation attempt and initiate the next steps in treatment.

Whether as team co-ordinator or as a team member, the anaesthetist contributes vital skills that may be necessary throughout the resuscitation phase – in particular, emergency airway management and vascular access.

The anaesthetist is best qualified to provide expert airway evaluation, establish manual ventilation and secure the airway by intubation, if necessary. Emergency intubation in the emergency room (ER) should be performed if patients are unable (or likely to become unable) to maintain their own airway, are in respiratory distress, in severe pain from thoracic or other injuries or have cerebral injury. In unconscious patients, intubation may be performed without pharmacological assistance. However, acutely distressed combative patients with signs of acute hypovolaemia, who are losing their airway, present a major challenge. Anaesthetic induction agents may vasodilate such a patient and precipitate profound hypotension. There is the ever-present risk of aspiration of gastric contents, and the possibility of cervical spine instability. In this situation, a rapid sequence induction with pre-oxygenation and cricoid pressure, using ketamine 0.25–0.5 mg/kg as the induction agent (to minimize vasodilatation), together with a short-acting muscle relaxant to ensure optimal intubating conditions, may be the technique of choice. Throughout intubation an assistant should provide counter-traction to the head to minimize risk of cervical spine injury at intubation. In the hypovolaemic patient who is peripherally shut down, rapid establishment of adequate venous access is vital. Since most deaths following thoracic trauma are due to exsanguination, this cannot be over-emphasized.

Classification

Chest trauma may be classified according to aetiology, i.e. non-penetrating, penetrating or both.

Non-penetrating chest trauma accounts for 90 per cent of peacetime chest trauma. It may be due to blunt injury (direct impact), deceleration injury (most commonly due to a motor vehicle accident) or crush injury, or a combination of all the above. A distinct type of non-penetrating lung injury, blast lung injury, is discussed separately.

Penetrating chest trauma is rare in peacetime and is responsible for only 10 per cent of thoracic injuries. Fifteen per cent of combat injuries involve the thorax, and of these 95 per cent are penetrating. Penetrating thoracic trauma may be secondary to low or high velocity bullet or shrapnel wounds, stabbing or impalement. It is important to obtain a clear history of the mechanism of injury, as this may be a guide to its severity. The greater the kinetic energy (KE) transferred to thoracic tissues by the penetrating object, the greater the tissue damage. Since $KE = MV^2/2G$ (where M = mass, V = velocity and G = acceleration due to gravity), the severity of injury depends on the mass and velocity of the penetrating object. Consequently, a high velocity bullet passing thorough the thoracic cavity causes damage that is not merely limited to the bullet track. The dissipation of high kinetic energy to the tissue leads to shock waves vibrating through the relatively non-compliant surrounding tissue, which results in tearing and shearing forces and widespread tissue damage. In contrast, a low velocity bullet may cause surprisingly little collateral tissue damage.

Penetrating thoracic trauma is managed non-operatively in the majority of adult patients.

Conditions arising from penetrating and non-penetrating injury

Conditions common to both penetrating and non-penetrating injuries include haemothorax, cardiac tamponade and pneumothorax.

Haemothorax

This occurs in 70–80 per cent of all chest trauma patients. Haemothorax may range from a minimal bleed, barely detectable on upright chest X-ray (< 500 ml), to a massive bleed where 30–40 per cent of the blood volume may accumulate in one hemithorax. In such a situation the patient will present with symptoms and signs of severe hypovolaemia. If the haemothorax is sufficient to compress lung volume, there may be symptoms of dyspnoea. On examination, in addition to the signs of hypovolaemia, there may be decreased expansion on the affected side, deviation of the trachea from the affected side (if the haemothorax is large), dullness to percussion and decreased breath sounds on the affected side. A haemothorax greater than 500 ml can be seen in a chest X-ray in the upright or decubitus position. Up to a litre of blood may be not seen in a supine portable chest X-ray, although it should be suspected if there is increased density in one hemithorax.

Having ensured the adequacy of respiration, intravenous access must be rapidly achieved and blood volume replacement expedited. The diagnosis is confirmed by placement of a chest drain. This allows the collapsed lung to be re-inflated, the size of the haemothorax to be determined and the rate of any ongoing haemorrhage to be monitored. Late onset haemorrhage, as can occur following some penetrating injuries, can also be observed. Chest drain insertion alone is usually the only intervention required for most patients. Haemothorax most commonly arises from damaged low-pressure pulmonary vessels, which frequently stop bleeding spontaneously. In the small number of patients with bleeding persisting at a rate greater than 200 ml/hour, urgent transfer to the operating room for thoracotomy should be expedited. Massive haemothorax (1000–1500 ml) is likely to be due to damage to a major arterial vessel such as hilar or mediastinal vessels or an intercostal artery. Since death from these injuries is most commonly due to exsanguination, it is vital to establish immediate intravenous access and aggressive blood volume replacement. Only *in extremis* is emergency room thoracotomy indicated. One large series suggested that an emergency room thoracotomy was only successful in 3.7 per cent of patients. This tiny band of survivors was found to have penetrating trauma and pre-operative signs of life. A total of 252 thoracotomies were performed for penetrating injuries (92 per cent), and 21 (8 per cent) were performed for blunt trauma. There were no neurologically intact survivors in the blunt trauma group, and only 10 (3.7 per cent) in the penetrating trauma group.

Cardiac tamponade

Following blunt or penetrating trauma, accumulation of blood within the pericardium can significantly compromise myocardial function.

The pericardium is a tight structure, but has sufficient volumetric reserve to permit the heart to increase its end diastolic size to accomplish an increased stroke volume if required. In cardiac tamponade, even 100–150 ml of blood within the pericardium will limit this reserve mechanism. In mild cardiac tamponade, cardiac output will be maintained adequately to meet the patient's needs. This dangerous condition may therefore not be recognized until demands are made on the heart to increase cardiac output in order to maintain mean arterial pressure, such as may occur during the vasodilatation accompanying induction of anaesthesia. Profound hypotension may then develop. In more severe cardiac tamponade, the ability of the heart to dilate sufficiently during diastole to maintain even a normal resting cardiac output may be compromised, and rapid haemo-dynamic decompensation may occur. It is important, therefore, for the anaesthetist to be acutely aware of the possibility of this condition in all thoracic trauma patients, especially those presenting to the operating room for anaesthesia.

The clinical signs of tamponade are elevated central venous pressure with normal pulmonary artery pressures. Heart sounds are soft, and there may be hypotension in severe cases. Beck's triad describes jugular venous distension, distant heart sounds and hypotension. The limitation of this is that hypo-tension may not initially be apparent. Kussmaul's sign describes the para-doxical filling of the jugular veins during inspiration. While theoretically interesting, this is difficult to elicit in the busy emergency room and in an unco-operative patient. The key to diagnosis is to have a high index of sus-picion for this condition in all chest injuries, especially if there is unexplained hypotension in the presence of normal or high central venous pressures. If time permits, the diagnosis can be confirmed by transthoracic echo; how-ever, in the haemodynamically-compromised patient it may be necessary to proceed directly to pericardiocentesis. To perform an emergency room pericardiocentesis, the patient is placed in the semi-sitting position and a 14 or 18 gauge cannula advanced from just beneath the xiphoid process in the direction of the left shoulder. The cannula is passed into the pericardium and the contents drained. If the V lead of the ECG is attached to the metal hub of the needle, sudden ST segment elevation may indicate that the needle has contacted myocardium and should be redirected. After aspiration of as little as 50–60 ml of blood, marked haemodynamic improvement may occur. It is prudent to leave the plastic portion of the cannula *in situ* for further drainage. Definitive treatment for tamponade by creating a pericardial window under local anaesthesia to allow drainage of the pericardial collection has been described. While this may be appropriate for chronic non-traumatic pericardial collections, it is generally not appealing in the acute situation. A full general anaesthetic to facilitate a thoracotomy to explore and treat the cause of the bleeding is the preferred choice. The principle of the anaesthetic management is to maintain a high central venous pressure and use an induction technique with which myocardial depression or reduction in systemic vascular resistance will be minimal. Ketamine is ideally suited for these objectives, but should be commenced in low dose, 0.25–0.5 mg/kg. Maintenance of a tachycardia may help to prevent reduction in cardiac output. The management of patients with tamponade can be summarized as being aimed at keeping the circulation 'fast, full and squeezed tight' until the pericardium is drained.

Pneumothorax

A pneumothorax occurs in 15–50 per cent of non-penetrating trauma and 80 per cent of penetrating trauma. Symptoms of pneumothorax depend on its size; in a small pneumothorax there may be no symptoms, whereas in a large pneumothorax the patient may have severe dyspnoea, cough and pleuritic chest pain. Signs may only be apparent in moderate to severe pneumothorax. There will be decreased chest movement and breath sounds on the affected side, together with hyper-resonance on percussion. Diagnosis is confirmed on an expiratory chest X-ray.

If the pneumothorax is secondary to penetrating trauma, the diagnosis may be immediately obvious, particularly if there is an open chest wall defect (termed a 'sucking' chest wound). Intrathoracic pressure immediately equals atmospheric pressure, and the lung collapses under its own elastic forces. As perfusion is still maintained to the collapsed lung, a large ventilation–perfusion inequality develops, with severe hypoxia. Emergency treatment involves placing an occlusive dressing over the defect, taped to the skin along three edges so that sucking of air into the thoracic cavity is reduced during inspiration and air is allowed to escape under the free edge. If the chest wound is smaller, air may initially enter and the defect then seal itself off. In either case, a chest drain should be placed and the defect closed as soon as possible.

If the pneumothorax is secondary to non-penetrating chest trauma, the mechanism is more difficult to establish. It is thought that an alveolus may rupture and air spread to the hilum and thence to the pleural cavity. Alternatively, there may be a tear involving a distal airway and the pleural space. The presence of rib fractures on the chest X-ray should create a high index of suspicion for development of a pneumothorax. In blunt trauma, there may be no obvious pneumothorax initially (the occult pneumothorax) but it may develop later on, particularly intra-operatively in a patient undergoing positive pressure ventilation or receiving nitrous oxide. For this reason, many anaesthetists insist on insertion of prophylactic chest drains on the affected side in patients with rib fractures undergoing anaesthesia. Nitrous oxide should be withheld.

Irrespective of whether the mechanism of injury is penetrating or non-penetrating, the great danger is the development of a tension pneumothorax. Air accumulates in the thoracic cavity and cannot escape. Intrathoracic pressure increases, leading to kinking of the great veins, and obstructs venous return to the heart. In addition, mediastinal structures are pushed to the opposite side and cause collapse of the contralateral lung. If untreated, cardiac arrest will rapidly occur. The diagnosis is based on clinical grounds and should not await a chest X-ray. Often this situation may suddenly develop intra-operatively, and should be suspected if there is a marked increase in airway pressures and falling oxygen saturation associated with profound hypotension. Neck veins are likely to be distended. Treatment involves immediate needle thoracostomy followed by placement of a chest drain.

Conditions due mainly to non-penetrating trauma

The history of the cause of injury may give clues as to the expected tissue damage.

A direct impact (blunt) injury

In the elderly patient, whose chest wall has become less compliant with age, a blunt chest injury usually results in chest wall damage, with fractured ribs, sternum and soft tissue injury. Intrathoracic organs may be surprisingly unscathed. The anaesthetic management will largely be directed to analgesia for rib fractures and flail chest. In younger patients, whose chest wall is more compliant, rib fractures may also occur, but contusion and laceration of intrathoracic structures may also ensue.

Rib fractures

This is the most common finding in chest trauma. The patient will have a history of blunt trauma and may complain of pain over the affected part. The sharp edge of the fractured rib may lead to pneumothorax, so vigilance must be maintained for development of this complication. Should such a patient require surgery for a thoracic or non-thoracic cause, it is prudent to place a prophylactic chest drain on the affected side.

Flail chest

This occurs if the patient has sustained rib fractures involving three or more ribs in two places on the same side. During normal spontaneous respiration, the resultant 'floating segment' moves in the opposite direction to the rest of the chest wall, leading to compromised respiratory function of the affected side. The chest X-ray should be carefully screened for underlying pneumothorax or haemothorax. In addition, there is often underlying contused pulmonary tissue. Flail chest does not seem to be any more frequently associated with great vessel, tracheobronchial or diaphragmatic injuries than simple rib fractures. This condition can be extremely painful for the patient, leading to rapid shallow breathing, atelectasis, poor clearance of pulmonary secretions and pneumonia. The majority of patients require mechanical ventilation for prolonged periods. Treatment may be either conservative or surgical. Conservative treatment centres on good quality analgesia, ideally with a regional block (see Chapter 17). Ongoing physiotherapy is important to help the patient to cough and clear secretions. Often, however, decreasing respiratory function and patient exhaustion make it necessary to intubate and ventilate the patient. Surgical treatment involving thoracotomy for internal fixation of these fractures has been described. This has been shown to reduce ventilator-dependent time and shorten intensive care unit (ICU) stay. In one series, in the surgical internal fixation group 80 per cent were weaned from the ventilator in 1.3 days, whereas in the ventilation-only group the average ventilation period was 15 days. Interestingly, chest infection was seen in 15 per cent of the internal fixation group compared with 50 per cent in the non-surgical group.

Pulmonary contusion

This is common in blunt chest trauma, but may also occur in association with high velocity penetrating injuries. It may be unilateral or bilateral. The passage of a shock wave through the pulmonary tissue leads to microscopic disruption at the alveolar–air interface. Alveolar haemorrhage and pulmonary parenchymal damage ensue, become maximal at 24 hours, and usually resolve over the following week.

The spectrum of injury can vary from mild to severe respiratory dysfunction. For several days oedema and lung stiffness may increase, mirrored by worsening dyspnoea, tachypnoea and deteriorating blood gases. The chest X-ray may show opacity in the peripheral lung near to the injured chest wall. Chest X-ray changes often lag 12–24 hours behind the clinical changes. Poor outcome (hospital stay > 7 days) can be predicted by signs of contusion on the admission chest X-ray, admission Pao_2/FiO_2 ratio of less than 250, and three or more rib fractures.

Severe pulmonary contusion may rapidly lead to respiratory dysfunction due to ventilation–perfusion mismatch in the injured area of lung. The magnitude of the resultant respiratory dysfunction will depend on the extent to which perfusion to the traumatized lung is maintained. In some patients hypoxic pulmonary vasoconstriction reduces perfusion of the traumatized pulmonary parenchyma, thereby reducing shunt fraction. In other patients this vasoconstrictor response in damaged tissue is not as pronounced, or may be absent, in which case shunt fraction increases with ensuing respiratory dysfunction. In severe cases of unilateral pulmonary contusion, differential lung ventilation may be beneficial by resting the injured lung. Major complications of severe pulmonary contusion are pneumonia, adult respiratory distress syndrome (ARDS) and empyema. Prolonged ventilation in the intensive care unit may be required.

Myocardial contusion

This is uncommon (< 10 per cent of emergency thoracotomy patients), and rarely directly contributes to death in blunt thoracic trauma. However, intra-operative mortality is significantly higher in patients with myocardial contusion, due generally to other serious intrathoracic injuries.

Although rare, this condition should be suspected in all severe blunt thoracic injuries, particularly in young people and especially if there is a fractured sternum. Over several hours the patient may develop tachycardia, atrial or ventricular arrhythmias and conduction abnormalities. There may be decreased left ventricular function secondary to myocardial wall motion abnormalities and mitral regurgitation secondary to papillary muscle dys-function and, in severe cases, pulmonary oedema may develop. Rarely, cases of myocardial rupture have been reported, and this may occur up to 1 week following the injury. Because of the anterior position of the right atrium and the right ventricle, these are the most frequently involved in rupture. Mortality of one chamber rupture is 60 per cent, and of two chamber rupture is 100 per cent.

Radionuclide angiography is probably the best diagnostic method at present. As this is impractical in the emergency room and intra-operatively, diagnosis of myocardial contusion is based on the history of severe blunt trauma when associated with the finding of tachycardia and other complex atrial or ventricular arrhythmias on the ECG. ST segments may be elevated, although normal ST segments do not exclude myocardial contusion. If the patient is stable, transoesophageal (TOE) or transthoracic echocardiography should be performed. This may show regional wall abnormalities or papillary muscle rupture with mitral or tricuspid incompetence. CK-MB enzyme fractions may be misleading.

Treatment is usually supportive, with management of arrhythmias and left ventricular failure. Intra-aortic balloon counter-pulsation may be required to off-load a severely contused heart.

Coronary artery injury

In a patient without previous history of coronary artery disease who appears to be developing clinical signs of myocardial infarction, the possibility of traumatic occlusion of the coronary arterial supply should be considered. If the patient's condition permits, coronary angiography should be performed and surgical revascularization expedited.

Decelerating injury

Following decelerating injury, the patient may have surprisingly little sign of thoracic wall damage but catastrophic internal organ damage. This stems from sudden motion of the heart, lungs and great vessels within the thorax, which continue to move after the chest wall has been brought to an abrupt halt. Massive sudden shearing forces account for the resulting injuries, which may include ruptured thoracic aorta, tracheo-bronchial rupture, cardiac contusions and pulmonary contusion or laceration.

Transected thoracic aorta

About 90 per cent of patients who sustain thoracic aortic transection have a complete thoracic aortic rupture and exsanguinate at the accident scene. The anatomical site of the tear is usually at the aortic isthmus. Of those who survive to reach the emergency room, the aortic adventitial layer may be intact. After initial formation of a sub-adventitial haematoma, during which there may be marked hypotension, the patient's haemodynamic condition may stabilize. Symptoms and signs of thoracic aortic transection include midscapular back pain (in the absence of thoracic spine fracture), unexplained hypotension, upper extremity hypertension, bilateral femoral pulse deficits and initial blood loss of greater than 750 ml via chest drains.

The chest X-ray is an important baseline examination, but a normal chest X-ray cannot exclude intrathoracic aortic injury. Mediastinal widening greater than 8 cm has a sensitivity of 92 per cent (i.e. only 8 per cent false negatives), but a specificity of less than 10 per cent (i.e. over 90 per cent false positives) in predicting transection. Other suggestive X-ray signs include deviation of the trachea, nasogastric tube or central venous pressure line, and blurring of the aortic arch. Since a widened mediastinum on the chest X-ray carries such a high sensitivity and low specificity, further evaluation is required. The investigation of choice is aortic angiography, although some centres use CT scanning. TOE may be used to confirm the site of injury, and is particularly useful in patients who are too unstable to undergo detailed radiological examination. For the definitive diagnosis of transected aorta, TOE yields a sensitivity of 63 per cent and a specificity of 84 per cent.

Anaesthesia for surgical repair of ruptured thoracic aorta

Pre-operatively, adequate intravenous access is established. Arterial pressures proximal and distal to the transection are monitored by cannulation of the right radial or brachial artery and a dorsalis pedis artery. If time permits, a pulmonary artery flotation catheter should be passed. This is especially important if there is evidence of pulmonary or myocardial contusions. In pulmonary contusion, excessive fluid overload may exacerbate pulmonary oedema in the contused areas. In myocardial contusion, left ventricular dysfunction may occur during the period of aortic cross clamping, and vasodilator or inotropic therapy will be needed. Anaesthesia is induced, taking care to choose techniques of induction and maintenance which minimize surges in blood pressure or heart rate. A left double-lumen endobronchial tube is passed, position confirmed by auscultation and fibre-optic bronchoscopy, and the patient placed in the right lateral position. Surgical access is usually through a left thoracotomy incision. After collapse of the upper lung to facilitate access to the descending thoracic aorta, the surgeon commences the aortic repair. Before doing so, the surgeon may decide to use a spinal cord protection technique. Commonly used surgical techniques and their anaesthetic implications are considered below.

In the clamp–repair technique, the surgeon clamps the aorta and performs the repair, if possible in less than 35 minutes. This is the spinal cord ischaemic period, beyond which paraplegia is very likely. The physiology of spinal cord blood flow during descending thoracic aorta cross clamping has been investigated in dogs. Such experiments have shown that during cross clamping of the descending thoracic aorta there is a marked increase in proximal mean arterial pressure (MAPp), central venous pressure (CVP) and cerebrospinal fluid pressure (CSFP). This increase in CSFP is thought to reflect increases in CVP. Cerebral blood flow does not increase, as autoregulation appears to compensate for the marked increase in cerebral perfusion pressure. During cross clamping, distal MAP (MAPd) is markedly reduced. Spinal cord perfusion pressure (SCPP) is dependent on MAPd and CSFP. (SCPP = MAPd-CSFP). During aortic cross clamping, MAPd is reduced and CSFP is increased, consequently reducing SCPP. Theoretically, reduction in CSFP would be beneficial for SCPP. Phlebotomy during aortic cross clamping has been shown in dogs to reduce CVP and also CSFP. However, it also reduced MAPp and MAPd and, because both MAPd and CSFP were reduced, no improvement in SCPP was shown. Clinically, vasodilators and phlebotomy may be used to reduce MAPp and CVP during cross clamping. Theoretically this would not improve SCPP, but it may be necessary during aortic cross clamping to prevent left ventricular failure, which may develop as a consequence of left ventricular dysfunction, secondary to myocardial contusion or ischaemic heart disease. If such a scenario is anticipated pre-operatively, use of partial pump bypass or a Gott shunt bypass may be preferable (see below).

In the partial pump bypass technique, prior to clamping the aorta the surgeon establishes perfusion of the lower body by a left atrial–femoral arterial partial bypass. In this technique, the left atrium and a femoral artery are cannulated and the lower body is perfused by a centrifugal pump. Since the blood does not have to go through an oxygenator, heparin can be withheld. The advantages of this technique are good operative field exposure, pre- and afterload reduction and maintenance of stable distal aortic perfusion without heparin. Alternatively, partial bypass via cannulation of the femoral vein and artery can be used with an oxygenator to maintain lower body perfusion.

In the Gott shunt bypass technique, the surgeon bypasses the rupture site within the chest without recourse to an extracorporeal circuit system. The shunt may be placed proximally into the left ventricle, the ascending thoracic aorta, the aortic arch or the descending aorta proximal to the rupture. The shunt is inserted distally into the descending thoracic aorta beyond the repair site or, if necessary, into the abdominal aorta or a femoral artery. This technique has been very successful in preventing spinal cord ischaemia in patients undergoing repair of descending thoracic aortic aneurysms.

Despite the use of protective measures, the most important factor in reducing post-operative paraplegia is a cross clamp time of less than 35 minutes.

Injury to the other great vessels

Injury to the other great vessels, arterial or venous, will lead to haemorrhagic shock, haemothorax or cardiac tamponade. Treatment involves rapid volume replacement, chest drain insertion and thoracotomy.

Tracheal and bronchial disruption

Most patients with tracheal and bronchial disruption do not survive to reach hospital. This is partly because major airway injury is usually accompanied by other catastrophically serious intrathoracic and spinal injuries. Most tracheobronchial injuries occur within 2.5 cm of the carina. The patient may have signs of acute dyspnoea, dramatically worsening surgical emphysema, haemoptysis and pneumothorax, which may be tensioning. If the lung cannot be re-inflated after insertion of chest drains, or there is a persistent air leak via the drains, a breach in the integrity of the airway should be strongly suspected. If the patient has been intubated with a single-lumen endotracheal tube, an air leak may become apparent on application of positive pressure, rendering ventilation difficult. The site of the tracheobronchial tear can be identified by fibre-optic bronchoscopy. The torn airway can be isolated by endobronchially intubating the intact bronchus, using a right or left endobronchial double-lumen tube as appropriate. If there is a small tracheal tear, a single-lumen endotracheal tube may be placed with the cuff distal to the wound site and the patient safely ventilated.

Blast lung injury

Perhaps the earliest accounts of this condition go back to the 18th century, when respiratory difficulties were noted in gunners in the British Navy who stood too close to a firing cannon. The condition was described as an adverse effect of 'the wind of the shot'. In 1924, Hooker first described 'air concussion' in blast victims as a specific condition, but it was only during the Second World War that the pathophysiology of blast lung injury was beginning to be understood.

The rapid conversion of solid or liquid explosive material to the gaseous phase gives rise to a massive increase in pressure and heat, resulting in the blast wave, which spreads radially from the explosive focus as the blast wave front. The blast wave rapidly reaches a peak (3–5 atmospheres), and then slowly (2–3 ms) declines to sub-atmospheric pressure. The physical characteristics of the blast wave may be described in terms of velocity, wavelength and amplitude. However, it is the magnitude of the positive amplitude of the blast wave that principally determines resultant blast lung injury. Blast wave amplitude rapidly declines with distance from the explosive focus, and may be further diminished by obstacles in the way. Injury to tissues caused by the blast wave itself is called primary blast injury. Moving radially from the explosive focus, three areas of reducing vulnerability to the effects of primary blast injury have been described. The area nearest to the explosion, where all victims will be instantly killed, is called the 'lethal zone'. Beyond this is the 'L-50 limit', where 50 per cent of victims will be instantly killed, and beyond this is the 'injury zone', in which instant death does not occur as a result of the primary blast wave, although the victim may still sustain significant injury. It is victims within the L-50 and injury zones who are likely to suffer from blast lung injury.

The incidence of bomb blast victims sustaining blast lung injury varies widely depending on circumstances. There is a much higher incidence of blast lung injury following an explosion in an enclosed space than following open air bombings. In open air bombings, victims generally suffer from secondary and tertiary blast injury. Secondary blast injury refers to tissue injury due to flying shrapnel and debris. Tertiary injury refers to injuries sustained by being hurled against a stationary surface, and may involve deceleration and blunt injury mechanisms as mentioned above. Finally, quaternary injury describes injury from scalds caused by intense heat and the inhalation of smoke and dust.

Pathophysiology of blast lung injury

Pulmonary parenchymal damage

When the blast wave front hits tissue that contains pockets of air, these pockets are compressed. As the blast wave passes, there is rapid expansion of these compressed gas pockets, resulting in secondary 'explosions' within gas-filled tissue. This is particularly important within the lung, but can also lead to rupture of gas-containing organs such as the gastrointestinal tract and the middle ear. If the pressure wave hits fluid-containing tissue such as alveolar capillaries, which are relatively non-compressible as compared with the relatively compressible gas filled alveoli, this leads to a pressure differential between the alveolar capillaries and the alveolar spaces and causes fluid to pass from the high pressure within the capillaries to the lower pressure within the alveoli. Fluid and blood accumulate within alveolar spaces, a process that is further enhanced by breaches in alveolar capillary integrity caused by the blast wave itself. Massive rupture of capillaries and extravasation of red cells leads to release of haemoglobin, which is subsequently oxidized to met-haemoglobin. This interacts with lipid hydroperoxides to produce ferryl-haemoglobin. This potent oxidant induces tissue damage directly by peroxidation reactions, and indirectly by depleting intrapulmonary anti-oxidant reserves (ascorbate, vitamin E, GSH). By these and other mechanisms, the clinical picture of worsening respiratory distress rapidly develops.

Arterial air embolism

Tears in small airways under pressure may lead to a unique form of air embolism due to alveolar–pulmonary venous fistulae through which air passes directly to the pulmonary veins and rapidly to the systemic circulation. If air emboli enter the coronary circulation, myocardial ischaemia and arrhythmias develop. This is thought to contribute to many of the deaths within the lethal zone of the blast. Such air emboli may also contribute to neurological deficit in bomb blast patients.

Clinical appearances of blast lung injury

Sometimes there may be no external sign of chest injury. Despite this, increasing hypoxia, dyspnoea, haemoptysis, myocardial ischaemia and confusion develop. Serial X-rays show development of uni- or bilateral pulmonary infiltrates, which may have a bat-wing appearance. Uni- or bilateral pneumothoraces may also be seen.

In respiratory distress, early intubation and ventilation is required. The mode of ventilation in these patients is a matter of debate, some authors suggesting that intermittent positive pressure ventilation (IPPV) in the immediate post trauma phase carries the theoretical risk of barotrauma and additional arterial air embolism. Such considerations have led some to advocate high frequency jet ventilation in these patients to reduce tidal volumes and airway pressures. Nevertheless, IPPV has been used satisfactorily in these patients, both intra-operatively and in the intensive care unit.

The preceding account has focused on blast lung injury as a syndrome. However, the victim is likely to have multiple trauma, both thoracic and non-thoracic.

General principles of anaesthesia for thoracic trauma

Pre-operative preparation

It may be impossible to obtain a previous medical history. Blood tests and arterial blood gas analysis are useful as baseline measurements, but by the time the result is available these may bear little relation to the current state of the patient.

Cause of death is usually exsanguination; large-bore cannulae including, if possible, a central venous pressure cannula should be inserted pre-operatively, and massive blood transfusion organized. This may lead to fluid overload, hypothermia, hypocalcaemia and coagulopathy. Progress with blood replacement should be monitored by CVP trends, and by checking blood samples regularly for arterial pH, ionized calcium, base excess, haematocrit, haemoglobin and clotting status. Intravenous fluid and patient warming devices should be used. It is always ideal to anaesthetize the euvolaemic patient, but for emergency thoracotomy the anaesthetist may not have this luxury. As mentioned previously in the section *Anaesthesia for surgical repair of ruptured thoracic aorta*, it may be advisable pre-operatively to pass a pulmonary artery flotation catheter, particularly if there is any risk of left ventricular dysfunction during aortic cross clamping.

Anaesthetic management

The patient is likely to have a full stomach; rapid sequence induction with pre-oxygenation and cricoid pressure is indicated. An anaesthetic technique of induction and maintenance should be chosen with which myocardial depression or systemic vasodilatation is minimal. In the hypovolaemic patient, induction with either ketamine 0.25–0.5 mg/kg or etomidate 0.2–0.3 mg/kg followed by suxamethonium to allow rapid optimal intubating conditions is recommended. During intubation, an assistant should provide counter-traction to the head, unless the cervical spine has been cleared radiologically. In pulmonary lacerations and contusions, such as those following gunshot wounds to the chest, haemorrhage into the bronchial tree frequently occurs. A double-lumen endobronchial tube should be placed to isolate the bleeding lung.

Post-operatively, it is appropriate to change the endotracheal tube to a single-lumen tube in the operating room and then transfer the patient to the intensive care unit.

The problems the patient faces post-operatively are multiple, but will stem from the primary pulmonary injury due to the trauma and then the super-imposed secondary systemic injury. Secondary lung injury may result from massive transfusion, fat embolism or sepsis. Renal dysfunction may arise as a result of hypotension, or in association with ARDS or sepsis.

KEY POINTS

- Trauma is the single greatest cause of death in young people. Chest trauma contributes to death in half of these.

- Chest trauma may be considered as penetrating, non-penetrating or both.

- Life-threatening consequences of chest trauma include tension pneumo-thorax, haemothorax and cardiac tamponade. Prompt institution of fluid resuscitation, chest drain placement and/or pericardiocentesis may be life saving.

- Thoracotomy is usually indicated for management of persistent haemo-thorax or repair of a ruptured airway.

- Anaesthetic management is aimed at prevention of spillage of blood into undamaged areas of lung, controlling ventilation by isolating damaged lung or airways, maintaining circulating blood volume and employing cardiovascularly stable techniques of anaesthesia.

- Surgery for transected thoracic aorta carries the risk of spinal cord ischaemia.

- Blast lung injury may occur in the absence of external signs of thoracic injury. It may complicate management in the already multiply injured patient.

- The patient with major thoracic trauma is at high risk of multiple organ failure.

Bibliography

Ahmed, Z. and Mohyuddin, Z. (1995). Management of flail chest injury: internal fixation versus endotracheal intubation and ventilation. *J. Thorac. Cardiovasc. Surg.*, **110(6),** 1676–80.

Brismar, B. and Bergenwald, L. (1982). The terrorist bomb explosion in Bologna, Italy. *J. Trauma*, **22(3),** 216–20.

Ciraulo, D.L., Elliott, D., Mitchell, K.A. and Rodriguez, A. (1994) Flail chest as a marker for significant injuries. *J. Am. Coll. Surg.*, **178(5),** 466–70.

Cohn, S.M. (1997). Pulmonary contusion: review of the clinical entity. *J. Trauma*, **42(5),** 973–9.

Devitt, J.H., McClean, R.F. and McClellan, B.A. (1993). Peri-operative cardiovascular complications associated with blunt thoracic trauma. *Can. J. Anaesth.*, **40(3),** 197–200.

Finucane, B.T. (1991). Thoracic trauma. In *Thoracic Anaesthesia* (J.A. Kaplan, ed.), pp. 463–84. Churchill Livingstone Inc.

Gebhard, F., Kelbel, M.W., Strecker, W. *et al.* (1997). Chest trauma and its impact on the release of vasoactive mediators. *Shock*, **7(5)**, 313–17.

Hoff, S.J., Shotts, S.D., Eddy, V.A. and Morris, J.A. Jr (1994). Outcome of isolated pulmonary contusion in blunt trauma patients. *Am. Surg.*, **60(2)**, 138–42.

Hunt J.P., Baker C.C., Lentz C.W. *et al.* (1996). Thoracic aorta injuries: management and outcome of 144 patients. *J Trauma.*, **40(4)**, 547–55.

Kram H.B., Appel P.L., Wohlmuth D.A. and Shoemaker W.C. (1989). Diagnosis of traumatic thoracic aortic rupture: a 10-year retrospective analysis. *Ann Thorac Surg.*, **47(2)**, 282–6.

Leibovici, D., Gofrit, O.N., Stein, M. *et al.* (1996). Blast injuries: bus versus open air bombings – a comparative study of injuries in survivors of open air versus confined space explosions. *J. Trauma*, **41(6)**, 1030–5.

Mazzorana, V., Smith, R.S., Morabito, D.J. and Brar, H.S. (1994). Limited utility of emergency department thoracotomy. *Am. Surg.*, **60(7)**, 516–21.

Peclet, M.H., Newman, K.D., Eichelberger, M.R. *et al.* (1990). Thoracic trauma in children: an indicator of increased mortality. *J. Pediatr. Surg.*, **25(9)**, 961–5.

Perchinsky, M.J., Long, W.B. and Hill, J.G. (1995). Blunt cardiac rupture. *Arch. Surg.*, **130**, 852–7.

Peterson, R.J., Tiwary, A.D., Kissoon, N. *et al.* (1994). Pediatric penetrating trauma: a 5-year experience. *Pediatr. Emerg. Care*, **10(3)**, 129–31.

Saletta, S., Lederman, E., Fein, S. *et al.* (1995). Transoesophageal echocardiography for the initial evaluation of the widened mediastinum in trauma patients. *J. Trauma*, **39(1)**, 137–41.

Shorr, R.M., Crittenden, M., Indeck, M. *et al.* (1987). Blunt thoracic trauma: analysis of 515 patients. *Ann. Surg.*, **206**, 200–5.

Stafford, P.W. and Harmon, C.M. (1993) Thoracic trauma in children. *Curr. Opin. Pediatr.*, **5(3)**, 325–32.

Verdant, A., Cossette, R., Page, A. *et al.* (1995). Aneurysms of the descending thoracic aorta: 366 consecutive cases resected without paraplegia. *J. Vasc. Surg.*, **21(3)**, 385–90.

Wagner, R.B., Slivko, B., Jamieson, P.M. *et al.* (1991). Effect of lung contusion on pulmonary hemodynamics. *Ann. Thorac. Surg.*, **52(1)**, 51–8.

12

Paediatric thoracic anaesthesia

S. J. B. Nicoll and R. Bingham

Introduction

This chapter begins by reviewing the physiology of one-lung ventilation in infants and children. Peri-operative care of the child undergoing thoracic surgery is discussed. Specific conditions and procedures and their anaesthetic implications are then presented in more detail. Although some of the material is covered in other chapters, it is appropriate to discuss it again here with the emphasis on paediatric anaesthetic practice. The chapter concludes with a brief review of the medical conditions of asthma and cystic fibrosis.

General principles

Physiology of one-lung ventilation in children

Most thoracic surgery is performed in the lateral decubitus position. In adult patients who are awake, breathing spontaneously and in the lateral position, gravity causes a vertical gradient in pulmonary blood flow and pleural pressure so flow (Q) and ventilation (V) are greatest in the dependent lung and the V/Q ratio is not altered to any great extent. In spontaneously breathing infants and children, however, the distribution of ventilation in response to gravity is the opposite of that seen in adults – that is, it is better to the non-dependent lung. Therefore, ventilation in infants and very young children with unilateral lung disease is optimized if they are positioned with their better lung uppermost. Perfusion, however, remains better in the dependent lung, which results in some V/Q mismatch and a reduction in Pao_2. These differences in ventilation may be due to the greater compliance of the chest wall seen in this age group. Functional residual capacity (FRC) is close to residual volume, so airway closure can occur during tidal ventilation in the dependent lung. This pattern is seen until around the age of 10 years, when there is a gradual transition to an adult pattern.

The effects of one-lung ventilation on pulmonary haemodynamics and gas exchange in neonates have been investigated using an animal model. Hypoxic pulmonary vasoconstriction may be age-dependent, and more pronounced in infants than adults. Normal neonates have a lower arterial oxygen tension (Pao_2) than adults, mainly due to greater inequalities in

V/Q ratios and impaired oxygen diffusion. Total lung volume, vital capacity and FRC are all less per unit body mass compared with those of a child over the age of 7 years. Metabolic rate and alveolar ventilation are both approximately twice the adult values. In theory, therefore, one-lung ventilation may critically interfere with gas exchange. A recent study using newborn domestic pigs, however, showed that the arterial oxygen saturation remained stable during one-lung ventilation (with a fractional inspired oxygen concentration of 1.0), and there were only slight increases in pulmonary artery pressure, intrapulmonary shunt and Pa_{CO_2}.

In practice, despite theoretical considerations, the ventilation and perfusion abnormalities in infants and small children may be ameliorated by careful monitoring of alveolar and arterial gas tensions and employing an increased FiO_2.

Pre-operative assessment

The pre-operative assessment should ascertain the child's baseline respiratory status and the degree of functional impairment present. In addition, it is important to determine whether any improvement can be obtained by pre-operative measures such as the use of bronchodilators, antibiotics and physiotherapy.

In addition to the routine pre-anaesthetic assessment, the history should concentrate on cough, dyspnoea, wheeze, exercise tolerance, recurrent infection, failure to thrive and weight loss. The drug history may include bronchodilators (including home nebulizers), current or recent steroids, antibiotics and oxygen dependence. The examination should follow the standard routine of inspection, palpation, percussion and auscultation. In particular, signs of respiratory distress such as tachypnoea, use of accessory muscles, stridor or wheeze and intercostal recession should be sought. A raised jugular venous pressure, right ventricular heave and hepatomegaly may indicate the presence of cor pulmonale. Other congenital abnormalities should be identified or excluded.

The following investigations should be considered:

- Full blood count
- Cross match
- Urea and electrolytes (U + E)
- Sputum for culture
- Chest X-ray
- Electrocardiograph (ECG) ± echocardiography
- Computerized tomography (CT)
- Pulmonary function tests
- Arterial blood gases.

A baseline haemoglobin should be checked for anaemia or, conversely, polycythaemia secondary to chronic hypoxia. The white cell count and differential may indicate active infection. Patients on chronic diuretic therapy should have their U + E checked. Arterial blood gas sampling is a painful invasive procedure and is rarely done pre-operatively in children, although a chronic respiratory acidosis may indicate an increased requirement for post-operative ventilation. Pulse oximetry is a useful non-invasive method of determining baseline oxygen saturation on air, and the response to supplemental oxygen. Pulmonary function test ranges are available for children, but co-operation tends to be poor in those under 5 years old.

The child's medical condition should be optimized and pre-operative drug therapy continued.

Monitoring

Surgical manipulation during thoracic surgery can cause sudden cardio-vascular compromise and difficulties with ventilation. All patients require routine minimal monitoring with an ECG, non-invasive blood pressure measurement, a pulse oximeter, gas analysis (including fractional inspired oxygen concentration (FiO_2), end-tidal carbon dioxide ($EtCO_2$) and anaes-thetic vapour), a peripheral nerve stimulator, a ventilator alarm and temperature measurement. In addition, more invasive monitoring should be considered for patients with complex pre-operative disease and those undergoing major surgery. An arterial line is useful, as it allows immediate observation of beat-to-beat changes in blood pressure and simplifies blood sampling for arterial gases, acid–base status and haematocrit. It is not neces-sary to measure central venous pressure (CVP) in all cases, but it may be used to assess intravascular volume in patients in whom major blood loss is anticipated, or if a requirement for inotropic support is anticipated. A pre-cordial or oesophageal stethoscope allows auscultation of the heart and breath sounds, and may help with early detection of bronchospasm and airway obstruction. Since an oesophageal stethoscope lies centrally, it cannot identify the site of a unilateral problem. Manual ventilation may allow changes in resistance and compliance to be identified quickly. Blood loss and urine output measurement may be helpful if significant haemor-rhage is expected.

Equipment

In any thoracotomy, as large an intravenous cannula as possible should be inserted to allow rapid transfusion, as there is the potential for considerable blood loss. One-lung ventilation is usually used during thoracic surgery in adults. Absolute indications for this include massive air loss (e.g. from a large bronchopleural fistula) or the risk of contamination of the unaffected lung (e.g. from bronchial haemorrhage, during bronchopulmonary lavage or from a lung abscess). It allows easier access for the surgeon, avoids the need for surgical retraction on the operated lung and minimizes damage. In adults and older children, this is usually achieved by using a double-lumen tracheal tube or, occasionally, an endobronchial tube or bronchial blocker. Double-lumen tubes are not readily available in sizes suitable for infants and small children.

Methods of lung separation in children

Surgical retraction

This is the simplest and commonest method, and is adequate for most purposes. This technique can result in airway obstruction, a reduction in cardiac output and, rarely, lung damage.

Double-lumen tubes (Tables 12.1 and 12.2)

1. Conventional small adult double-lumen tubes for children over 12 years, e.g. 35 French.
2. Small paediatric double-lumen tubes: Mallinckrodt make 28 or 32 French paediatric BronchoCaths. These are left-sided tubes; the smallest right-sided tube made by Mallinckrodt is a 35 French.
3. Marraro bilumen tube: this consists of two separate uncuffed tubes of different lengths attached laterally to each other. Each lumen is circular rather than D-shaped. A larger tube size than normal can be used, because the tubes are uncuffed. When the Marraro tube is made from tubes with different diameters, the bronchial lumen is always larger to reduce gas loss. Both tubes end in a lip shape, with the bronchial tube having a Murphy's eye. There is no carinal hook. It is available in sizes suitable for premature babies from 1500 g upwards to 5 year old children.

Bronchial blockade

With a bronchial blocker in place, obstruction of the non-ventilated

Table 12.1 Approximate suggested age ranges and sizes for Marraro Bilumen tubes. When the sizes of the lumen differ, the larger is the bronchial lumen

Age	Approximate size (ID mm)
Premature baby 1400–2500 g	2 + 2
Newborn 2500–4000 g	2.5 + 2 2.5 + 2.5
1 month	2.5 + 2.5
6 months	3 + 2.5
12 months	3.5 + 3

Table 12.2 Sizes and approximate suggested ages for double-lumen and Univent tubes

Tube type	Size	Tracheal lumen (OD m)	Bronchial lumen (OD m)	Approx. age (years)
Double-lumen	28	9.3–9.5	7.3–7.5	10
Double-lumen	32	10.6	N/A	12
Double-lumen	35	11.6	9.5	over 12
Univent	3.5	7.5–8	N/A	8
Univent	4.5	8.5–9	N/A	10

bronchus results in lung collapse from absorption atelectasis. Bronchial blockade can be achieved by using:

1. A conventional single-lumen tracheal tube passed endobronchially on non-operative side.
2. A tracheal tube plus Fogarty embolectomy catheter, balloon-tipped radiology catheter or modified Foley catheter passed beyond the tip of the tube in the trachea into the bronchus to be occluded.
3. A modified tracheal tube, e.g. Univent tube. This has an additional small lumen, containing a bronchus blocker with a suction channel, that can be advanced blindly or under direct vision using a fibre-optic scope. It is advanced past the end of the larger lumen into the bronchus, which is then obstructed by inflating a balloon. Fuji Systems Corporation now make these tubes in sizes 3.5 and 4.0 mm internal diameter (Table 12.2).

Analgesia

Post-thoracotomy pain is severe, and providing effective, safe analgesia in infants and children is difficult. Pulmonary complications may be reduced when patients are able to breathe deeply, cough and move around. The methods available include:

- Opioids – by systemic infusion or intermittent injection.
- Single shot or continuous paravertebral infusion of local anaesthetic.
- Single shot or continuous thoracic extradural infusion of local anaesthetic/opioid.
- Continuous intrapleural infusion of local anaesthetic.
- Single shot or continuous intercostal nerve block.

Optimal analgesia is usually obtained by using a combination of techniques. Non-steroidal anti-inflammatory drugs (NSAIDs) such as diclofenac and ibuprofen have a morphine-sparing effect, and are given to most children in the absence of a specific contraindication such as asthma or renal impairment. They are not routinely used in infants under 1 year old. Paracetamol may given instead of, or in addition to, NSAIDs. These drugs can be administered orally or rectally.

Traditionally, systemic opioids have been used to provide pain relief despite potential problems with respiratory depression. Opioid infusions used alone or in combination with regional analgesia remain the commonest way of managing post-operative pain after a thoracotomy. Morphine can be given intravenously or subcutaneously in a dose range of 10–30 μg/kg per hour. Children over the age of 5–6 years can usually manage a patient-controlled analgesia pump. Younger children require nurse controlled analgesia. In the latter technique, a low dose background infusion (0–20 μg/kg per hour) is often run in addition to the bolus doses of morphine (10–20 μg/kg). These children require close monitoring and supervision so that side effects such as sedation, respiratory depression and nausea and vomiting are either prevented or recognized and treated promptly.

All the regional anaesthetic techniques have potential problems; technical difficulties siting the catheter and failure to provide complete analgesia are the commonest.

Paravertebral catheters can be inserted under direct vision into the extrapleural paravertebral space at the time of surgery. In a recent study, 90 per cent of infants received effective analgesia using this method; the 10 per cent failure rate was due to catheter blockage.

Extradural analgesia can be used with the catheter inserted at the caudal, lumbar or thoracic level. Placing the catheter at the level of the surgical incision reduces the total dose of local anaesthetic required, but the risk of dural puncture, vascular damage and neurological damage is theoretically higher. It is often easy to advance an epidural catheter to the appropriate level from the lumbar region in infants and small children. In infants under 6 months the caudal route can also be used for this purpose.

Extradural opioids have some advantages over local anaesthetic agents, as there is no motor, sensory or sympathetic block. When given in combination with local anaesthetic, lower doses of both drugs can be used, with a resultant reduction in side effects. With certain opioids (e.g. morphine) the quality of analgesia may be better, the duration of action longer, the total dose reduced and the incidence of side effects fewer compared with the same drug given parenterally. Extradural administration of opioids is not without risk. Side effects of extradural opioids include sedation, respiratory depression, nausea and vomiting, pruritus and urinary retention. Pruritus and urinary retention may be reversed by giving naloxone 0.5 μg/kg intravenously. Respiratory depression should be managed by stopping the infusion and giving naloxone 4 μg/kg intravenously.

Intrapleural local anaesthetic can be given via a catheter placed directly between the visceral and parietal pleura at the time of surgery. Intrapleural infusion of bupivacaine has been shown to be variably effective, with inadequate analgesia if the patient is sitting up due to rapid run off of local anaesthetic. This does not occur if the local anaesthetic is retained in an extrapleural paravertebral pocket.

Single shot intercostal blocks have been a popular method of analgesia for many years, because they are easy to perform and free from opioid-type side effects. However, analgesia is limited to the duration of local anaesthetic activity. In an effort to overcome this, continuous intercostal nerve blocks have been attempted. These can be achieved by placing two catheters subpleurally under direct vision into posterior intercostal spaces at the time of surgery. This technique does not provide complete analgesia, and is associated with high levels of systemic local anaesthetic absorption.

Specific conditions

Conditions associated with gas trapping

Congenital lobar emphysema

Over-distension of a lobe due to air trapping compresses the surrounding normal lung tissue and causes mediastinal shift. It is usually unilateral; the left upper lobe is the commonest site, then right middle lobe and right upper lobe. The male to female ratio is 2 : 1, and congenital lobar emphysema usually presents between birth and 6 months of age. The aetiology is unknown in around 50 per cent of cases. Obstruction of the bronchus supplying the affected lobe may be extrinsic (e.g. by the pulmonary artery or lymph nodes), or due to bronchial stenosis or bronchomalacia. Congenital heart disease is associated in 10–15 per cent of cases; usually a ventricular septal defect, patent ductus arteriosus or an absent pulmonary valve.

The clinical presentation is usually respiratory distress with tachypnoea, wheeze and cyanosis or recurrent chest infections in the early neonatal period. There may be severe hypoxia due to a combination of the emphysematous lobe and compression atelectasis.

The chest X-ray may show an emphysematous lobe, mediastinal shift and compression atelectasis. The differential diagnosis includes post-pneumonic pneumatocele, pulmonary cystic disease, congenital diaphragmatic hernia, foreign body inhalation and pneumothorax. The presence of bronchial and vascular markings should help distinguish between a pneumothorax and congenital lobar emphysema.

Bronchoscopy may occasionally be required to exclude intraluminal obstruction by a foreign body as the underlying cause, but is usually unnecessary and may be dangerous. Lobectomy is the management of choice and is usually curative; however, some infants develop further areas of emphysematous lung post-operatively.

Bronchogenic cyst

Bronchogenic cysts can present at any age, but are usually seen in older children. Cysts are unilocular and filled with fluid and/or air. They lie in the parenchymal tissue or adjacent to the tracheobronchial tree, but do not communicate with it. Some patients may be asymptomatic with the cyst being found on chest X-ray, whilst others present with cough and recurrent chest infections. Occasionally, respiratory distress from bronchial obstruction occurs. Chest X-ray and computerized tomography are useful in making the diagnosis. Differential diagnoses include mediastinal mass, congenital lobar emphysema and lung abscess.

Cysts are removed, as they represent a potential focus for infection and can cause cardiovascular compromise, respiratory distress and life-threatening airway obstruction. Open thoracotomy is usually required, although thoracoscopic resection is possible.

Anaesthetic technique

There is a theoretical risk of deterioration associated with the use of nitrous oxide (N_2O) and controlled ventilation. Although this risk has probably been over-emphasized, caution is advised. Gas-filled spaces within the body may expand significantly when nitrous oxide diffuses into them, and it is therefore best avoided until the emphysematous lobe or cyst has been removed. Positive pressure ventilation may also cause expansion of an emphysematous lobe and mediastinal shift. Some authors recommend spontaneous ventilation until the bronchus is controlled, but this may result in inadequate ventilation. In practice, paralysis and gentle positive pressure ventilation with low inflation pressures is well tolerated.

Pulmonary parenchymal problems

Lung abscess

Lung abscesses are now uncommon. They may be due to a primary bacterial infection, for example with staphylococci or klebsiella, or secondary to aspiration of a foreign body. There is usually a history of fever, cough and weight loss, although there may be minimal clinical signs in children compared with adults. The diagnosis is usually made using a combination of a chest X-ray, CT scan and blood cultures. The chest X-ray may show single or multiple abscesses and, possibly, an air–fluid level. Primary abscesses are treated with antibiotics, secondary require surgical drainage. Soiling of other areas of lung is a risk during surgery; therefore, one-lung anaesthesia may be required.

Sequestered lobe

Embryonic and non-functioning lung tissue is sequestered from normal lung, and receives its blood supply from the aorta or one of its branches. This tissue can be intralobar or extralobar and usually consists of multiple cysts, which become infected. Intralobar sequestration may present late with recurrent chest infections or lung abscess. Occasionally the sequestered tissue communicates with the oesophagus, although this rarely remains patent. If a fistula persists between the abnormal tissue and the oesophagus, there may be severe respiratory distress. Management is by lobectomy, with division of the fistula if present. Blood loss from aberrant arteries can be severe. The condition is associated with other congenital abnormalities in around 50 per cent of cases, and around half the cases are diagnosed in the first year of life.

Bronchiectasis

Dilated bronchi due to inflammation lead to recurrent chest infections. Bronchiectasis is associated with cystic fibrosis, recurrent lower airway disease, recurrent chronic aspiration or aspiration of a foreign body. Children present with a persistent cough and purulent sputum. It is commonest in the left lower lobe, lingula or right middle lobe, but is often more diffuse. These patients should be managed with antibiotics and chest physiotherapy with postural drainage. Anaesthesia may be required for bronchoscopy and lobectomy. As with a lung abscess, there is the potential for contamination from infected material. Bronchial blockers or a double-lumen tube may be required to prevent contamination of the healthy lung. If possible, surgery should be delayed until the child is older.

Other conditions

Congenital diaphragmatic hernia

This condition is included here because the primary pathology is intra-thoracic, although the surgery is normally performed via a laparotomy incision. There are several types; the commonest is a left postero-lateral hernia through the foramen of Bochdalek or pleuro-peritoneal sinus. The incidence of congenital diaphragmatic hernia is 1 in 4000, but the perinatal mortality rate is 1 in 2000 live births. The high mortality rate in this condition is due to pulmonary hypoplasia, which occurs mainly on the affected side but often on the opposite side as well. This is particularly severe when the abdominal viscera herniate early during fetal development leading to a combination of hypoplasia and atelectasis. Herniation through the foramen of Morgagni is not associated with severe hypoplasia. The prognosis depends on the degree of hypoplasia and severity of any associated abnormalities. The leading causes of death are:

- Associated anomalies – for example, malrotation, cardiac, renal or neurological
- Pulmonary hypoplasia and unrelenting pulmonary hypertension
- Iatrogenic barotrauma
- Bleeding – usually if extracorporeal membrane oxygenation (ECMO) is used.

Congenital diaphragmatic hernia may be diagnosed antenatally by ultrasound. Clinical signs in the neonate include respiratory distress (cyanosis, tachypnoea and intercostal recession), mediastinal shift, absent breath sounds on the affected side and the classic scaphoid abdomen. There may be severe hypoxia, hypercapnia and acidosis. The chest X-ray is diagnostic, showing bowel in the chest and mediastinal shift with compression of the contralateral lung. This may sometimes be mistaken for congenital lobar emphysema.

Surgical repair of congenital diaphragmatic hernia was formerly an emergency procedure with a high mortality rate. It is now agreed that early surgery does not convey any advantage, and has an adverse effect on pulmonary mechanics. Most centres opt for a period of stabilization. The mortality rate for this procedure is around 50 per cent. Factors associated with a poor outcome include the presence pre-operatively of high inflation pressures above 40 cmH$_2$O, CO$_2$ retention and acidosis. In addition, around 15 per cent of cases develop a transitional circulation with pulmonary hypertension. When pulmonary arterial pressure (PAP) becomes supra-systemic, blood shunts away from the lungs through the ductus arteriosus. If the right ventricle fails, right atrial pressure is higher than left so blood shunts through the foramen ovale, which leads to progressive hypoxia and acidosis. This can be monitored using echocardiography. These neonates die from critical hypoxia unless pulmonary vascular resistance can be reduced. Various pharmacological vasodilators have been used, e.g. tolazoline, sodium nitroprusside, glyceryl trinitrate and prostacyclin, but coincidental systemic hypotension compounds the problem by encouraging right to left shunting and reducing myocardial perfusion. Nitric oxide (NO) is a selective pulmonary vasodilator that has been used in an attempt to reduce PAP and the requirement for ventilatory support or ECMO. Despite initial reports that nitric oxide produces immediate improvements in oxygenation, a recent study has shown that inhaled nitric oxide did not reduce the need for ECMO or the mortality rate. ECMO has been used pre-operatively as a bridge until the PAP is reduced, and there are some reports of successful repair on ECMO. In a comparative study between Boston and Toronto, conventional mechanical ventilation (CMV) with ECMO as rescue produced an overall survival equivalent to CMV with high frequency oscillatory ventilation (HFOV) rescue. Neither HFOV or ECMO has significantly improved outcome, but the introduction of permissive hypercapnia has. Formerly, aggressive hyperventilation and alkalosis were used in an attempt to reduce pulmonary hypertension and right-to-left shunting. Permissive hypercapnia is thought to increase survival because it limits ventilator-induced lung damage and preserves alveoli.

Anaesthetic technique

Most infants are ventilated pre-operatively, and surgery is performed when they are stable. For those who are not, care should be taken to avoid gut distension with bag and mask ventilation. A nasogastric tube or Repogle double-lumen sump tube should be placed early and put on continuous drainage. The infant is paralysed and ventilated, with the inflation pressure kept as low as possible. Intra-operatively, anaesthesia is commonly maintained using an opioid-based technique (e.g. fentanyl 10 μg/kg) since postoperative ventilation is usual. A volatile agent may be added as required. A pneumothorax can occur in the contralateral lung at any time; this should be considered if there is any deterioration in the child's condition. No attempt should be made to re-expand the ipsilateral lung. Postoperatively, primary pulmonary hypertension can be a problem (see above).

These infants can do well following successful repair, as the number of alveoli continues to increase until about the age of 8 years.

Oesophageal atresia and tracheo-oesophageal fistula

Oesophageal atresia, plus or minus a fistula, has an incidence of 1 in 3000 live births. There are five different types. Between 30 and 50 per cent have associated anomalies; congenital cardiac disease, the VATER syndrome (cardiac, vertebral, renal and anorectal abnormalities), laryngo- or tracheo-malacia, cleft lip and palate. Oesophageal atresia is associated with maternal polyhydramnios, premature labour and low birth weight. The diagnosis should be suspected at birth if the baby drools saliva, or chokes and regurgitates when first fed. Inability to pass a 10 FG catheter down the oesophagus into the stomach confirms the diagnosis. A plain X-ray will show the radio-opaque catheter in the blind upper pouch. With a distal tracheo-oesophageal fistula, a gas bubble may be seen in the stomach. Contrast should not be used in these studies, as there is a risk of aspiration and subsequent pneumonitis. A fistula without atresia may be more difficult to diagnose. Once the diagnosis has been made, a Repogle tube (double-lumen sump tube) should be inserted into the upper pouch and continuous low-pressure suction applied. These neonates are at constant risk of aspiration and pulmonary infection, and should be managed actively with physiotherapy, antibiotics, and early surgery to try and avoid pulmonary complications. Those with infant respiratory distress syndrome and low pulmonary compliance may need urgent fistula ligation to prevent gastric distension. Gastrostomies are not performed routinely, and should only be required in patients in whom a primary anastomosis is impossible. Pre-operative echocardiography should be performed routinely to exclude congenital heart disease.

Anaesthetic technique

There are several potential problems during this procedure:

- Increased risk of aspiration
- Positive pressure ventilation causing gas to pass through the fistula into the stomach
- Gastric distension leading to hypoventilation and an inadequate venous return
- Airway obstruction from surgical manipulation and secretions.

Traditionally, awake intubation has been advocated as a means of avoiding the theoretical problem of being unable to ventilate the lungs in a paralysed patient. Recently, however, it has been recognized that not only is awake intubation unpleasant, but that neuromuscular blockade increases the compliance of the chest and therefore enhances pulmonary ventilation.

Following suction to the upper pouch, an inhalational induction is usually performed. Intubation is accomplished under neuromuscular blockade, usually with suxamethonium. Gentle hand ventilation is used to minimize gastric distension. Following intubation, it may be necessary to alter the position of the tube tip, or angle of the bevel, to optimize ventilation and avoid gastric distension. Anaesthesia is usually maintained with a volatile agent, and the patient paralysed with atracurium. Opiates can be used freely if post-operative ventilation is planned. Tracheal obstruction is common during dissection of the fistula, and hand ventilation at this stage aids early detection. Many surgeons employ a trans-anastomotic nasogastric tube, which replaces the Repogle tube before completion of the oesophageal anastomosis.

All cases should be managed in an intensive care unit post-operatively. Around half will need to be ventilated electively, particularly those with a tight anastomosis. Analgesia can be provided using a systemic morphine infusion or epidural catheter introduced via the caudal route. The latter technique is particularly useful in those expected to be self-ventilating post-operatively.

Anastomotic leaks and strictures are the most frequent surgical complications. Tracheomalacia occurs post-operatively in around 10–20 per cent of patients due to poor stability of the tracheal wall (see below).

The mortality rate in infants with surgically repaired oesophageal atresia and tracheo-oesophageal fistula has fallen, but respiratory complications (e.g. wheeze and lower respiratory tract infection) are common amongst survivors. Pulmonary function tests may show minor obstructive and restrictive defects.

Tracheomalacia

Abnormal flaccidity of the tracheal wall causes collapse, particularly when pressure gradients are high. It may be congenital (very rare) or associated with tracheo-oesophageal fistula or extrinsic compression from vascular anomalies or mediastinal masses. It is most commonly acquired following prolonged intubation or tracheostomy. Children may present with stridor, a persistent cough and chest infection. They tend to obstruct when crying or agitated, and may require nasal CPAP or even a tracheostomy. There is a tendency to try and avoid surgery, if possible, as tracheal wall rigidity improves with age.

Bronchomalacia

Collapse of a mainstem bronchus may be primary or secondary, and may occur in association with tracheomalacia. Primary bronchomalacia is commoner on the left side. Secondary bronchomalacia results from extrinsic compression of the bronchus by the heart, a bronchogenic cyst or vascular ring. It also occurs in ex-premature babies who have received long-term ventilatory support. It plays a role in the development of congenital lobar emphysema. During normal quiet breathing, the pleural pressure remains negative. During forced expiration, the pressure surrounding the bronchus becomes positive. In bronchomalacia a loss of rigidity allows the soft part of the bronchus to collapse, which results in a loud wheeze, retained secretions and chest infections. All patients are symptomatic in the first 6 months, with cough and harsh, low-pitched monophonic wheeze. The diagnosis is normally made by bronchoscopy or tracheobronchography, as signs are not normally obvious on a chest X-ray. Flexible or rigid bronchoscopy with the patient breathing spontaneously will show dynamic collapse of a narrow segment of bronchus.

The medical management includes chest physiotherapy with postural drainage, nebulized ipratropium bromide and CPAP, which may need to be delivered via a tracheostomy. Surgical management includes broncho-pexy or insertion of an endobronchial stent. Gradual improvement occurs with age, but severely affected patients never have a normal exercise tolerance.

Mediastinal masses

Masses can occur in the anterior, middle or posterior mediastinum. Anterior and middle mediastinal masses are usually lymphomatous (Hodgkin's disease or non-Hodgkin's lymphoma), and impair respiratory function by compression or deviation of the trachea, bronchi and great vessels. Cardio-vascular system dysfunction may occur due to compression of the heart, pulmonary artery, superior vena cava (SVC) or the presence of a pericardial effusion. Posterior tumours are usually neuroblastomas, which do not impair respiratory function. Steroids or radiotherapy should be used if possible to shrink the mass prior to anaesthesia. However, this may prevent an accurate tissue diagnosis, so it is sometimes necessary to anaesthetize the child with clinical symptoms and signs of airway and/or great vessel obstruction. Symptoms associated with anterior mediastinal masses include: cough when supine, orthopnoea, dyspnoea at rest, wheeze, stridor, and SVC obstruction. Respiratory symptoms, and possibly SVC obstruction, are much commoner in children with non-Hodgkin's lymphoma. Orthopnoea is the symptom most predictive of peri-operative airway obstruction. SVC obstruction is usually insidious in onset. Clinical signs include dilatation of collateral veins and oedema of the upper chest and neck. Ominous clinical signs are positional dyspnoea, marked pulsus paradoxus and syncope on performing a Valsalva manoeuvre.

Pre-operative assessment includes chest X-ray, CT (which may require sedation or anaesthesia and therefore not be possible), magnetic resonance imaging and echocardiography. Echocardiography may show a pericardial effusion, distortion of the heart and great vessels and impaired function. Flow–volume loops are useful in predicting problems, but young children may not co-operate. Children with mediastinal lymphomas have both obstructive and restrictive defects on pulmonary function testing. Pulmonary function is significantly decreased in patients with non-Hodgkin's lymphoma, children who present with respiratory symptoms and those with very large masses (mediastinal mass ratio > 45 per cent). The extent of tracheal compression correlates with the size of the mediastinal mass.

Anaesthesia may be required for a variety of procedures such as biopsy, staging laparotomy, lumbar puncture and instillation of intrathecal drugs, bone marrow aspirate and trephine and insertion of long-term vascular access. Superficial tissue biopsies in older children should be done under local anaesthetic if possible.

Anaesthetic technique

Heavy sedative premedication should be avoided. Patients should be induced in the position they find most comfortable. It may be necessary to have intravenous access in a lower limb vein in case of severe SVC obstruction. An inhalational induction is optimal in cases with large airway obstruction. The airway can obstruct at any time in the peri-operative period. Complete airway obstruction may follow neuromuscular blockade, and spontaneous ventilation may need to be maintained. A long uncut tracheal tube and rigid bronchoscope should be immediately available. The bronchoscope can be used to bypass the obstruction and ventilate the patient, as well as for diagnosis. Particular care should be taken when positioning the patient; change of the patient's position to the lateral or prone position may be required.

Cardiovascular system collapse can also occur and, in extreme cases, the chest may need to be opened. The patient may need to remain intubated post-operatively until the mass is shrunk with chemo- or radiotherapy.

Specific techniques

Bronchoscopy

Paediatric bronchoscopy can be performed using a rigid or flexible broncho-scope. Indications may be diagnostic or therapeutic, and include examin-ation of the airway, biopsy, excision or laser of lesions, removal of a foreign body or inspissated secretions and broncho-alveolar lavage. A flexible bronchoscope is often used for diagnostic purposes because it is able to reach more peripheral areas. A rigid bronchoscope may be necessary for some therapeutic purposes.

There are several possible techniques for bronchoscopy.

Rigid ventilating bronchoscope (e.g. Storz)

Rigid ventilating bronchoscopes are commonly used, as they combine good optical qualities with continuous airway control and anaesthesia delivery. A selection of lengths and diameters are available, suitable for children of all ages. Optical telescopes incorporating a fibre-optic light source are used with it. An instrument channel enables the operator to pass suction catheters or a range of small forceps with the telescope in place. If larger forceps are required, however, the main channel must be used without the telescope. A sidearm with a 15 mm connector allows oxygen and anaesthetic gases to be given via an anaesthetic breathing system. Ventilation can be spontaneous, assisted or manual via this closed system. The telescope occupies most of the lumen of the smaller scopes, resulting in a reduced cross-sectional area for gas flow and increased resistance. This can lead to impaired ventilation or gas trapping. The tele-scope may need to be intermittently removed and the proximal opening occluded to allow adequate ventilation.

Fibre-optic bronchoscopy via a laryngeal mask airway

General anaesthesia via a laryngeal mask airway provides good conditions for fibre-optic bronchoscopy and broncho-alveolar lavage in infants and children. Following inhalational or intravenous induction of anaesthesia, a laryngeal mask airway is inserted. Spontaneous, assisted or controlled ventilation is possible. The fibre-optic bronchoscope is then passed through the laryngeal mask airway via a connector with a gas-tight seal. A 3.5 mm flexible scope with a 1.2 mm suction channel will pass through the smallest (size 1) laryngeal mask airway. This gives a good view of the glottis and trachea under dynamic conditions if the patient is breathing spontaneously. In addition, the airway resistance is much less with the bronchoscope in place than with a tracheal tube.

Rigid Negus bronchoscope with Sanders injector

This is used as an alternative to spontaneous or manual ventilation. It employs jets of oxygen at pipeline pressures (410 kPa) to entrain air by the Venturi principle. A 19 SWG injector is used for the child, infant and suckling bronchoscopes. There is a potential for inadequate ventilation in patients with high airway resistance or reduced lung compliance, which is more likely when the smallest scopes are used. Furthermore, during foreign body removal there is a risk of propelling the object deeper into the respiratory tract.

Insufflation of oxygen via catheter to an apnoeic patient

This technique is rarely used in paediatric practice due to high oxygen consumption in childhood and infancy.

Anaesthetic technique

Atropine premedication helps to reduce secretions and block vagal reflexes; it is more effective given intramuscularly. This is particularly important in spontaneously breathing techniques, where topical anaesthesia to the vocal cords (lignocaine 3–5 mg/kg of 10 per cent spray) is essential. An inhalational induction with halothane or sevoflurane is optimal in upper airway obstruction; alternatively, the intravenous route may be used. Mask CPAP may be required to maintain a patent airway after induction in infants with laryngo- or tracheomalacia. Spontaneous respiration may need to be maintained during bronchoscopy in cases of airway obstruction and foreign body removal, for assessment of the vocal cords and in dynamic lesions. Anaesthesia is usually maintained with 100 per cent oxygen and halothane or sevoflurane to provide jaw relaxation and sufficient depth of anaesthesia for the bronchoscope to be tolerated and normal ventilatory movements to be observed.

Anaesthesia for foreign body removal

Aspiration of foreign bodies is relatively common in children. Occasionally this results in obstruction to the larynx or trachea, and this is clearly an acute medical emergency. More often, however, the object lodges more distally and presents either because the event was witnessed or, later, with signs of obstruction of segmental bronchi such as infection or wheeze. The foreign body may be visible on chest X-ray, but it is often radiolucent. A common X-ray finding is either hyperinflation or collapse of lung tissue distal to the point of impaction of the object.

The general principles of anaesthesia are as above. Unless there is acute respiratory distress, this is not an emergency and the child can be fasted and premedicated with atropine. The rigid ventilating bronchoscope is most commonly used in conjunction with a spontaneous ventilation technique. Typically, an inhalation induction is performed and anaesthesia deepened with halothane or sevoflurane in oxygen until the laryngeal reflexes are suppressed. The larynx is then topically anaesthetized with lignocaine spray. Temporary tracheal intubation may be useful at this point to ensure airway control until the bronchoscope is in place. Anaesthesia is then maintained through the bronchoscope side-arm, using assisted spontaneous ventilation if necessary. The procedure itself may be protracted, particularly if the object is friable. If the object is too large to be retrieved via the lumen of the bronchoscope, it may be necessary to withdraw it and the scope as a unit. If the object is accidentally released in the trachea or larynx during this process, total airway obstruction may occur and it may become necessary to push the object back down the trachea beyond the carina in order to ventilate effectively. If the object has been in place for a long period, large amounts of infected material may be present beyond the obstruction, and suctioning, positioning and even bronchial blockade may be necessary to prevent soiling of healthy lung tissue. Inhaled peanuts pose a particular hazard because of the chemical pneumonitis associated with irritation of the airways caused by vegetable oils. The bronchus in contact with the peanut and airways distal to it become inflamed and oedematous and thus the respiratory symptoms may be disproportionate to the actual area of lung obstructed. Furthermore, if the peanut fragments during removal and the pieces are dissipated by positive pressure ventilation, a widespread pneumonitis may result.

Protracted airway manipulation may itself result in mucosal oedema, and a short course of dexamethasone should be considered.

Post-operatively, oxygen therapy, physiotherapy and antibiotics may also be required, depending on the nature of the foreign body and the degree of lung involvement.

Thoracoscopy

Thoracoscopy (and video-assisted thoracoscopy) is increasing in popularity in paediatric practice, because it allows intrathoracic procedures to be undertaken without the need for a thoracotomy. It may reduce surgical trauma, post-operative pain and hospital stay. Indications are either therapeutic or diagnostic. Therapeutic indications include drainage of empyema, pleurodesis, assessment and treatment of pneumothorax, drainage of clotted haemothorax, sympathectomy and resection of a mediastinal tumour or cyst. Diagnostic indications include pleural biopsy, pulmonary biopsy, mediastinal tumour biopsy and pleural nodule biopsy.

Certain problems are specific to thoracoscopy. Special instruments are needed in children under 2 years of age, instruments can be adapted in the 2–8 year age group, and conventional equipment is used in children over 8 years. Thoracoscopy is unsuitable in children under 6 months or less than 8 kg in weight due to the small size of the pleural space, high respiratory frequency and reduced compliance. Between the ages of 4 and 12 years, selective intubation or endobronchial blockers will be required. Double-lumen tubes can be used over the age of 10 years.

Intra-operative complications include poor visualization, bleeding from an intercostal artery and difficulty with suturing. These may require conversion to an open operation. Recurrence of the original problem may also occur, particularly with pneumothoraces and cysts.

Medical conditions

Asthma

Asthma is the commonest chronic childhood disease. It is increasing in incidence, and the mortality rate in all age groups is rising. The incidence of sudden death in children is also increasing, particularly in children with at least one ITU admission for an acute severe asthmatic episode.

Recent discoveries concerning asthma include the following:

1. There is a genetic contribution to asthma.
2. NO is found in expired air, and levels are higher in asthmatics. This correlates with eosinophils in the sputum, and is reduced by treatment with inhaled steroids. NO could be used as a marker of airway inflammation in asthmatics.
3. Vascular engorgement of the airway wall plus an increase in smooth muscle shortening are important factors in airway narrowing, rather than an absolute increase in the amount of smooth muscle.

Anaesthetic management of asthmatic children

Points to note include the following:

- Premedication: anxiolysis is best provided with agents that are minimally respiratory depressant, e.g. benzodiazepines
- Inhaled bronchodilators should be continued peri-operatively
- Additional steroid cover may be required
- Light anaesthesia is the commonest cause of bronchospasm
- Propofol and ketamine are the intravenous induction agents of choice
- All volatile agents are bronchodilators; they may be used for induction, maintenance and for the management of acute asthmatic episodes
- Neuromuscular blocking agents that do not release histamine, such as vecuronium and cis-atracurium, should be used
- Anaesthetic gases should be humidified, as breathing cold dry air can trigger bronchospasm
- Management of intra-operative bronchospasm includes deepening anaesthesia and administering 100 per cent oxygen and inhaled or intravenous bronchodilators.

Following anaesthesia in healthy children and children with well-controlled asthma there is a similar fall in FEV_1 and PEFR, which is maximal in the early post-operative period. This is not associated with any clinical problem.

Cystic fibrosis

Cystic fibrosis is the commonest inherited progressive, eventually fatal, disease in Caucasians. Obstruction of exocrine glands leads to multisystem disease. It either presents in the neonatal period with meconium ileus or, later, with recurrent chest infections and malabsorption.

Viscous tracheobronchial secretions and defective mucociliary transfer lead to airway obstruction, chronic infection and tissue destruction, with the development of bronchitis, bronchiolitis, bronchiectasis and bronchial hyper-reactivity. Gas trapping and hyperinflation are characteristic. Chronic hypoxia and hypercapnia result in pulmonary hypertension and right heart failure, and these patients may be reliant on hypoxic respiratory drive. Chronic resistant *Pseudomonas* colonization is almost universal. Pneumothorax is rare in children with cystic fibrosis, but becomes increasingly common in adolescents and adults. The only treatment for end-stage disease is lung or heart/lung transplantation. The disease does not recur in the transplanted tissue. Occasionally, surgery is required in the perinatal period, including laparotomy for meconium ileus, meconium peritonitis or intestinal atresia. Older children may need bronchoscopy, broncho-alveolar lavage, thoracoscopy for recurrent pneumothorax, lobectomy, pleurectomy, ileostomy, porto-caval shunt, injection of varices, nasal polypectomy, vascular access for chronic antibiotic therapy and lung transplantation.

Anaesthetic management of children with cystic fibrosis

Points to note include the following:

- Pulmonary and nutritional status should be carefully assessed prior to anaesthesia
- Active infection at the time of surgery should be excluded
- Sedative or opioid premedication should be used cautiously
- Intravenous access may be difficult
- Inhalational induction can be slow due to areas of V/Q mismatch, coughing and laryngospasm
- Physiotherapy should be performed following induction
- Pneumothorax may occur, especially during one-lung anaesthesia
- Disposable or sterilized equipment should be used
- Humidified oxygen, nebulized saline and beta agonists should be used to promote clearance and reduce the viscosity of secretions
- Effective analgesia may facilitate adequate physiotherapy (regional analgesia may be optimal)
- Post-operative intensive care may be required.

Bibliography

Azarow, K., Messineo, A., Pearl, R. *et al.* (1997). Congenital diaphragmatic hernia – a tale of two cities: the Toronto experience. *J. Ped. Surg.*, **32**, 395–400.

Bandla, H.P.R., Smith, D.E. and Kiernan, M.P. (1997). Laryngeal mask airway facilitated fibre-optic bronchoscopy in infants. *Can. J. Anaesth.*, **44**, 1242–7.

Bosenberg, A.T., Bland, B.A.R., Schulte-Steinberg, O. and Downing, J.W. (1988). Thoracic epidural anesthesia via caudal route in infants. *Anesthesiology*, **69**, 265–9.

de-Campos, J.R., Andrade-Filho, L.O., Werebe, E.C. *et al.* (1997). Thoracoscopy in children and adolescents. *Chest*, **111(2)**, 494–7.

Hammer, G.B., Brodsky, J.B., Redpath, J.H. and Cannon, W.B. (1998). The Univent tube for single-lung ventilation in paediatric patients. *Paed. Anaesth.*, **8**, 55–7.

Hatch, D. and Fletcher, M. (1992). Anaesthesia and the ventilatory system in infants and young children. *Br. J. Anaesth.*, **68**, 398–410.

Hogman, M. and Hedenstierna, G. (1998). Pathophysiology of asthma. *Curr. Opin. Anaesthesiol.*, **11**, 61–6.

Karmaker, M.K., Booker, P.D., Franks, R. and Pozzi, M. (1996). Continuous extrapleural infusion of bupivacaine for post-thoracotomy analgesia in young infants. *Br. J. Anaesth.*, **76**, 811–15.

King, D.R., Patrick, L.E., Ginn-Pease, M.E. *et al.* (1997). Pulmonary function is compromised in children with mediastinal lymphoma. *J. Ped. Surg.*, **32(2)**, 294–300.

May, H.A., Smyth, R.L. and Romer, H.C. (1996). Effect of anaesthesia on lung function in children with asthma. *Br. J. Anaesth.*, **77**, 200–2.

13

Lung volume reduction surgery (LVRS)

M. Gressier, V. Piriou, A. Schweizer and J. Neidecker

Introduction

In 1958, two definitions of emphysema emerged. First, it was defined as a condition of the lung characterized by an increase, beyond the normal, in the size of air spaces distal to the terminal bronchiole either from dilatation or from destruction of their walls. The second definition was a condition of the lung characterized by abnormal permanent enlargement of air spaces distal to the terminal bronchiole, accompanied by the destruction of their walls and without obvious fibrosis.

In 1962, the World Health Organization and the American Thoracic Society limited the term 'emphysema' to the enlargement of any part, or all, of the acinus, accompanied by destruction of respiratory tissue.

Emphysema is present in 20–25 per cent of patients with chronic obstructive pulmonary disease (COPD).

This disease represents an important cause of socio-professional disability, and is the fourth highest cause of mortality in occidental countries. Some toxic factors and a genetic predisposition are incriminated, especially smoking, which causes alveolar destruction (mainly at the upper lobes (typically centrilobular emphysema), while alpha-1 antitrypsin deficiency is associated with lesions that predominantly involve the lower lobes.

In 1957, Brantigan introduced the technique of lung volume reduction (LVRS) to treat patients with severe respiratory insufficiency due to non-bullous emphysema. LVRS consisted of the resection of inflated non-functional areas of the lung. The technique was abandoned because of frequent complications related to prolonged air leaks, and a high early mortality rate.

Recently LVRS has been reintroduced, but with technical modifications such as the buttressing of staples lines with bovine pericardial strips to reduce air leaks, and bilateral parenchymal reduction via median sternotomy.

The purpose of LVRS is:

- To achieve a reduction in pulmonary hyperinflation, allowing the diaphragm to recover a more physiological configuration to assume its respiratory work.

- To achieve an improvement in maximal expiratory airflow, resulting from an increase of lung elastic recoil and enlargement of airway diameter.

Surgical procedures

Several surgical techniques can be used for LVRS, and these are described below.

Standard median sternotomy

This is the most frequent procedure that permits a bilateral LVRS in a supine patient. It provides a good exposure of both lungs, and allows visual inspection and palpation of the lung tissue except for the left lower lung lobe. Once a standard median sternotomy is performed, the side with the worst pre-operative lung function (identified by chest computerized tomography (CT) and lung perfusion scans) is operated on first. The pleura is incised sequentially in order to keep the non-operated lung in place. The lung is deflated, and one-lung ventilation instituted to the other side. After a few minutes, the most pathological areas remain distended while the less emphysematous lung regions become atelectatic.

These inflated regions, because of poor or absent pulmonary blood flow, have previously been identified on the differential ventilation–perfusion scan and chest CT. They correspond to the target areas for resection. Multiple non-anatomical peripheral wedge resections are performed by successive applications of the linear stapling device buttressed with polytetrafluoro-ethylene or a xenopericardial patch. For upper lobe disease (the most common situation for smokers) a 'hockey stick' or a 'U-shaped' excision will allow the remaining lung to fill the apical portion of the operated hemi-thorax. For diseases of the bases, basilar segments of the lower lobes with the distal part of the lingula or middle lobe are resected to allow the diaphragm to rise adequately. In some patients there is a mixture of bullous and non-bullous areas, but the majority of patients have diffuse changes with no apparent bullae. The goal is to excise approximately 20–30 per cent of the lung volume, focusing on the most diseased areas. The lung is reventilated and carefully checked for air leaks and for adequate thoracic cavity filling by the remaining parenchyma. To reduce air leaks, techniques such as 'pleural tent', 'pleural talc poudrage' or fibrin glue instillation can be used. When the first side is completed, the procedure is repeated on the opposite side.

Chest tubes are placed and connected to a chest drainage system using low-pressure suction.

This bilateral surgical approach can also be performed via bilateral thoracosternotomy or 'clamshell' incision; the skin is incised in the infra-mammary crease in a curvilinear fashion, and bilateral thoracosternotomy is performed through the fourth intercostal space.

Video-assisted thoracoscopy (VAT)

VAT has been used to perform lung volume reduction unilaterally or, more frequently, bilaterally.

The patient is placed in the lateral decubitus position. Generally, the worst side is operated on first. Three trocars are placed within the chest cavity on the operated side. In addition to selective lung ventilation, some teams occasionally use carbon dioxide insufflation at 10 mmHg pressure to facilitate lung collapse. Lung volume is reduced by 20–30 per cent by resection of the most diseased areas, using videoscopic linear staplers without buttressing material. Bullectomy or laser pneumoplasty have been concomitantly performed by some surgical teams, but with little benefit, excessive morbidity and significant mortality.

Two chest tubes on each side are placed through the trocar holes and connected to a chest drainage system using low-pressure suction.

Recent studies did not find significant differences between the incidence of air leakage, the duration of chest tube drainage and median hospital stay for VAT or median sternotomy approaches.

Thoracotomy

Muscle sparing anterior thoracotomy is not as painful as postero-lateral thoracotomy. It can be used in cases of predominant unilateral emphysema. In addition, some surgeons convert VAT to thoracotomy because of extensive adhesions, which may create air leaks after dissection.

Resections of selected target areas as well as chest cavity drainage are performed in a similar way to the median sternotomy approach.

Whatever the chosen surgical technique, the resected lung tissue from patients undergoing LVRS must undergo histopathological examination. This may show undiagnosed pre-operative lesions such as interstitial fibrosis, non-caseating granulomatosis, chronic inflammation or unsuspected neoplasia.

Pathophysiologic mechanisms of functional improvement after LVRS

It is paradoxical to propose lung resection in patients with chronic respiratory insufficiency, particularly as thoracic surgery induces a transient, but significant, decrease in pulmonary function. In addition, a FEV_1 smaller than 0.8 l has often been considered as a contraindication to any major thoraco-abdominal surgery.

In the particular case of LVRS, a secondary improvement may occur as a result of the surgical procedure. Several mechanisms have been suggested to explain this improvement, related to increased elastic recoil, improved respiratory muscle function and cardiac performance.

Destruction of lung parenchyma, resulting in loss of elastic recoil and tethering open of small airways, is a prominent feature of centrilobular emphysema. Progressive hyperinflation represents an attempt to maintain airway patency as tidal respiration is displaced towards higher functional residual volume. Typically, the distribution of emphysema is heterogeneous; the most diseased areas remain inflated throughout the respiratory cycle and act as a dead-space volume, which compresses the better-preserved areas in which shunting occurs.

It has been shown that, by resecting these functionally inert areas, both elastic recoil and expiratory driving pressure increase, whereas the resistance to airflow and intrinsic positive end expiratory pressure (PEEPi) decrease. Although there is no strong correlation between changes in elastic recoil and spirometric indices, patients with significant post-operative improvement in exercise capacity also demonstrate higher elastic recoil.

Better ventilation–perfusion matching is expected after removal of dead-space areas, and could explain the small increase in Pao_2 that is observed in some patients.

In patients with severe emphysema, dyspnoea is more related to respiratory muscle dysfunction than to airflow limitation. Hyperinflation flattens and shifts the diaphragm downwards and results in a lower inspiratory force, increased work of breathing and progressive muscular weakening and fatigue.

By resecting 20–30 per cent of the lung volume, the recovery of the normal dome-shaped form of the diaphragm can be achieved with significant increase in generation of transdiaphragmatic pressure and a sparing effect on the energy requirements for breathing.

Hyperinflation and auto-PEEP impede venous return and cardiac pre-load. Very high PEEPi levels, such as during exercise, may cause an increase in pulmonary artery pressure and direct compression of cardiac chambers ('breath-stacking' or pulmonary tamponade).

Using two-dimensional echocardiography, improvement of right ventricular ejection fraction has been demonstrated as a result of better atrial filling and, possibly, lower right ventricular afterload after LVRS.

Evaluation and selection of patients

Currently, there are three therapeutic options for managing patients with COPD (Fig. 13.1):

1. Pulmonary rehabilitation associated with optimal medical management.
2. Lung transplantation – due to the lack of donors, this is reserved for patients with severe respiratory insufficiency ($FEV_1 < 20$ per cent predicted) and who are less than 65 years old.
3. LVRS – generally, emphysematous patients are candidates for this procedure. They should have severe respiratory insufficiency ($FEV_1 < 35$ per cent predicted), which implies major limitations for daily activities and a poor quality of life.

Pre-operative evaluation has to select patients likely to benefit from LVRS (Table 13.1). Those with too a high a risk of morbidity or mortality will

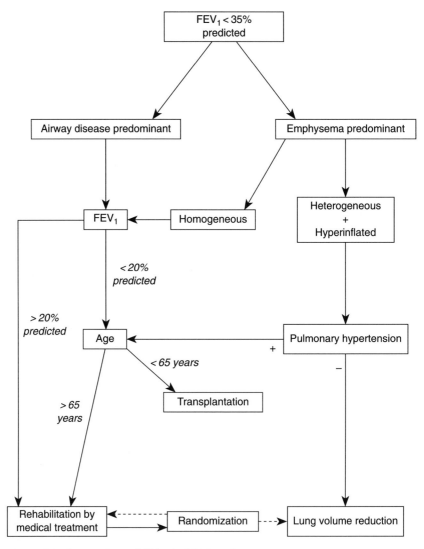

Figure 13.1 Therapeutic possibilities in COPD patients.

be excluded. A randomized trial (National Emphysema Treatment Trial) comparing LVRS to maximal medical therapy began in the USA in December 1997. The study mandates a period of pulmonary rehabilitation for all patients prior to randomization. Patients are then randomized to receive either LVRS or continuation of medical management. The study, which is expected to last 7 years, will enrol over 4000 patients.

Table 13.1 Inclusion criteria for patients for lung volume reduction surgery

- Hyperinflated and heterogeneous emphysema
- Severe dyspnoea in spite of optimal medical treatment
- No smoking (cessation > 6 months)
- Age < 75 years
- High motivation and acceptance of pulmonary rehabilitation programme and risks of morbidity and/or mortality
- Marked airflow limitation: FEV_1 < 35 per cent predicted
- Marked thoracic hyperinflation and trapped gas: RV > 250 per cent, TLC > 125 per cent (measured by plethysmography)
- Alveolar gas exchange: 20 per cent < TLCO < 50 per cent predicted
- $Paco_2$ < 7.3 kPa (55 mmHg)
- Adequate arterial oxygen tension with nasal cannula oxygen supplementation if necessary
- Adequate cardiovascular function:
  - normal left heart function
  - no significant coronary artery disease
  - mean PAP < 4.7 kPa (35 mmHg), systolic PAP < 5.8 kPa (45 mmHg)
- Oral corticosteroids at a dose < 10–15 mg of prednisolone equivalent
- Acceptable nutritional status (BMI)

FEV_1, forced expiratory volume in 1 second; RV, residual volume; TLC, total lung capacity; TLCO, transfer capacity of the lung for carbon monoxide; $Paco_2$, arterial carbon dioxide tension; PAP, pulmonary artery pressure; BMI, body mass index

Assessment (Table 13.2)

Morphological evaluations

Postero-anterior and lateral inspiratory and expiratory chest radiographs are used to evaluate thoracic hyperinflation with flattened diaphragms and enlarged retrocardiac and retrosternal air spaces. The chest radiographs may also suggest the overall severity and relative distribution of emphysema. Other abnormalities such as marked scarring, cancer, pleural or cardiac diseases may be found on the films. A fibre-optic bronchoscopy is performed to look for expiratory collapse or a neoplastic lesion. It also allows assessment of inflammation and infection, and biopsies and bacteriological samples can be taken.

A chest CT scan and lung perfusion scans provide detailed information on the severity and distribution of emphysema. They allow specification of pulmonary disease patterns (panacinar or centrilobular and homogeneous or heterogeneous emphysema) and lobe predominance, and localization of non-functional pulmonary areas.

Physiological testing

Pulmonary function tests

Spirometry evaluates airways obstruction and reversibility with β_2-adrenergic receptor agonists. Lung volumes are measured by plethysmography and gas dilution to evaluate trapped air. Diffusing capacity for

Table 13.2 Pre-operative assessment for lung volume reduction surgery

Pulmonary imaging

- chest radiographs (postero-anterior and lateral)
- chest computed tomography (high-resolution)
- dynamic magnetic resonance imaging (diaphragm and chest wall studies)
- lung ventilation/perfusion scans

Pulmonary function test

- spirometry and flow–volume loops
- plethysmography (lung volumes and Raw)
- diffusing capacity
- arterial blood gases at rest and exercise
- pulmonary compliance and lung recoil pressure
- transdiaphragmatic pressure
- dyspnoea indices – oxygen supplementation

Exercise capacity test

- Six-minute walk test
- VO$_2$ max

Cardiac tests

Quality of life

---

carbon monoxide allows an evaluation of the damage to pulmonary capillary bed. Arterial blood gases are measured with oxygen supplementation if necessary, with the patient at rest. These tests can be repeated after exercise to evaluate the respiratory reserve.

Pulmonary compliance and specific airway conductance are measured to provide a baseline for comparison with post-operative values. Characteristics of emphysema are an increase in static pulmonary compliance, a decrease in lung recoil pressure at a given lung volume and a modified shape of the static pressure–volume curve.

Transdiaphragmatic pressure measurement before and after LVRS allows an evaluation of diaphragmatic function and its improvement.

Pulmonary function assessment is completed by dyspnoea analysis, using a visual analogue scale or the American Thoracic Society's modified Medical Research Council Score (with grades 0 to 4) (Table 13.3). An assessment of quality of life before and after the procedure may be made using standard questionnaires such as the Nottingham Health Profile or St George's Hospital Respiratory Questionnaire.

Exercise capacity tests

The aim of these tests is to evaluate physical status and functional results to quantify improvement after the procedure.

Two tests can be used:

- A 6-minute walk test to assess functional capacity is easy to perform, but may not achieve the limits of exercise tolerance in all patients.

Table 13.3 Modified Medical Research Council dyspnoea scale*

Grade	Symptoms
0	Not troubled with breathlessness except with strenuous exercise
1	Troubled by shortness of breath when hurrying on the level or walking up a slight hill
2	Walks slower than people of the same age on the level because of breathlessness, or has to stop for breath when walking at own pace on the level
3	Stops for breath after walking about 100 m or after a few minutes on the level
4	Too breathless to leave the house, or breathless when dressing or undressing

*The task group official statement of the American Thoracic Society (1982). *Am. Rev. Respir. Dis.*, **126**, 952–6

- A maximal oxygen consumption (VO_2 max.) test using direct measurement is performed on a cycle ergometer or treadmill, and allows quantitative and qualitative assessment of the physiological determinants of maximal exercise performance.

After LVRS, and during rehabilitation, a regular evaluation of the functional improvement of patients is of interest. Nevertheless, the latter test is not as good a predictive test of operative morbidity and mortality in LVRS as it is for evaluation of lung resectability in patients with lung cancer (predicted post-operative VO_2 max. 10 ml/kg per min indicates inoperability). The reason for this is that LVRS improves respiratory mechanics (e.g. diaphragm function) and, consequently, post-operative VO_2 max., whereas lung cancer surgery does not.

Cardiovascular function tests

Cardiovascular assessment is essential because of possible associated heart disease, particularly coronary artery disease, which is frequent in former smokers.

Exercise ECG testing cannot always detect ST segment and T wave changes, because of the patient's inability to exercise until heart rate limits.

Transthoracic echocardiography may not provide accurate information because of pulmonary hyperinflation resulting in poor visualization of cardiac cavities. Coronary artery disease diagnosis using dobutamine stress echocardiography has the same limitation. Coronary angiography and right heart catheterization are therefore mandatory to evaluate ventricular function, pulmonary artery pressure and ischaemic heart disease.

Biventricular ejection fraction and left ventricular end-diastolic volume may be measured by radionuclide ventriculography, and dipyridamole thallium scans used to evaluate coronary disease.

Pre-operatively, bronchodilator, steroid and antibiotic regimens should be optimized and, because of the patients' generally poor nutritional status and lack of condition, a rehabilitation programme should be commenced.

Patients should be instructed in the breathing and muscular exercises planned for the early post-operative period.

Anaesthetic management

In addition to the routine anaesthetic assessment using the information from the tests outlined above, the anaesthetist should pre-operatively ascertain the patient's respiratory and cardiovascular reserve. Surgery should be delayed until acute exacerbations of COPD, infection or cardiac failure are controlled.

The method of post-operative analgesia (ideally a thoracic epidural), the possibility for an extended period of ventilatory support and the respiratory rehabilitation programmed should be explained to the patient.

Steroids, antibiotics, bronchodilators, diuretics and any cardiovascular medication should be continued peri-operatively and adjusted to obtain optimum response.

Anaesthetic technique

The anaesthetic technique will be influenced by the surgical approach (median sternotomy, thoracotomy or VAT), but should utilize agents that permit rapid return of spontaneous respiration and protective airway reflexes combined with good analgesia. Much of the intra-operative management centres on the optimization of ventilation in relation to airway pressures, expiratory time and lung isolation.

The specific anaesthetic problems presented by patients for LVRS are as follows:

- The potential for rupturing emphysematous bullae by application of IPPV. This may impair ventilation intra-operatively as a result of gas leakage from the airways and lung collapse due to pneumothorax, or may cause cardiovascular instability if a tension pneumothorax develops. Post-operatively, prolonged air leaks have been associated with significant morbidity following LVRS.
- The potential for gas trapping during IPPV in patients with COPD. This may result in pulmonary hyperinflation and, by impairing venous return to the heart, cause cardiovascular instability.
- The need to avoid post-operative ventilation, if possible, in order to obviate the risks of barotrauma and the development of ventilatory dependence and nosocomial infection.
- The possibility of coronary disease.

Premedication

Sedative premedication should be cautiously prescribed because of its deleterious effects in patients with limited respiratory reserve. The majority of the patients are lightly premedicated with a benzodiazepine. Some patients do not receive any premedication on the ward, to avoid the risk of unexpected pre-operative respiratory depression.

Monitoring

Standard patient monitoring is used. Facilities to monitor capnography curves and continuous spirometry to display flow–volume or pressure–volume loops should be available. Invasive arterial and central venous pressure monitoring is essential.

In addition, pulmonary artery catheterization with either continuous or intermittent cardiac output measurements and mixed venous oxygen saturation (SvO_2), or SvO_2 combined with right ventricular ejection fraction assessment, may be recommended.

Alternatively, cardiac function can be evaluated using transoesophageal echocardiography.

Induction of anaesthesia

If a thoracic epidural is to be used, it should ideally be inserted with the patient awake. Thereafter, induction of general anaesthesia is performed, preferably using short-acting agents such as propofol (1.5–2 mg/kg) or etomidate. Opioids (sufentanil or fentanyl) are given in low doses. Non-depolarizing neuromuscular blocking agents (vecuronium 0.1 mg/kg or atracurium 0.6 mg/kg) are used for muscular relaxation. Neuromuscular transmission is monitored quantitatively. After cautious manual ventilation, a left-sided double-lumen endotracheal tube is placed. Because of emphysema, correct tube position may be difficult to assess by auscultation. The accurate position of the tube is best confirmed by fibre-optic bronchoscopy. In case of difficult intubation, the Univent tube may be helpful. Just after intubation, bacteriological examination is performed on sputum obtained during bronchoscopy.

Maintenance of anaesthesia

General anaesthesia is maintained by using a continuous infusion of propofol (4–6 mg/kg per hour). Caution needs to be exercised if volatile agents are used to maintain anaesthesia because of the frequency of gas leaks from the lungs during LVRS, leading to the possibility of awareness.

Nitrous oxide should not be used because it increases intra-alveolar pressure, leading to rupture of bullae and pneumothorax. It may also increase pulmonary vascular resistance.

Choosing anaesthetic agents with the least deleterious effects on gaseous exchange and airway resistance is important. An increased airway resistance may induce rapid development of PEEPi, leading to the haemodynamic instability. In addition, haemodynamic impairment can be worsened by hypoxia. Anaesthetic induction with propofol provides lower respiratory resistance after endotracheal intubation in comparison to etomidate or thiopental. Furthermore, propofol may prevent fentanyl-induced broncho-constriction. A comparison of propofol with isoflurane for maintenance of anaesthesia in patients with COPD shows similar effects on arterial blood gases and pulmonary mechanics. However, in contrast to inhaled anaesthetics like isoflurane, which inhibit hypoxic pulmonary vasoconstriction, propofol does not diminish hypoxic pulmonary vasoconstriction or produce a significant increase in intrapulmonary shunting during one-lung ventilation.

Management of ventilation

There are two essential goals:

1. To limit hyperinflation by using the appropriate manual or mechanical ventilatory support.
2. To avoid hypoxia in relation to one-lung ventilation and ventilation–perfusion mismatching, especially when the patient is in the lateral decubitus position. It is important to emphasize that pulmonary and cardiovascular function may be impaired, with little reserve for compensation.

The monitoring added to microprocessor-controlled ventilators may be useful in analysing and reducing hyperinflation, particularly when measurement of PEEPi is available. In order to limit dynamic hyperinflation, mechanical ventilation can be initiated with a reduced tidal volume (6–8 ml/kg), a decreased respiratory rate (10–12 breaths per min.) and inspiratory–expiratory time ratio (1 : 4–1 : 5).

The peak inspiratory pressure should be as low as possible (<25–30 cmH$_2$O).

Intermittent disconnection from the ventilator to permit prolonged expiration is recommended to prevent gas trapping.

All parameters should be adjusted to optimize arterial blood gases, respiratory parameters and the appearance of the lungs when the chest is opened. Permissive hypercapnia (PaCO$_2 < 8.5$ kPa) is advocated to avoid hyperinflation and to counteract haemodynamic instability.

Prior to one-lung ventilation, FiO$_2$ is set to 1.0 to limit hypoxia. Optimized ventilation–perfusion matching during one-lung ventilation is a challenge, especially in severe heterogeneous emphysema associated with multiple ventilation–perfusion mismatching areas.

Other than dynamic hyperinflation, commonly encountered problems include bronchospasm, sputum retention with mucous plugging, and pneumothorax on the non-operative side.

Frequent suctioning, possibly aided by flexible bronchoscopy, and the use of bronchodilator nebulizers may be required.

An acute tension pneumothorax on the non-operative side produces a sudden increase in inspiratory pressure associated with rapid haemodynamic alteration and gas exchange decompensation. Immediate detection and treatment are required, particularly in the case of VAT or thoracotomy, where visual observation is not possible. The operated lung is re-inflated and manually ventilated, while a rapid chest drainage is performed on the opposite side. However, a similar clinical picture may be caused by a mucus plug or endotracheal tube displacement.

As the 'worst' lung is operated on first, particular attention is essential when re-inflating the reduced lung. Over-inflation may cause rupture close to the staple lines, and should be avoided. Hypoxia may become a rather more difficult problem while the 'best' lung undergoes surgery. Ventilation is applied now to the reduced lung, with a lower tidal volume to avoid air leaks. The permeability of the alveolo-capillary membrane may be increased, leading to pulmonary oedema. Consideration should be given to the use of colloids for fluid replacement to maintain plasma osmolality, and to the administration of diuretics.

Extubation

Extubation may be problematical because of pulmonary function impairment induced by anaesthesia, pulmonary oedema, severe emphysema, pain and air leaks.

At the end of surgery, if immediate extubation is not possible, the double-lumen endotracheal tube is replaced by a single-lumen tube. It may also be useful to perform a fibre-optic bronchoscopy in order to remove secretions and take samples for bacteriological examination.

After LVRS, pulmonary areas adjacent to the suture line are particularly fragile and can be damaged by mechanical ventilation, coughing or the application of suction to chest tubes. Therefore, immediate post-operative extubation and limited suction on the chest drains (usually $-10\,cmH_2O$) are recommended by most authors. Early extubation also reduces the risks of development of nosocomial pneumonia.

Post-operatively, a decrease of auto-PEEP and improved respiratory mechanics will decrease the work of breathing. This decrease, together with adequate pain control and the use of short-acting anaesthetic agents, will facilitate spontaneous breathing in a normothermic patient.

Many patients can be successfully extubated despite a $Paco_2$ of around 7.5 kPa and a pHa of around 7.20–7.25. Triantafillou reports an initial $Paco_2$ (immediately after extubation) of greater than 8.5 kPa in 50 per cent of patients, and greater than 10 kPa in 25 per cent of patients.

Patients with significant respiratory acidosis can benefit from continuous positive airway pressure (CPAP) and PSV via a face mask.

Most sternotomy and VAT patients are reported to be successfully extubated immediately after the surgical procedure. However, patients undergoing thoracoscopic laser resection appear to require post-operative mechanical ventilation for several days.

After extubation, the conscious patient is immediately placed in an upright sitting position to facilitate diaphragmatic movement. Humidified oxygen is administered by facemask or nasal cannulae at the lowest possible concentration to maintain SpO_2 ranging from 90–92 per cent and preserve respiratory drive.

Pain control is particularly important, together with physiotherapy, in preventing sputum retention, atelectasis and infection. Epidural analgesia is the method of choice, combined with paracetamol and non-steroidal anti-inflammatory drugs in the absence of contraindications.

Early post-operative management

Epidural analgesia is continued for 4–5 days. Low concentrations of local anaesthetics (e.g. bupivacaine 0.125 per cent) with opioids (e.g. morphine, about 0.1 mg/kg per day) are continuously administered post-operatively according to the clinical situation and visual analogue scale for pain and the rate of infusion adjusted as required.

Blood gases are monitored in order to assess Pa_{O_2} and Pa_{CO_2} and acid–base status. Results can be abnormal for several days, with low Pa_{O_2} and markedly increased Pa_{CO_2}.

Blood loss and air leakage must be closely monitored. Chest drains are removed when blood loss is minimal and air leakage ceases. Their post-operative management should be conducted cautiously, because there is a high risk of air leakage for several days.

Fluid balance is maintained, aimed at avoiding an increase in lung water content. Patients are generally kept on the dry side to avoid pulmonary oedema; thus intravenous crystalloid infusion is restricted.

Vasopressors and/or catecholamines may be required, according to the clinical haemodynamic situation.

Antibiotics, bronchodilators and steroids are continued post-operatively, together with antithrombotic and stress ulcer prophylaxis. Steroids are progressively tapered to the pre-operative dose. Physiotherapy, incentive spirometry and fibre-optic bronchoscopy to clear mucous plugs, if required, are important features of post-operative care. Fibre-optic bronchoscopy is, however, not suitable for routine pulmonary hygiene because broncho-spasm, hypersecretion and mucosal oedema can occur and worsen hypoxia. If clearance of secretions is a problem, suctioning via a mini-tracheostomy should be considered.

The patient should be mobilized early, and pulmonary rehabilitation started. The aims of early mobilization and rehabilitation include weaning from supplemental oxygen, increasing exercise tolerance with the help of a treadmill or ergometric bicycle, retraining the diaphragm and improving musculoskeletal strength.

Assessment of the nutritional state is essential because emphysema patients have a poor nutritional status. Patients unable to start adequate early oral nutrition are temporarily placed on parenteral nutrition.

Morbidity and mortality

During the post-operative period, the most common complication is pro-longed air leakage. This may occur in 50 per cent of the cases for a period exceeding 7 days, and results in an extended hospital stay and more compli-cated pulmonary rehabilitation because chest drainage is prolonged. Avoid-ance of suction on the chest tubes reduces the risk of this complication. Indeed, the negative pressure applied at the tip of the chest drain, which is in contact with the surface of the fragile emphysematous lung, can damage it. If a pneumothorax greater than 30 per cent is diagnosed on chest radiograph, or there is marked subcutaneous emphysema, suction is required. Cooper *et al.* (1996) reported that around 20 per cent of their last 50 patients required chest drain suction. In cases of modest persisting air leak beyond a week, a Heimlich valve may be safely connected to the chest drain to facilitate patient mobility and discharge from the hospital.

Few patients require re-operation because of air leak worsening and leading to progressive respiratory failure, or because of intrathoracic bleeding.

A second major complication that can occur at any time during the post-operative course and requires the continuation of mechanical ventilation (or a return to it) is chest infection. This should be treated aggressively from the appearance of the first signs.

Cardiovascular morbidity is limited if the screening process of the patients is correct. However, myocardial infarction or ischaemia are reported in the literature as a cause of death (< 2 per cent). Post-operative cardiac arrhythmia may occur, as in any thoracic procedure.

The overall mortality rate is reported to be below 10 per cent, or even below 5 per cent, according to the different surgical teams. These results are surprising when considering the patient population has a high probability of post-operative complications due to age and respiratory insufficiency. Strict selection of patients and intensive training of the teams have contributed to these encouraging results.

KEY POINTS

- LVRS is one of the developing surgical treatments for severe pulmonary emphysema. The goals are a reduction in pulmonary hyperinflation, allowing the diaphragm to regain a more physiological configuration and work more efficiently, and an improvement in maximal expiratory airflow. This can initially be attributed to the increase in lung elastic recoil and to the secondary effect of dilatation of the airways, resulting in increased airway conductance.

- Surgery may be performed using a sternotomy, VAT or thoracotomy. The operation consists of non-anatomic resection of multiple regions of destroyed lung, either uni- or bilaterally.

- Anaesthesia for LVRS is challenging because of the severity of pulmonary disease together with the poor general condition of the patients. General anaesthesia is chosen in combination with thoracic epidural analgesia.

- One-lung ventilation must be used, and dynamic hyperinflation should be avoided by using deliberate hypoventilation with permissive hypercapnia.

- Extubation should be performed as soon as possible.

- Post-operatively, adequate physiotherapy and pulmonary rehabilitation, adequate pain control and close control of air leaks are mandatory. The most specific complication is prolonged air leaks.

Bibliography

American College of Chest Physicians and American Association of Cardiovascular and
Pulmonary Rehabilitation, Pulmonary Rehabilitation Guidelines Panel (1997). Pulmonary rehabilitation: joint ACCP/AACVPR evidence-based guidelines. *Chest*, **112**, 1363–96.

Brantigan, O.C., Mueller, E. and Kress, M.B. (1959). A surgical approach to pulmonary
emphysema. *Am. Rev. Resp. Dis.*, **80**, 194–202.

Conacher, I.D. (1997). Anaesthesia for the surgery of emphysema. *Br. J. Anaesth.*, **79**, 530–
38.

Cooper, J.D., Patterson, G.A., Sundaresan, R.S. *et al.* (1996). Results of 150 consecutive
bilateral lung volume reduction procedures in patients with severe emphysema.
J. Thorac. Cardiovasc. Surg., **112**, 1319–29.

DeSouza, G., deLisser, E.A., Turry, P. and Gold, M.I. (1995). Comparison of propofol
with isoflurane for maintenance of anesthesia in patients with chronic obstructive
pulmonary disease: use of pulmonary mechanics, peak flow rates, and blood gases.
J. Cardiothorac. Vasc. Anesth., **9**, 24–8.

Giebler, R.M., Scherer, R.U. and Peters, J. (1997). Incidence of neurologic complications
related to thoracic epidural catheterization. *Anesthesiology*, **86**, 55–63.

Keller, C.A. and Naunheim, K.S. (1997). Peri-operative management of lung volume reduction patients. *Clin. Chest Med.*, **18**, 285–300.

Kellow, N.H., Scott, A.D., White, S.A. and Feneck, R.O. (1995). Comparison of the effects
of propofol and isoflurane anaesthesia on right ventricular function and shunt fraction
during thoracic surgery. *Br. J. Anaesth.*, **75**, 578–82.

Krucylak, P.E., Naunheim, K.S., Keller, C.A. and Baudendistel, L.J. (1996). Anesthetic
management of patients undergoing unilateral video-assisted lung reduction for treatment of end-stage emphysema. *J. Cardiothorac. Vasc. Anesth.*, **10**, 850–3.

Liu, S., Carpenter, R.L. and Neal, J.M. (1995). Epidural anesthesia and analgesia. Their
role in post-operative outcome. *Anesthesiology*, **82**, 1474–506.

National Heart, Lung and Blood Division (1985). The definition of emphysema. Report
of a National Heart, Lung, and Blood Institute, Division of Lung Diseases workshop.
Am. Rev. Resp. Dis., **132**, 182–5.

Triantafillou, A.N. (1996). Anesthetic management for bilateral volume reduction surgery.
Sem. Thorac. Cardiovasc. Surg., **8**, 94–8.

Yusen, R.D., Lefrak, S.S. and Trulock, E.P. (1997). Evaluation and pre-operative
management of lung volume reduction surgery candidates. *Clin. Chest Med.*, **18**, 199–224.

Zollinger, A., Zaugg, M., Weder, W. *et al.* (1997). Video-assisted thoracoscopic volume
reduction surgery in patients with diffuse pulmonary emphysema: gas exchange and
anesthesiological management. *Anesth. Analg.*, **84**, 845–51.

Zollinger, A. and Pasch, T. (1998). Anaesthesia for lung volume reduction surgery. *Curr.
Opin. Anesth.*, **11**, 45–9.

14

Anaesthesia for pulmonary thrombo-endarterectomy

W. C. Wilson and A. Vuylsteke

Introduction

In the United States, between 500 000 and 600 000 patients develop pulmonary emboli annually. Approximately 150 000 of these patients die within 1 hour, either from a single haemodynamically catastrophic embolic event or as a result of recurrent, less clinically apparent emboli. These statistics may be an underestimate, as pulmonary embolism was unsuspected in 70 per cent of patients in whom it was shown to be the principal cause of death at autopsy. The vast majority of patients surviving pulmonary embolism will dissolve their embolic clots and go on to lead a fairly normal life (anticoagulation therapy with heparin or warfarin will restore pulmonary blood flow within 1–4 weeks). However, 0.1–0.5 per cent of the survivors have massive unresolved pulmonary emboli, and these 500–2500 patients will go on to develop the classic picture of chronic thrombo-embolic pulmonary hypertension (CTEPH) each year.

CTEPH comprises a broad spectrum of disease. Typically, these patients experience a major deep venous thrombosis (DVT) and a subsequent pulmonary embolism, which goes undetected initially but leaves some residual sequelae of dyspnoea upon exertion. The embolism resolves and the patient enjoys a subsequent 'honeymoon' period, followed in months to years by deterioration.

The reason that some patients (0.1–0.5 per cent of survivors) go on to develop CTEPH is not well understood, but it may partly be due to the fact that many of the acute episodes go undetected clinically and are thus untreated. No clear dysfunction of the fibrinolytic system has yet been identified; both the plasminogen activator activity and inhibitor activity are typically within the normal range in these patients. Furthermore, antithrombin III, protein C and protein S are abnormal in less than 1 per cent of patients with CTEPH. The only prothrombotic factor that has been identified in a high proportion of this patient population is the lupus anticoagulant, which is present in approximately 10 per cent of patients with CTEPH.

The majority of patients who develop CTEPH present for medical evaluation late in the course of the disease. This is partly because few of these patients recall an obvious history of DVT or pulmonary embolism.

Furthermore, early signs of pulmonary hypertension may be subtle and the progression of the disease is often insidious.

Diagnostic evaluation and surgical selection

Once CTEPH is considered, the diagnostic work-up is straightforward. Major goals are:

1. To quantify the degree of pulmonary hypertension
2. To search for the aetiology or contributing factors (such as a hyper-coagulable state)
3. To verify that the emboli are proximally located, ensuring surgical accessibility.

The diagnostic evaluation of CTEPH is discussed below.

Physical examination

Physical examination typically demonstrates evidence of right heart failure: peripheral oedema, hepatomegaly and jugular venous distension. Pericardial and pleural effusions and ascites are occasionally encountered. Precordial examination reveals a right ventricular heave and a unique murmur associated with CTEPH. This distinctive murmur is heard over the lung fields rather than solely over the precordium, and is caused by turbulent flow through partially obstructed or recanalized pulmonary vessels. The significance of this murmur unique to CTEPH is that it is not present in primary pulmonary hypertension, the major differential diagnostic entity.

Laboratory findings

Routine laboratory tests should include measurement of haematocrit, as this may be elevated due to secondary polycythaemia. Renal function tests are typically normal until late in the disease process, when there may be elevations in blood urea nitrogen and uric acid. Liver function tests may be elevated in a non-specific pattern reflecting hepatic congestion. Prothrombin time and partial thromboplastin time are usually normal. However, an unexpected prolongation of the activated partial thromboplastin time should trigger consideration of the presence of lupus anti-coagulant or other anti-phospholipid antibodies such as anti-cardiolipin antibodies.

Another important pre-operative consideration for the anaesthetist is the patient's history of prior exposure and response to heparin. Some of these patients develop heparin-induced anti-platelet antibodies; this necessitates the scrupulous avoidance of heparin during cardiopulmonary bypass and the use of heparin-free flush in the invasive monitoring lines. Anticoagulation for patients who have developed heparin-induced anti-platelet antibodies has been managed with administration of iloprost (a prostacyclin analogue) or heparinoid.

Chest radiography typically demonstrates clear lung fields. Indeed, there may be relative oligaemia in certain lobes of the lungs, reflecting the diminished pulmonary blood flow. There may also be asymmetry in the size of the central pulmonary arteries. A greater diameter of the left main pulmonary artery shadow compared to that of the aorta is a subtle finding invariably seen with CTEPH. In addition, evidence of right atrial and right ventricular hypertrophy (best appreciated on the lateral chest X-ray) is almost universally noted.

In contrast to acute pulmonary embolism, which has characteristic electrocardiogram (ECG) changes (e.g. S1Q3 pattern), the ECG with CTEPH may be normal but usually shows non-specific evidence of right ventricular hypertrophy and strain.

Pulmonary function tests (PFTs) will demonstrate a decreased carbon monoxide diffusing capacity and a moderate restrictive defect. The decreased carbon monoxide diffusion capacity is a combination of both decreased membrane diffusion and decreased capillary blood volume. The restrictive defect may in part reflect scarring of the lung in areas that have suffered prior infarction. Severe restrictive patterns are an indication of pulmonary vascular hypertension of interstitial aetiology. Obstructive patterns may also be seen; the obstruction may result from bronchial hyperaemia related to the large bronchial arterial collateral circulation in these patients. Arterial blood gas analysis may reveal a fairly normal resting Pao_2 but there is an increased alveolar–arterial oxygen gradient, which will widen further with exercise. Dead space ventilation is often increased, and also worsens with exercise. Minute ventilation is typically elevated to compensate for the increased dead space ventilation. When multiple inert gas elimination technique (MIGET) is performed, moderate ventilation perfusion (V/Q) abnormalities are observed.

The diagnosis of CTEPH is most often initially made on echocardiography and V/Q scanning. The echocardiogram typically demonstrates right atrial and right ventricular enlargement, and occasionally proximal clots are seen. There may be severe compression of the left ventricle due to impingement from the hypertrophic right heart. Tricuspid regurgitation is typically observed. Echocardiography may, however, grossly underestimate the degree of pulmonary hypertension in these patients, especially at rest.

V/Q scanning typically demonstrates lobar and segmental defects. This is in contrast to V/Q scan results obtained in patients with primary pulmonary hypertension, which are typically normal or demonstrate patchy subsegmental abnormalities. It should be noted that V/Q scans are notorious for dramatically underestimating central pulmonary vascular obstruction in patients with CTEPH.

Right heart catheterization demonstrates the severity of pulmonary vascular hypertension at rest. If the pulmonary artery pressures are only modestly elevated at rest, repeat measurements are made following exercise. Right heart pulmonary angioscopy may further help to evaluate and quantify the extent of proximal disease.

Pulmonary angiography has been the most important invasive diagnostic modality, providing characteristic patterns including the following:

- Irregular arterial contours
- Abrupt cut-off or narrowing of vessels
- Pulmonary artery webs and bands
- Pouch defects
- Obstruction of lobar or segmental arteries at their point of origin.

In patients at risk for coronary artery disease (typically patients over 35 years of age), coronary angiography is also performed.

Recently, CTEPH patients have been evaluated with spiral computerized axial tomographic (CT) scans and magnetic resonance imaging (MRI) as well as pulmonary angiography, currently the gold standard. Interestingly, the spiral CT scan has been shown to be diagnostically equivalent to, and in some cases superior to, pulmonary angiography and, at this stage of technical advancement, distinctly better than MRI for evaluating pulmonary thrombo-embolic disease. The advantages of spiral CT scan are that it is non-invasive and that the required contrast is administered intravenously rather than intra-arterially, as required for angiography. Distal thrombus, however, is still best characterized by pulmonary angiography. Furthermore, over 600 pulmonary angiograms have been completed with non-ionic contrast at the University of California San Diego Medical Center (UCSD) without a single fatality.

Selection and preparation for surgery

The decision to proceed to pulmonary thrombo-endarterectomy (PTE) is typically made by the chest physician, in consultation with the surgeon, after evaluation of all the pre-operative data. The criteria used at Papworth and UCSD are as follows:

- The presence of pulmonary vascular obstruction which is haemodynamically significant; the majority of patients have a pulmonary vascular resistance (PVR) greater than 300 dynes.sec.cm^{-5}
- Thrombi must be proximally located, but may extend into the main lobar and segmental arteries; emboli that are further distal are not subject to endarterectomy
- There must be no significant co-existing disease
- The patient and the family must be willing to accept the morbidity of the procedure; this is currently 5–7 per cent.

Pre-operatively, the patient will undergo placement of a Greenfield inferior vena cava filter to protect against embolic recurrence.

Surgical technique and management

The surgical approach to patients with CTEPH involves a median sternotomy and cardiopulmonary bypass with deep hypothermic circulatory arrest (DHCA). Although used in the past, thoracotomy is a sub-optimal approach. Median sternotomy allows for treatment of both pulmonary arteries and, by definition, CTEPH involves both pulmonary arterial systems. The use of cardiopulmonary bypass with periods of complete circulatory arrest provides the bloodless operative field necessary for complete meticulous lobar and segmental dissection.

Following median sternotomy, cardiopulmonary bypass is established with ascending aortic cannulation and trans-atrial cannulation of the superior and inferior vena cavae. The patient is immediately cooled following initiation of cardiopulmonary bypass, and a temporary pulmonary vent is inserted. A left ventricular vent is inserted through the right upper pulmonary vein when the heart fibrillates.

Immediately after cross-clamping the aorta, at a core temperature of 20°C, 1000 ml of cold cardioplegia solution is administered into the aortic root. Additional myocardial protection is afforded by placing a cooling jacket around the heart. Cooling to 20°C typically takes 45–60 minutes, and the length of time is related to the size of the patient as well as the perfusion flow rate. Topical cold saline is not used in the PTE procedure, as it has been associated with excessively high rates of phrenic nerve injury when combined with the profound systemic hypothermia needed for DHCA.

An incision is made in one of the pulmonary arteries, the pulmonary endarterectomy plane is established and dissection continues while still on cardiopulmonary bypass until bronchial artery back-bleeding impairs good visualization. At this point, circulatory arrest is imperative. Bronchial arterial back flow in these patients is frequently substantial, and complete repair cannot be accomplished without circulatory arrest. However, in some unfortunate patients with significant distal disease, there may be very little back-bleeding during the endarterectomy. Trivial back-bleeding is associated with a poor prognosis, and indicates that significant segments of endarterectomized pulmonary vessels are still partially obstructed (due to distal disease). Subsequently, PVR will remain high and there is an increased risk of reperfusion pulmonary oedema through the very few adequately endarterectomized segments.

Circulatory arrest is limited to 20-minute episodes to promote neurological protection. With experience, an entire unilateral endarterectomy can be accomplished within this time frame. If additional arrest time is necessary to complete the endarterectomy, reperfusion is carried out at 18°C until the venous saturation returns to 90 per cent, or for a minimum of 10 minutes. At the completion of the endarterectomy, reperfusion is re-established while the first pulmonary artery incision is closed.

The other pulmonary artery is incised and a repeat endarterectomy procedure is initiated as described above for the other side. Following completion of the second endarterectomy, a small incision (approximately 1 cm in length) is made in the right atrium near the junction of the atrium and the inferior vena cava. This incision allows inspection and repair of the atrial septum if a defect is present. Any additional procedures that may be required, such as coronary artery bypass grafting or valve replacement, can be performed during the rewarming period.

Anaesthetic management

Pre-induction preparation

Premedication is with a lightly sedative dose of benzodiazepine. On arrival in the operating theatre, the patient is positioned supine on the operating table. ECG, pulse oximetry and invasive arterial monitoring are established, and a large-bore peripheral venous cannula is placed prior to induction. At UCSD, electro-encephalography monitoring (EEG) electrodes are placed on the patient's head bilaterally, and the EEG is followed throughout the procedure.

Patients who are haemodynamically unstable, or are considered to be likely to decompensate and become severely cardiovascularly compromised in response to administration of anaesthetic drugs, should have a pulmonary artery catheter placed prior to induction. In the majority of cases the pulmonary artery catheter can be placed following induction, as the haemodynamic status of the patient is usually known and the haemodynamic target goals are already defined (see below).

Haemodynamic considerations and the pre-cardiopulmonary bypass period

Although a small percentage of patients with CTEPH presenting for PTE will have associated left ventricular pathology (< 10 per cent), the vast majority do not. Haemodynamic assessment and decision making should concentrate upon the right ventricle rather than the left (which is usually normal but empty). The patient with CTEPH has right ventricular pathology equivalent to that seen in patients with aortic stenosis; the right ventricle is thick, hypertrophic and chronically stressed. The coronary artery blood supply to this right ventricle is constantly at risk, and must be maintained. The vast majority of these patients will manifest evidence of right-sided heart failure, and are classified as New York Heart Association (NYHA) classifications III and IV. Patients with right ventricular end-diastolic pressures (RVEDP) greater than 14–16 mmHg tend to have more evidence of right-sided failure and are sicker. Furthermore, these patients do not tolerate induction of general anaesthesia as well as those with RVEDP less than 12 mmHg. Thus inotropes such as dopamine should be started pre-operatively, and vasopressors such as phenylephrine should always be available for increasing the systemic vascular resistance and maintaining the perfusion pressure to the right coronary artery.

Pre-operative data of particular importance to the anaesthetist when planning the induction sequence and pre-cardiopulmonary bypass goals include the cardiac catheterization information regarding cardiac output, PVR and the patency of coronary vessels. Additionally, knowledge of the presence of an atrial septal defect is useful. Patients with known atrial septal defect may have worsening of right-to-left shunt through the atrial septal defect when PVR increases. Many consider patients with CTEPH to have a fixed PVR because of mechanical obstruction due to the clots. However, PVR can be made worse at induction and post-induction by factors that increase PVR in normal patients (e.g. hypoxia, hypercarbia, acidosis, pain and anxiety).

Induction of anaesthesia

Once monitoring and venous access are established, pre-oxygenation and intravenous induction commences. Those with decreased right ventricular function (right RVEDP > 16 or cardiac index (CI) < 1.5) should receive pre-induction dopamine running at 3–5 μg/kg per minute. Dopamine is rarely needed if RVEDP is < 10 and CI > 2.5, and is optional in intermediate cases. Differing induction agents have been successfully used. At UCSD, etomidate 0.2 mg/kg and fentanyl 25–50 μg/kg are titrated to haemodynamic response. At Papworth, propofol infusion is started at 3 mg/kg per hour and fentanyl 15 μg/kg is given over a few minutes. A small dose of midazolam (0.02 mg/kg) can be given at the start of induction, but higher doses should only be administered if the patient remains haemodynamically stable. Phenylephrine or metaraminol administration is frequently necessary in order to maintain coronary artery perfusion pressure by keeping the mean arterial pressure in the 75–85 mmHg range. Phenylephrine has been shown to improve right ventricular performance in patients with pulmonary hypertension. The relaxant of choice is pancuronium, which provides profound and prolonged relaxation yet maintains haemodynamic stability.

Post-induction and pre-cardiopulmonary bypass period

Following induction and intubation with a single-lumen tube, anaesthesia is maintained using propofol at 3 mg/kg per hour by infusion. Air/oxygen at a FiO_2 sufficient to maintain a normal Pao_2 is used for ventilation. Tidal and minute volumes are adjusted to maintain normocapnia whilst avoiding high airway pressures.

A second invasive arterial monitoring is established via a femoral arterial line, as arterial pressure may be significantly underestimated because of the prolonged cooling and rewarming phases associated with DHCA.

A pulmonary artery flotation catheter and transoesophageal echo (TOE) probe are placed and baseline measurements made. The TOE study begins with a cardiac survey, starting with the short axis view, moving to a four-chamber view, and then evaluating the tricuspid valve. The aortic valve and pulmonary outflow tract is viewed looking at both the right and left pulmonary arteries (clots are frequently seen here). Once this survey is completed, attention is turned to the atrial septum to determine the presence of an atrial septal defect. Agitated saline is administered in a 10 ml bolus through the right atrial CVP port; air bubbles can be seen entering the left atrium if an atrial septal defect is present. TOE is more sensitive and specific than surface echocardiography, but still misses a few atrial septal defects (75 per cent sensitive and 95 per cent specific).

Temperature should be measured at the tympanic membrane or nasopharynx and rectum and bladder to quantitate thermal gradients at various sites. The pulmonary artery catheter will give an accurate measure of blood temperature, but this can vary by as much as 10°C from the true core temperature during rapid cooling and warming.

Haemodilution is utilized to decrease blood viscosity, optimize capillary blood flow and promote uniform cooling. The high pre-operative haematocrit in most CTEPH patients allows for venesection of two or more units of blood, and this can be completed before initiation of cardiopulmonary bypass. Haematocrit is maintained at 18–25 per cent during cooling and DHCA.

Cardiopulmonary bypass period

The patient is immediately cooled following initiation of cardiopulmonary bypass. When the temperature descends to approximately 30°C, the heart rate begins to slow and Osborne waves are seen on the ECG. Soon after, the heart will begin to fibrillate.

Systemic cooling is achieved using a cardiopulmonary bypass flow of 4–5 l per minute. A gradient of 10°C is maintained between the arterial blood and the bladder/rectal temperature. The patient's head is covered with ice bags for further neuroprotection. During the cooling phase, venous saturation increases. Saturations of 80 per cent are typically encountered at 25°C and up to 90 per cent at 20°C. Phenytoin is administered intravenously during cooling at a dose of 50 mg/kg (maximum dose of 1 gm). A few minutes before the first episode of DHCA, at a temperature of 18–20°C, thiopentone is administered via the cardiopulmonary bypass pump until the EEG becomes iso-electric (typically after 500–1000 mg of thiopentone).

Deep hypothermic circulatory arrest

Any flushing of arterial or venous lines during DHCA is strictly forbidden as this may allow air, debris or warm saline to be infused into the cerebral circulation during the period of no-flow, with potentially disastrous consequences. Just after circulatory arrest is established the lungs are ventilated to push residual blood out of the pulmonary veins and bronchial vessels, allowing the surgeon to operate temporarily in a bloodless field. The pulmonary artery catheter is withdrawn while the pulmonary artery is opened and re-positioned before closure of the pulmonary artery incision.

Post-DHCA and post-rewarming

Once the PTE is completed, the aortic cross clamp is removed and full perfusion flow restored during rewarming. Methylprednisone 500 mg (to stabilize membranes and decrease reperfusion pulmonary oedema) and mannitol 12.5 g (to promote diuresis, thus leading to increased haematocrit, and for its free radical scavenger effects) are administered. A 10°C core-peripheral gradient is maintained during rewarming (warming more rapidly may promote egress of air bubbles from the blood). Rewarming times are variably related to the patient's weight and systemic perfusion, typically requiring 90–120 minutes to rewarm to a rectal temperature of 36.5°C. In the event that systemic vascular resistance is increased at this time, an infusion of sodium nitroprusside is started to promote uniform warming by allowing increased flows on cardiopulmonary bypass. The haematocrit is slowly raised to 30 per cent by using ultra-filtration. In some centres a left atrial monitoring line is inserted under direct vision, and is used to monitor precisely the left-sided filling pressure in the early post-operative period.

The heart generally begins to beat spontaneously with a bradycardiac rhythm as the blood temperature approaches 25°–30°C. Cardioversion will be necessary if ventricular fibrillation occurs. Prior to termination of cardiopulmonary bypass, 20 mg of frusemide is given to reduce lung water content and calcium chloride is administered if the measured ionized calcium is low.

Separation from cardiopulmonary bypass

When the core temperature reaches 35°C, lung ventilation is commenced and dopamine is administered at 3–5 g/kg per minute. Sinus rhythm at a rate of 80–100 bpm should optimally be achieved, and it may be necessary to pace the heart electrically.

Prior to separation from cardiopulmonary bypass, the patient's temperature should be 36–37°C. Inspired oxygen concentration should then be increased above 60 per cent, and the tidal volumes set at approximately 20 per cent above pre-operative values. PEEP at 5 cmH$_2$O is typically added at this time. An increased respiratory rate may be required because of the paradoxically increased dead space that occurs in the immediate post-operative period. End-tidal CO$_2$ is thus a poor measure of ventilatory adequacy in these patients.

Prior to and during separation from cardiopulmonary bypass, TOE is used to evaluate cardiac filling, left and right ventricular function and air emboli. The TOE typically reveals immediate post-PTE architectural changes of the left and right ventricles. There is usually much less distension of the right ventricle with less impingement of the left ventricle. The pulmonary artery diastolic pressure is usually significantly decreased from pre-operative values. Cardiac output measurement typically reveals an index double that of the pre-operative value, and a PVR at quarter of the pre-operative value.

The anaesthetist should check the airway for any frothy sputum or bleeding, as severe pulmonary hypertension and reperfusion pulmonary oedema may begin to manifest at this time in some cases.

The post-cardiopulmonary bypass period

Heparin is reversed with protamine. Any autologous blood that has been removed prior to cardiopulmonary bypass and not used to increase the haematocrit during rewarming is re-administered.

If frothy sputum is noted in the endotracheal tube, this is suctioned and increasing amounts of PEEP are applied (escalating to a maximum of 10 cmH$_2$O). If frank blood exudes via the endotracheal tube, fibre-optic bronchoscopy may be required to evaluate the source of bleeding.

Surgical haemostasis is attained and the chest closed with pleural and mediastinal drains in place. Fresh frozen plasma and platelets may be required to aid coagulation following cardiopulmonary bypass.

The use of blood salvage techniques such as cell savers is recommended throughout the procedure.

Post-operative care

Post-operative management of the PTE patient is similar to that following cardiac operations. The two major post-operative complications that are unique to the PTE patient are reperfusion pulmonary oedema and pulmonary arterial steal.

Reperfusion pulmonary oedema is a localized form of high permeability (non-cardiogenic) lung injury, a form of adult respiratory distress syndrome (ARDS). This typically occurs within the first 24 hours, but may appear up to 72 hours following PTE. The severity can range from mild to fulminant. In its most severe form, reperfusion pulmonary oedema begins immediately after cardiopulmonary bypass, in the operating room, as described above. The most interesting aspect of reperfusion pulmonary oedema following PTE is that the areas of lung most involved correlate with those segments that have been endarterectomized to the greatest degree. Management of reperfusion pulmonary oedema is mainly supportive, with pressure-controlled, inverse-ratio ventilation used judicially to improve V/Q mismatch and shunting. Inhaled nitric oxide can help to improve oxygenation.

Pulmonary artery steal represents a post-operative redistribution of pulmonary arterial blood away from the previously well-perfused segments into the newly endarterectomized segments. Whether the cause is due to inability of the newly endarterectomized segments to auto-regulate or whether there are secondary small vessel changes in the previously open segments has not been clarified. However, long-term follow-up in the majority of patients suggests a remodelling process of the pulmonary vascular bed.

Outcome

The majority of patients will have immediate improvement in their pulmonary artery pressure and PVR following endarterectomy. This is documented in the published experience of UCSD, with pre-operative PVR and pulmonary artery pressures averaging 901 dynes.sec.cm^{-5} and 46 mmHg respectively, decreased to 261 dynes.sec.cm^{-5} and 28 mmHg post-operatively. Gas exchange may take longer to improve. The long-term improvements result from a combination of improved auto-regulation and normalization of vascular permeability. In addition, resolution of pulmonary hypertensive changes within the pulmonary vascular bed is seen and remodelling of the right ventricular hypertrophy continues to occur over weeks to months. Both V/Q and cardiac output improve and return to normal. The majority of patients who were initially NYHA class III and IV status return to NYHA class I and II, and are able to resume normal activities.

All patients are maintained on life-long anticoagulation with warfarin. Although thrombo-embolic recurrence has been detected in a few patients in whom anticoagulation therapy was discontinued or allowed to fall below therapeutic levels, there have been no documented occurrences of recurrent thrombo-embolic events in patients who have been maintained on adequate anticoagulation. Patients frequently have psychiatric changes, which can range from paranoia to euphoria, and (more rarely) focal neurological deficits.

PTE is a potentially curative procedure for CTEPH. Although probably less than 1500 of these operations have been performed worldwide, there has been progressive annual improvement in operative outcome. At UCSD, the mortality of the first 388 cases was 10.8 per cent, of the next 150 was 5.3 per cent, and currently the mortality is down to 5 per cent. Patients with severe disease (PVR > 1100 dynes.sec.cm^{-5} and PAP > 50 mmHg) have a higher risk of operative mortality.

Patients who do not undergo PTE have a uniformly poor prognosis, with their only alternative being lung transplantation. Compared to lung transplantation, PTE offers a lower surgical mortality rate, better long-term survival, and fewer chronic complications.

KEY POINTS

- CTEPH is still under-diagnosed, but is a highly disabling disease.

- PTE offers a promising alternative to lung transplantation for patients suffering from CTEPH.

- Operative management of PTE includes cardiopulmonary bypass and DHCA.

- Complications are mainly due to reperfusion injuries resulting from cardiopulmonary bypass and DHCA.

- Careful monitoring and support of the right heart is a key issue in the management of patients for PTE.

Bibliography

Auger, W.R., Fedullo, P.F., Moser, K.M. *et al.* (1992). Chronic major vessel thrombo-embolic pulmonary artery obstruction: appearance at angiography. *Radiology*, **182(2)**, 393–8.

Bergin, C.J. (1997). Chronic thrombo-embolic pulmonary hypertension: the disease, the diagnosis and the treatment. *Semin. Ultrasound CTMR*, **18(5)**, 383–91.

Bergin, C.J., Sirlin, C.B., Hauschildt, J.P. *et al.* (1997). Chronic thrombo-embolism diagnosis with helical CT and MR imaging with angiographic and surgical correlation. *Radiology*, **204(3)**, 695–702.

Dalen, J.E. and Alpert, J.S. (1975). Natural history of pulmonary embolism. *Prog. Cardiovasc. Dis.*, **17(4)**, 257–70.

Fedullo, P.F., Auger, W.R., Channick, R.N. *et al.* (1995). Chronic thrombo-embolitic pulmonary hypertension. *Clin. Chest Med.*, **16(2)**, 353–74.

Hartz, R.S., Byrne, J.G., Levitsky, S. *et al.* (1996). Predictors of mortality in pulmonary thrombo-endarterectomy. *Ann. Thorac. Surg.*, **62(5)**, 1255–9.

Jamieson, S.W., Auger, W.R., Fedullo, P.F. *et al.* (1993). Experience and results with 150 pulmonary thrombo-endarterectomy operations over a 29-month period. *J. Thorac. Cardiovasc. Surg.*, **106(1)**, 116–26.

Kapitan, K.S., Buchbinder, M., Wagner, P.D. *et al.* (1989). Mechanisms of hypoxemia in chronic thrombo-embolic pulmonary hypertension. *Am. Rev. Respir. Dis.*, **139(5)**, 1149–54.

Levinson, R.M., Shure, D. and Moser, K.M. (1986). Reperfusion pulmonary oedema after pulmonary artery thrombo-endarterectomy. *Am. Rev. Respir. Dis.*, **134(6)**, 1241–5.

Moser, K.M., Auger, W.R. and Fedullo, P.F. (1990). Chronic major vessel thrombo-embolic pulmonary hypertension. *Circulation*, **81(6)**, 1735–43.

Olman, M.A., Marsh, J.J. and Lang, I.M. (1992). Endogenous fibrinolytic system in chronic large-vessel thrombo-embolic pulmonary hypertension. *Circulation*, **86(4)**, 1241–8.

Olman, M.A., Auger, W.R., Fedullo, P.F. *et al.* (1990). Pulmonary vascular steal in chronic thrombo-embolic pulmonary hypertension. *Chest*, **98(6)**, 1430–4.

Rubinstein, I., Murray, D. and Hoffstein, V. (1988). Fatal pulmonary emboli in hospitalized patients. An autopsy study. *Arch. Intern. Med.*, **148(6)**, 1425–6.

Tanabe, N., Okada, O., Nakagawa, Y. *et al.* (1997). The efficacy of pulmonary thrombo-endarterectomy on long-term gas exchange. *Eur. Respir. J.*, **10(9)**, 2066–72.

15

Lung transplantation

I. D. Conacher

Introduction

Long-term survival after lung transplantation for end-stage pulmonary disease only became feasible in the late 1980s. Previous efforts faltered because of inappropriate selection of patients, ineffective immunotherapy and poor donor organ preservation. The quality of donor lungs remains the single most important factor for long-term survival. As the lungs are particularly susceptible to contusion and oedema during resuscitation and management of catastrophic states, there is a paucity of suitable organs. There is, therefore, a tendency to use single lung transplantation (Fig. 15.1) to benefit as many patients as possible rather than using a heart-lung or double lung block for a single recipient, even though this may not be the most physiologically appropriate solution for a particular pulmonary pathology. However, the better the matching of the operation to a cure of the pathophysiology, the less the peri-operative complications and the better the prognosis. Living related donors have been used, but have made little impact on the supply of lungs except in paediatrics.

The tracheal anastomosis necessary for double lung transplant operations remains problematical and is more likely to dehisce than bronchial anastomoses; many surgeons thus prefer the sequential single lung operation for conditions requiring replacement of both lungs. The use of cardiopulmonary bypass (CPB) is more an issue nowadays of the specialist training and preference of the surgeon conducting the operation than one of concerns about the effects of anticoagulation, fluid load and cellular damage on transplant organ function – as was the case previously, when CPB techniques were less well developed (Table 15.1).

Early organ failure is due to reperfusion (re-implantation) injury or infection. The development of obliterative bronchiolitis is the main cause of late organ failure. This complex disease is probably a low-grade rejection process. The influence of anaesthesia on any of these processes is unknown. Survivors of lung transplantation have a significant incidence of problems with airway anastomoses. Laser resection of granulation tissue may be required, and stents of various kinds may need to be inserted.

(a)

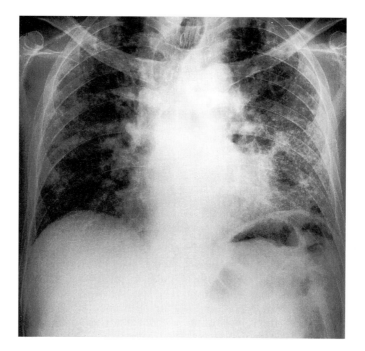

(b)

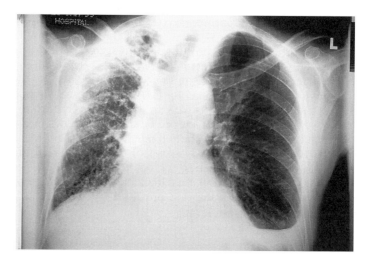

Figure 15.1

(a) Chest X-ray of patient with pulmonary fibrosis pre-transplant.
(b) Chest X-ray of same patient post-transplant (left single lung).

Table 15.1 Indications for lung transplantation and intra-operative respiratory management technique

Lung transplant type	Primary indication	Secondary indication	Respiratory management
Single	• Pulmonary fibrosis (e.g. histiocytosis X)	• Emphysema • Pulmonary hypertension (mild)	• One-lung ventilation
Sequential single	• Emphysema • Infective lung (e.g. cystic fibrosis)		• One-lung ventilation • One-lung ventilation with cardiopulmonary bypass
Double	• Emphysema • Infective lung (e.g. cystic fibrosis)		• Cardiopulmonary bypass
Heart–lung	• Pulmonary hypertension		• Cardiopulmonary bypass

Surgical procedure

Initially, pneumonectomy is necessary. For single lung procedures, a standard antero-lateral thoracotomy is used for access. A standard sternotomy is usual for bilateral pulmonary resections and heart-lung transplantation, but the transverse sternotomy ('clam-shell') is proving increasingly popular for double lung procedures, either carried out *en bloc* or as sequential single lung. Cannulation for CPB takes place at this stage for heart-lung and double lung procedures. For double lung transplants some surgeons prefer to remove the first lung without CPB, but cannulate and institute bypass to conduct the second pneumonectomy. Sequential single lung transplant is increasingly being performed without CPB. The first implanted lung is ventilated on completion of anastomoses, and the second pneumonectomy and transplant then performed. The transplant lung is anastomosed in the sequence pulmonary veins and pulmonary artery, and finally bronchial anastomosis is carried out. Flushing out of the perfusate and air must be conducted before vascular integrity is complete.

Anaesthetic management

Pre-operative assessment

Patients on transplant waiting lists are extensively investigated, but deterioration tends to be rapid, and their state may have significantly altered by the time a suitable donor organ is available. Investigations worth reviewing immediately pre-operatively are simple pulmonary function tests and blood gases. Echocardiographic assessment of right heart function, in those not anticipated to require CPB for the transplant operation, is useful. Chest X-rays, computerized tomography (CT) and ventilation–perfusion scans should be evaluated for changes in lung structure, such as the presence of bullae, infection, oedema or pleural effusions. Most patients presenting for lung transplantation are cachetic and short of breath at rest despite optimal medical therapy, fitness training programmes and dietary regimens. Protocols for administration of antibiotics, immunosuppressants and anti-coagulants should be checked and adhered to.

Anaesthetic technique and monitoring

For single lung transplants, the techniques of anaesthesia for major pulmon-ary resection and establishment of one-lung ventilation are fundamental. Most United Kingdom centres use double-lumen tubes to achieve this, but the use of bronchus blockers and the combination of tracheal tube with integral blocking device (Univent tube) is proving increasingly popular. This is because confirmation of optimal positioning of endobronchial devices, without compromising oxygenation, is relatively easy with modern fibre-optic bronchoscopes.

As the anaesthetic techniques for lung transplantation are adapted from the time-honoured ones of thoracic anaesthesia, there is little practical objection to the use of modern volatile agents to maintain anaesthesia. Air–oxygen mixtures should be used; nitrous oxide should be avoided. Some advocate the use of total intravenous anaesthesia.

Cardiorespiratory instability is particularly likely to occur on induction of anaesthesia. This is particularly evident on application of IPPV, the onset of one-lung ventilation, pulmonary artery clamping and section, and when the transplanted lung is allowed to function. Most of these events relate to changes in pulmonary haemodynamics. Obtaining the necessary infor-mation to make the therapeutic decisions to cope with these changes is awkward, as pulmonary artery flotation catheters may intrude into the surgical field. Solutions to the dilemma include ignoring it (except in those with pre-operative right heart dysfunction or pulmonary hypertension), using main pulmonary artery pressure monitoring and measuring mixed venous oxygenation, or siting a flotation catheter in the distal pulmonary artery of the ventilated lung. Transoesophageal echocardiography intra-operatively is proving valuable in assessing cardiac filling and performance in situations where pulmonary artery catheterization is not feasible.

Low-compliant lung conditions, such as pulmonary fibrosis, rarely pre-sent a problem with regard to ventilatory support. Higher inflation pressures and respiratory rates will usually result in adequate gas exchange during one-lung ventilation while pneumonectomy and transplant of the opposite lung are conducted. Emphysematous lungs may be problematical to venti-late; gas trapping with the development of dynamic hyperinflation is likely unless a ventilatory pattern with low inflation pressures and prolonged expiratory times is employed. A moderate degree of permissive hypercapnia is commonly accepted as a worthwhile risk in such cases.

It would appear that a lack of specific pulmonary vasodilators has not hampered the success of lung transplantation. A variety of vasodilators with systemic effects, including nitrates, nitroprusside, theophyllines, prosta-glandins and alpha-blockers, have been and still are used. Nitric oxide has yet to make a significant clinical impact. Hypotensive events are best treated with sympathomimetic agents.

Aprotonin is commonly used prophylactically to reduce blood loss in infective conditions, and in those in whom pleural adhesions are anticipated to be extensive. Adhesions are particularly marked in those patients who have had previous pulmonary surgery such as pleurodesis, pleurectomy or lobectomy.

The sectioning of lymphatic drainage results in excess fluid accumulating in the alveoli or pulmonary interstitium. This can only be controlled by alteration of intravascular osmolality. Urine flow should be promoted with dopamine and/or diuretics if necessary. Volume replacement should be cautious, primarily with colloid. The CPB circuit, if CPB is to be used, should be primed with a moderately hyperosmolar solution. Deliberate water extraction, with in-line haemofiltration, is worth conducting before termination of CPB.

Post-operative care

As the failing organ has been replaced by one of normal function, recovery can be rapid. A straightforward, uncomplicated single lung transplant can progress though an intensive care unit almost as rapidly as an uncomplicated pneumonectomy. It is possible to extubate at the end of the operation, but the majority of patients require up to 48 hours of post-operative positive pressure ventilation and stabilization before weaning. A transplanted single lung has a different compliance to the native lung, and the effect of this is particularly marked in emphysema. In order to ensure that the transplant lung is not compromised by an over-inflated native lung, double-lumen tubes, blockers and differential lung ventilation may be required if an early return to spontaneous respiration is not achieved.

There is a theoretical problem of a large ventilation–perfusion mismatch as a result of single lung transplantation in recipients with pulmonary hypertension; in practice, this has rarely proved to be the case.

The routine pain-relieving techniques of thoracotomy and sternotomy are adequate, as discussed in Chapter 17. Epidural analgesia is the method of choice, particularly for the transverse 'clam-shell' sternotomy and for those patients less able to undertake physiotherapy or weakened by perioperative complications. In some centres the epidural catheter is sited prior to weaning from ventilatory support; care should be taken to correct coagulopathy if CPB has been used for the transplant.

If lung transplant recipients require non-pulmonary or emergency surgery, regional anaesthetic blocks and general anaesthetic techniques employing spontaneous respiration will avoid the complications associated with differential pulmonary compliances. Volume replacement must be conducted cautiously, as recipients have difficulty clearing excess lung water. Aspiration can occur without activating the cough reflex as a consequence of denervation of the lung.

KEY POINTS

- The techniques of thoracic anaesthesia are fundamental to, and readily adapted for, lung transplantation.

- Bilateral lung transplant may be conducted as sequential single lung or implantation of a double lung block.

- CPB is used in some cases; the choice depends on surgical preference and the recipient's cardiorespiratory reserve.

- Intra-operative monitoring should include pulmonary artery catheterization (if possible) or transoesophageal echo, as the accumulation of excess lung water occurs easily in transplant recipients and haemodynamic instability may be difficult to manage.

- Ventilatory patterns need to be adjusted peri-operatively to take account of the patient's pathology, particularly emphysema.

- The differential pulmonary compliances that are a result of single lung transplantation can prove problematical post-operatively.

- Pain control is best achieved by thoracic epidural, particularly for the transverse sternotomy that is sometimes used for double lung transplantation.

- Regional and spontaneous respiration techniques are safest in recipients requiring anaesthesia for emergency and non-pulmonary surgery.

Bibliography

Boscoe, M.J. (1996). Anaesthesia for heart-lung and lung transplantation. In *International Practice of Anaesthesia* (C. Prys-Roberts and B.R. Brown, eds), pp. 1/67, 1–15. Butterworth Heinemann.

Bracken, C.A., Gurkowski, M.A. and Naples, J.J. (1997). Lung transplantation: historical perspectives, current concepts and anesthetic considerations. *J. Cardiothorac. Vasc. Anesth.*, **11,** 220–41.

Conacher, I.D. (1997). Anaesthesia for the surgery of emphysema. *Br. J. Anaesth.*, **79,** 530–8.

Raffin, L., Michel-Cherque, M., Sperandio, M. *et al.* (1992). Anesthesia for bilateral lung transplantation without cardiopulmonary bypass. *J. Cardiothorac. Vasc. Anesth.*, **6,** 409–17.

Simpson, K.P. and Garrity, E.R. (1997). Peri-operative management in lung transplantation. *Clin. Chest Med.*, **18,** 277–84.

Walsh, T.S. and Young, C.H. (1995). Anaesthesia and cystic fibrosis. *Anaesth.*, **50,** 614–22.

16

Common peri-operative problems and complications: pulmonary haemorrhage/empyema/ bronchopleural fistula/persistent air leaks

L. Doolan and P. Clarke

Pulmonary haemorrhage

Introduction

The practising thoracic anaesthetist encounters pulmonary haemorrhage either as a complication of a specific surgical procedure (e.g. bronchoscopy, biopsy) or as part of a team dealing with an acute airway haemorrhage.

Generally, massive haemoptysis is easily recognized when it occurs and is defined as expectorating 600 ml or more of blood in 24 hours. Mortality rates range from 12 per cent to greater than 50 per cent with conservative management. Bleeding rates of greater than 600 ml in 16 or less hours are associated with mortality of approximately 75 per cent. Although surgical treatment carries a significant mortality of 15–20 per cent, it should be considered in cases of continued bleeding rather than allowing a patient's condition to deteriorate and then having to operate. Ideally, if the patient's condition is stable, massive haemoptysis is managed conservatively, with subsequent surgical intervention when the patient's general condition has been optimized and suitability for surgery better evaluated.

Massive haemoptysis is usually from systemic bronchial arteries rather than the low-pressure pulmonary arterial system. Carcinoma, infective or inflammatory lung disease, bronchiectasis, trauma and post-surgical bleeding are the most common causes. In tuberculosis, bleeding can occur from bronchial vessels or a Rasmussen's aneurysm of the pulmonary artery; copious bleeding associated with tuberculosis is now less commonly seen due to the lower incidence of the disease in developed countries.

The amount of bleeding has no relationship to the gravity of the underlying pulmonary lesion, and heavy bleeding may be associated with mild bronchiectasis or even a ruptured bronchial artery in patients with systemic hypertension.

One of the most common emerging causes of massive pulmonary haemorrhage is pulmonary artery rupture from pulmonary artery catheterization. This complication is more likely to occur in patients who are older or have clotting defects or pulmonary hypertension, and when the catheter is placed distally and the balloon hyperinflated. Strict protocols must be applied in intensive care units and operating rooms to minimize pulmonary artery complications from pulmonary artery catheters. In particular, emphasis should be placed on slowly inflating the balloon to the minimum volume required to achieve a 'wedge position'. Catheter migration to the periphery of the lung is so fast that the catheter may be wedged whilst the balloon is still being inflated, thus rupturing the pulmonary artery.

Airway haemorrhage from pulmonary artery catheter-induced pulmonary artery rupture may be classified as small (< 15 ml blood), moderate (> 15–30 ml) or large (continued blood loss). In general, if pulmonary haemorrhage occurs the pulmonary artery catheter should be withdrawn centrally and **not** inflated. Intermittent positive pressure ventilation (IPPV) with positive end expiratory pressure (PEEP) may tamponade the bleeding. Reversal of anticoagulants or treatment of an underlying clotting abnormality should commence if indicated.

Surgical management

The cornerstone of initial management of pulmonary haemorrhage is bronchoscopy to clear the airway, localize the site of bleeding and institute local control measures. This is best achieved by a combination of rigid and fibre-optic flexible bronchoscopy under general anaesthesia. Initial clearing of the major airways is followed by irrigation with 10 ml aliquots of normal saline or diluted adrenaline and further suction. The fibre-optic broncho-scope can be used for tamponade if bleeding is from a segmental bronchus. If the bleeding is controlled, the patient can be evaluated for other necessary procedures. However, if the bleeding continues, isolation of the 'normal' lung should be performed expeditiously. Once the normal lung has been protected from aspiration, and if the patient is deemed to be operable, definitive surgical treatment can proceed. An algorithm for the management of pulmonary haemorrhage is outlined in Figure 16.1.

In those patients who are not suitable for lung resection but who continue to bleed (particularly from cavities in the lung, which are almost always fed by bronchial arteries), embolization of the bronchial artery under radiographic control is an alternative. This needs to be performed during active bleeding, as the radiologist is dependent on seeing the blush at the end of the vessel for precise identification. Experience and skill are required as the first branch of the bronchial artery goes to the spinal cord and, if compromised, the spinal cord may be damaged.

Anaesthetic management

Patients are transported to the operating room sitting up, to maximize functional residual capacity, with supplementary oxygen.

Arterial cannulation for continuous blood pressure monitoring and placement of one or two large-bore intravenous cannulae is advisable. Central venous cannulation is an advantage, but should only be undertaken if the patient can be positioned head down without the risk of spilling blood into the normal airways.

The anaesthetist should select those drugs with which he or she is most familiar to deal with these acutely ill patients. After anaesthetic induction, initial paralysis for bronchoscopy and clearing of the airway should be

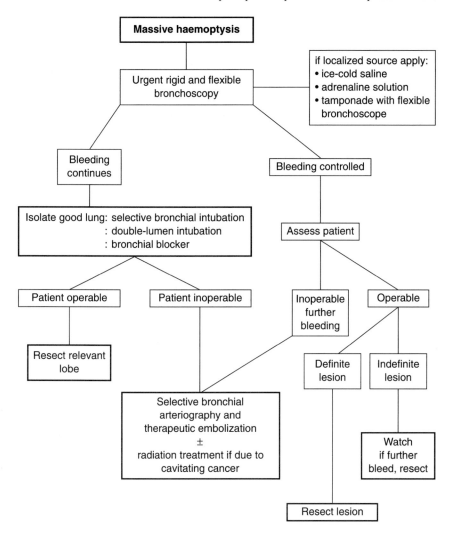

Figure 16.1 Algorithm for the management of acute airway haemorrhage.

with suxamethonium, which has a rapid onset and provides the best conditions for intubation. Maintenance of anaesthesia during bronchoscopy is by an intravenous agent, e.g. propofol. The agents used for subsequent anaesthesia and paralysis, if a more definitive operation is required, are a matter of personal choice, but should be aimed at minimizing haemodynamic disturbance and the prompt recovery of spontaneous respiration and protective airway reflexes at the end of the procedure.

High-volume suction must be available to the anaesthetist at all times for the removal of blood clots, particularly when surgical bronchoscopy is finished and control of the airway is passed solely to the anaesthetist.

Following bronchoscopy, lung isolation is required prior to thoracotomy, if this is indicated. There are several options for achieving this:

1. Bronchial blocking (e.g. with a Foley catheter) to the affected lung via a single-lumen tube.
2. Using a combination endotracheal tube and bronchial blocker placed under bronchoscopic control (e.g. the Univent tube).
3. Selective endobronchial intubation of the non-bleeding lung.
4. Use of a double-lumen endobronchial tube to allow isolation and ventilation of either lung as required.

Airway haemorrhage associated with bronchoscopy

Moderate haemorrhage following bronchoscopy and biopsy is not uncommon. The anaesthetist or surgeon must maintain direct vision of the bleeding area in the bronchus and suction blood away until the patient is awakening and able to cough. Only then should the bronchoscope be removed.

Following removal of the bronchoscope, the patient is positioned affected side down to confine any blood to that lung and prevent soiling of the unaffected lung. The patient is transferred to the recovery room breathing oxygen by mask. When able to cough on command, the patient is turned affected side up to encourage drainage of any accumulated blood. Drainage is further facilitated by coughing or oral suction.

Occasionally, recovery room patients may present *in extremis* following bronchoscopy and biopsy. This is usually due to a carinal clot blocking both main bronchi, and requires immediate treatment and removal of the clot via a rigid bronchoscope. Bronchoscopic equipment should be available in the recovery room, as expeditious removal of the asphyxiating carinal clot is life-saving. Following removal of the clot and assessment of bleeding, the patient is sat up and encouraged to cough. These manoeuvres will effectively deal with this problem in the vast majority of cases. Should the bleeding be continuous and massive, the patient should be treated as outlined in Figure 16.1.

Empyema

Introduction

Empyema was first described over 2400 years ago by Hippocrates, who observed that patients with suppuration in the pleural space that discharged spontaneously through the skin did better than those who continued to languish with fevers. He noted that linen packing of the wound allowed drainage of pus yet prevented inflow of air into the chest.

The first deliberate incision for drainage of an empyema was described by Serefeddin Subuncoglu in his book *Imperial Surgery*, written in 1465. Further advances were slow, mainly because of the difficulty of diagnosis and failure to distinguish between an effusion and empyema.

Earlier diagnosis was made possible by the description of percussion by Auenbrugger in 1761 and auscultation by Laennec in 1816. The bacterial nature of infection was established by Robert Koch in the middle of the nineteenth century, and diagnostic aspiration of the chest by Thomas Davies in 1835. Radiology of the chest, which followed Roentgen's discovery of X-rays in 1895, further refined diagnosis. Open drainage of empyema, which followed the development of anaesthesia, initially carried a high mortality. This trend was reversed when the importance of closed drainage was established by Graham, following studies of soldiers in the First World War. As anaesthetic and surgical techniques improved, death rates fell.

Operations for chronic empyema, usually due to inadequate treatment in the acute stage, began in the latter part of the nineteenth century. A variety of unroofing and destructive procedures were performed. Decortication of a chronic empyema was first proposed by Delorme in 1894.

Refinements in radiology, with the introduction of computerized tomographic (CT) scanning and, more recently, magnetic resonance imaging (MRI), have simplified the early diagnosis of empyema. The pathophysiological progress of empyema has been defined as follows:

- Stage 1   Development of an effusion, usually exudative in nature.
- Stage 2   Accumulation of fibropurulent fluid, bacterial multiplication within the fluid, development of loculation and a fibrinous pleural peel on the lungs.
- Stage 3   Organizational stage with development of a thick membrane entrapping the lung. If untreated, the natural history is erosion into the lung creating a bronchopleural fistulae, or spontaneous drainage via the chest wall (*empyema necessitans*).

Following improvements in surgical and anaesthetic techniques the incidence of empyema after lung resection has fallen. The Austin and Repatriation Medical Centre group (Melbourne, Australia), in a series of 543 lung resections since 1992, had an empyema rate of less than 4 per cent.

Surgical procedure

The principles of surgery for empyema are to obliterate the infected pleural space and to fully re-expand the lung. Stage 1 empyema only requires insertion of an intercostal drain and underwater sealed drainage. Stage 2 empyema is best managed by video-assisted thoracoscopic surgical techniques. If the trapped lung cannot be adequately freed, an open decortication may be required. This is the procedure of choice for Stage 3 empyemas. Some patients, however, will be too old or frail for a full decortication, or have an associated medical condition precluding major surgery. These patients are better managed by rib resection and tube drainage, although at the cost of permanently impaired pulmonary function.

Decortication is usually performed in the full lateral decubitus position using a postero-lateral or muscle sparing thoracotomy, as discussed in Chapter 6. The aim of the procedure is to peel the outer membrane on the chest wall and lung completely, allowing full re-expansion of the lung. Resection of a rib facilitates location of the correct plane. There is often significant blood loss during the procedure, and it may be difficult to avoid superficial damage to the lung with consequent air leak. At least two chest drains connected to underwater sealed drainage are left *in situ* at the end of the procedure.

In the past, if the opportunity to manage an empyema early was missed, it was considered advisable to delay surgical intervention for 6 weeks to allow the fibrous peel to mature and thus be detached more easily from the lung. More recently, early treatment has shown that this caution was not necessary.

Bronchopleural fistula

Introduction

A bronchopleural fistula is the term used for a communication between the trachea or bronchi and the pleural cavity. It may arise as the result of trauma, infection, inflammation or carcinoma breaching the integrity of the tracheobronchial tree. Whereas bronchopleural fistula was formerly a common sequelae of untreated empyema, it is now more often a rare post-operative complication of lobectomy or pneumonectomy. Predisposing factors for the formation of a bronchopleural fistula include residual carcinoma following pulmonary resection, previous radiotherapy, underlying inflammatory lung disease, gross pleural contamination and sputum culture positive for tuberculosis. Leaving a long dependent stump at operation may be a causal factor, as secretions pool in it and become infected. Bronchopleural fistula usually occur within the first 2 weeks following surgery, but may present some years later, particularly after pneumonectomy.

The development of an acute bronchopleural fistula is marked by the onset of pyrexia, dyspnoea and subcutaneous emphysema, and the development of a productive cough expectorating serosanguinous fluid. A wheezy nocturnal cough is a particularly suggestive symptom. The relative severity of symptoms depends on the size of the fistula. Large fistulae may cause flooding of the bronchi with pleural fluid or result in a large air leak, producing severe dyspnoea and subcutaneous emphysema; small fistulae may have a more subtle combination of the symptoms listed above, present insidiously, and be mistaken for pneumonia, cardiac failure or bronchospasm.

The diagnosis of bronchopleural fistula is confirmed by X-ray (with contrast being introduced into the pleural cavity), CT scanning and bronchoscopy. Classically, following pneumonectomy or lobectomy, serial X-rays may demonstrate a falling fluid level in the residual cavity (Fig. 16.2).

Prompt diagnosis and treatment of bronchopleural fistula is crucial in preventing overspill of fluid and the development of inflammation and infection in the contralateral lung, which is often otherwise healthy.

Surgical management

Bronchopleural fistulae resulting from inflammatory or cavitating lesions and small bronchopleural fistulae following lobectomy are usually managed conservatively with chest drainage and antibiotic therapy.

At bronchoscopy, a definitive diagnosis of post-pneumonectomy or post-lobectomy bronchopleural fistula can be made if fluid is seen exuding into the bronchial stump. Small bronchopleural fistulae can be sealed via the bronchoscope, using tissue glue thickened with preserved bone chips.

(a)

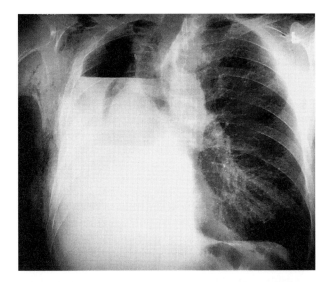

(b)

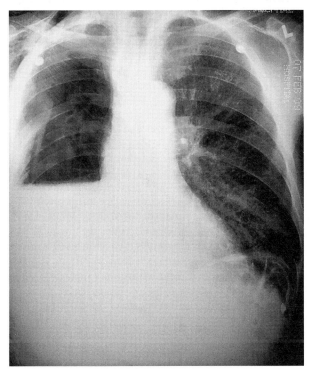

Figure 16.2

(a) Chest X-ray 1 month post-pneumonectomy showing partial
filling of right hemithorax with 'space' fluid and mediastinal
shift.
(b) Chest X-ray of the same patient 4 days later showing drop in
'space' fluid level and centralization of the mediastinum.

Persistent bronchopleural fistulae that do not heal after conservative measures and attempted bronchoscopic closure, or larger bronchopleural fistulae, will require surgical closure. Very occasionally, the bronchopleural fistula may be of such a magnitude as to cause respiratory embarrassment, necessitating immediate intubation and ventilatory support.

Surgical closure of bronchopleural fistulae following pulmonary resection is achieved by re-thoracotomy and re-suturing of the bronchial stump. Reinforcement of the closure may be required, using intercostal muscle flaps or omental grafts. Obliteration of residual space by thoracoplasty or using muscle or omental flaps may also be necessary.

Anaesthetic management

Patients presenting with bronchopleural fistula have compromised pulmonary function, either as a result of their underlying disease or as a result of pulmonary resection. Relatively healthy areas of the lung may have been damaged by overspill of pleural fluid, and the patient may be bacteraemic or frankly septic. Often, little pre-operative optimization can be achieved other than to ensure that fluid resuscitation is in progress and appropriate antibiotics commenced, and that a functioning chest drain is in place.

The patient should be maintained sitting upright with the diseased hemithorax dependent and transported to theatre in this position.

In general, premedication is to provide anxiolysis and is tailored to the patient being co-operative and able to cough and clear secretions.

The specific problems of anaesthetizing patients with bronchopleural fistula are:

- Prevention of overspill of fluid into the lung(s).
- Obtaining control of the distribution of ventilation; application of positive pressure will result in the leak of gas from the tracheobronchial tree, rendering ventilation at best inefficient and at worst impossible. If the chest drain is not functioning adequately, this may also result in the build up of pressure in the thorax, with displacement of fluid into the bronchi or mediastinal shift.
- The potential for iatrogenic enlargement of the bronchopleural fistula during passage of an endobronchial tube or bronchus blocker.

The options available to the anaesthetist are:

- Bronchoscopy and intubation under local anaesthesia.
- Bronchoscopy and intubation under general anaesthesia maintaining spontaneous respiration.
- Bronchoscopy and intubation with a muscle relaxant and general anaesthesia.

The safest option is the use of local anaesthesia for intubation, and the technique for this is described below. Intubation under general anaesthesia using a double-lumen tube can be difficult without administration of a muscle relaxant; this is also discussed below. A double-lumen tube is of choice for isolation of a bronchopleural fistula and protection of the 'healthy' lung, provided that it is passed under direct vision using a fibre-optic bronchoscope, with the endobronchial limb correctly positioned to the side contralateral to the fistula. A double-lumen tube permits the best access to suction the affected side. The ability to apply positive pressure to the affected side may also aid in the localization of the fistula by the escape of gas bubbles, if required.

Whichever technique of intubation is chosen, it is important to maintain the patient upright and with the affected side dependent until successful intubation has been achieved.

Suction apparatus should be available at all times. The greatest risk of tracheal flooding and overspill occur during initial tracheal instrumentation, opening of the chest and surgical manipulation of the lung.

The affected side and the 'healthy' lung should be suctioned repeatedly during the procedure and prior to extubation.

Bronchoscopy and intubation under local anaesthesia

Patients are encouraged to rinse their mouth with topical viscous lignocaine, or to breathe 1–2 ml of 2 per cent lignocaine via an acorn nebulizer or equivalent. This is followed by bilateral internal laryngeal nerve blocks with 2–3 ml 1.5 per cent lignocaine injected in the area of the thyrohyoid membrane (Fig. 16.3). A successful block causes a 'squeaking' voice. A pharyngeal plexus block is performed by using the laryngoscope like a spatula to expose the tonsillar fossae on either side. Using a guarded

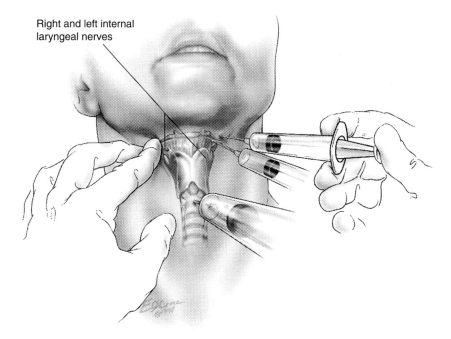

Right and left internal laryngeal nerves

Figure 16.3 Technique for internal laryngeal nerve block and intra-tracheal injection.

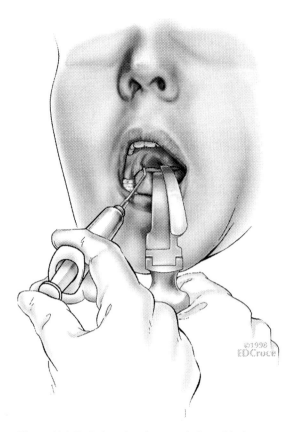

Figure 16.4 Technique for pharyngeal plexus block.

needle, 1–2 ml 1.5 per cent lignocaine with adrenaline 1 : 100 000 is injected at the mid-point of the posterior tonsillar pillar (palatopharyngeal fold). The use of the guarded tonsillar needle is important to avoid injury to the internal carotid artery (Fig. 16.4). Aspiration prior to injection of local anaesthetic to eliminate intravascular injection is mandatory.

The spectrum of blocks is completed with an intratracheal injection of 4 per cent lignocaine (2–3 ml) via a 23 gauge needle (Fig. 16.3). The trachea is punctured with a 23 gauge needle attached to a 5 ml syringe. The intra-tracheal position is confirmed by aspiration of air. The patient is instructed to take a deep breath in and then to breathe out. At the end of expiration, the anaesthetist rapidly injects lignocaine into the trachea and immediately withdraws the needle to minimize the chance of it breaking when the patient coughs upon injection of the lignocaine.

This combination of blocks, topical anaesthesia and sedation, using a benzodiazepine and opioid, allows gentle bronchoscopic assessment of the fistula, or placement of a double-lumen endotracheal tube to isolate the affected lung from the non-affected lung.

Intubation under general anaesthesia with spontaneous ventilation

As instrumentation may cause further disruption of the infected and inflamed lower airway, resulting in a large air leak and inability to ventilate the patient, the maintenance of spontaneous ventilation during intubation is an important safety factor.

If chosen, general anaesthesia is induced with the patient sitting tilted to one side with the good lung uppermost. Posture as for transport to the operating room is thus used to minimize the risk of lung soiling or flooding.

The choice of anaesthetic agent is mainly based on individual preference. The principles are to anaesthetize the patient to a level that enables intubation, whilst preserving spontaneous ventilation. Agents that depress ventilation (e.g. opioids) should initially be avoided. A combination of oxygen and inhalational anaesthetic agent with topical local anaesthetic spray to the larynx provides suitable conditions. The addition of a low dose of intravenous induction agent often enhances intubating conditions.

To achieve appropriate conditions for intubation requires both care and patience. Selection of the appropriate-sized endobronchial or double-lumen tube may be aided by reference to the previous anaesthetic history. Patients presenting with empyema and bronchopleural fistula are often unwell and malnourished, with limited respiratory reserve. They are sensitive to the haemodynamic side effects of anaesthetic agents, and appropriate drugs (e.g. atropine or vasopressor) therefore need to be immediately available.

Following intubation and lung isolation, patients are placed in a supine position and then turned to a lateral position for the definitive surgery. Suction must be available during this movement, and the position of the bronchial blocker, endobronchial tube or double-lumen tube re-checked.

It is safest to allow the patient to continue to breathe spontaneously until the chest is opened and the bronchial fistula controlled. Small doses of opioid may be titrated as required.

Some anaesthetists administer muscle relaxant to minimize the risk of coughing or muscle movement due to diathermy at this stage. The risk of a tube slipping or being displaced during dissection is judged to be minimal by those anaesthetists who are prepared to pass from spontaneous ventilation to respiratory paralysis prior to the surgeon being in a position to control a massive air leak via an open bronchopleural fistula.

Intubation under general anaesthesia and muscle relaxant

Intravenous induction and intubation using a rapidly acting muscle relaxant, such as suxamethonium, is advocated by some clinicians for anaesthesia for bronchopleural fistula.

Whilst intravenous induction of anaesthesia is appealing to some patients for its swiftness, intravenous induction and relaxant general anaesthetic may put patients with bronchopleural fistula at additional risk. If the anaesthetist is unable to achieve rapid lung isolation, the consequences for the patient may be dire. It is our view that this method of induction and tube placement should be reserved for those in whom intubation under local anaesthetic or spontaneously ventilating general anaesthetic are not possible.

Persistent air leaks

Introduction

Persistent air leaks may complicate a primary spontaneous pneumothorax or a pneumothorax secondary to emphysema or trauma, or may occur following thoracic surgical procedures. Air leaks are common after lung resection, and normally seal with conservative therapy. If an air leak persists for more than 1 week or causes respiratory embarrassment, patients are considered for more invasive measures. Of 423 lobectomies performed by the Austin and Repatriation Medical Centre group, 79 (18.6 per cent) had an air leak for longer than 7 days. Prolonged air leaks occur following the opening of incomplete fissures during surgery, or surgical injury to the lung in association with underlying lung disease such as emphysema.

Conservative management by pleural drainage with suction vents excess air and maintains negative intrapleural pressure to allow pulmonary expansion. If suction greater than 50 cmH$_2$O (7 kPa) does not achieve full lung expansion, this indicates the need for repositioning of chest drains or a check bronchoscopy to exclude a bronchial lesion. It should be noted that application of suction to pleural drains can worsen or prolong air leakage, and should be used judiciously. The progress of lung re-expansion should be followed by sequential chest X-rays.

Massive air leak may progress to surgical emphysema. Air dissects the fascial planes and extends to the face and, eventually, the limbs. Surgical emphysema of the chest may occur if chest drains are improperly positioned, with side holes located subcutaneously.

Surgical procedure

Surgical management aims to fully re-expand the lung, seal the air leak and remove lesions likely to result in recurrrence of pneumothorax. This may involve simple suturing or stapling of bullae or lung parenchyma, pleurodesis, pleurectomy or decortication, and these may be performed by open thoracotomy or VATS, as discussed in the relevant chapters.

Anaesthetic management

The aims of the anaesthetic management of patients presenting for surgery with persistent air leak are to control loss of gas from the respiratory tract and prevent expansion of air spaces.

These aims can be achieved by isolation of the affected lung by endo-bronchial intubation or blockade, and the avoidance of the application of intermittent positive pressure ventilation (IPPV) until lung isolation is achieved and/or the chest is opened. Alternatively, high frequency jet ventilation (HFJV) may be used to limit airway pressure during ventilation, as discussed in Chapter 18. Nitrous oxide tends to diffuse into air spaces and expand their size, and is best avoided.

Anaesthesia should be tailored to achieve spontaneous ventilation at the end of the procedure. Post-operative IPPV may perpetuate air leak from the lungs but, if required, the use of a pressure controlled mode of ventilation with the avoidance of PEEP or the use of HFJV may be beneficial. Occasionally, continued loss of ventilatory gas from one lung necessitates the use of differential lung ventilation.

KEY POINTS

Pulmonary haemorrhage

- Massive haemorrhage is defined as expectoration of more than 600 ml of blood in 24 hours.

- Bronchial arteries are the common source of haemoptysis.

- Pulmonary artery rupture and haemorrhage may be caused by pulmonary artery catheterization; initial management is to remove the pulmonary artery catheter to a central position and apply PEEP.

- Surgical management of pulmonary haemorrhage is initially by bronchoscopy, localization of the bleeding point and control of bleeding by conservative measures if possible.

- The principles of anaesthesia for pulmonary haemorrhage are the use of posture and suction to prevent soiling of the 'good' lung and, if required, endobrochial intubation or broncial blockade to isolate the bleeding lung.

Bronchopleural fistulae and empyema

- Principles of surgery are to obliterate the infected pleural space and fully re-expand the lung.

- Bronchopleural fistulae are most commonly a post-operative complication, and usually occur within 2 weeks of surgery.

- Bronchopleural fistulae present with sudden onset cough with expectoration of infected fluid and an associated sudden reduction of the space–fluid level on chest X-ray.

- The principles of anaesthesia are control of air leak and protection of the good lung from soiling.

- Intubation under local anaesthesia is the safest option.

- Times of major risk for lung flooding are tracheal instrumentation, opening of the chest and surgical manipulation of the lung.

- Isolation of the lung is best achieved with the use of a double-lumen tube.

Persistent air leaks

- Persistent air leaks are common after lung resections.

- The initial management is conservative; by pleural drainage.

- Prolonged air leak is often initially treated by VATS.

- The principles of anaesthesia are the control of gas leakage by lung isolation and the prevention of expansion of pneumothoraces.

- Pressure controlled ventilation, HFJV or differential lung ventilation may be of value in controlling gas leak if ventilation is required post-operatively.

Bibliography

Bobrowitz, I.D., Ramakrishna, S. and Shim, Y.S. (1983). Comparison of medical v. surgical treatment of major hemoptysis. *Arch. Int. Med.*, **143**, 1343.

Conlan, A.A. (1985). Massive hemoptysis – diagnostic and therapeutic implications. *Surg. Ann.*, **17**, 337.

Conlan, A.A., Hurwitz, S.S., Krige, L. *et al.* (1983). Massive hemoptysis: Review of 123 cases. *J. Thoracic Cardiovasc. Surg.*, **85**, 120.

Eggers, C. (1923). Radical operation for chronic empyema. *Am. Surg.*, 77, 327–53.

Feeley, T.W., Keating, D. and Nahimura, T. (1988). Independent lung ventilation using high frequency ventilation in the management of a bronchopleural fistula. *Anesthesiology*, **69**, 420–2.

Freixinet, J., Canalis, E., Rivas, J.J. *et al.* (1997). Surgical treatment of primary spontaneous pneumothorax with video-assisted thoracic surgery. *Eur. Respir. J.*, **10**, 409–11.

Greenfield, L.J. (1984). *Complications in Surgery and Trauma*. J.B. Lippincott.

Jiménez-Merchàn, R., Garcia-Diaz, F. and Arenas-Linares, C. (1997). Comparative retrospective study of surgical treatment of spontaneous pneumothorax. *Surg. Endosc.*, **11**, 919–22.

Lauckner, M.E., Beggs, I. and Armstrong, R.F. (1983). The radiological characteristics of bronchopleural fistula following pneumonectomy. *Anaesthesia*, **38**, 452–6.

McCollum, W.B., Mattox, K.L., Guinn, G.A. and Beall, A.C. (1975). Immediate operative treatment for massive hemoptysis. *Chest*, **67**, 152.

Opie, J., Vaughn, C., Comp, R. *et al.* (1992). Endobronchial closure of a post-pneumonectomy bronchopleural fistula. *Ann. Thorac. Surg.*, **53**, 686.

Paulson, D.M., Scott, S.T.M. and Sethi, G.K. (1980). Pulmonary hemorrhage associated with balloon flotation catheters. Report of a case and review of the literature. *J. Thoracic Cardiovasc. Surg.*, **80**, 453.

Roberts, A.C. (1990). Bronchial artery embolization therapy. *J. Thorac. Imaging*, **5**, 60–72.

Roth, M.D., Wright, J.W. and Bellamy, P.E. (1988). Gas flow through a bronchopleural fistula. Measuring the effects of high frequency jet ventilation and chest tube suction. *Chest*, **93**, 210–13.

Scuderi, P.E., Prough, D.S., Price, J.D. and Comer, P.B. (1983). Cessation of pulmonary artery catheter-induced endobronchial hemorrhage associated with the use of PEEP. *Anesth. Analg.*, **62**, 236.

Sehhat, S., Oreizie, M. and Moinedine, K. (1978). Massive pulmonary hemorrhage: Surgical approach as a choice of treatment. *Ann. Thoracic Surg.*, **25**, 12.

Shamji, F.M. and Vallieres, E. (1991). Airway hemorrhage. *Chest Surg. Clin. N. Am.*, **1(2)**, 255–89.

17

Pain control following thoracic surgery

I. Hardy and S. Ahmed

Post-thoracotomy pain

Post-thoracotomy pain is one of the most intensely painful surgical experiences. Its control and abolition is therefore of paramount importance. In order to ensure satisfactory post-operative recovery and comfort, adequate analgesia must be provided with minimal impairment of respiratory function and minimal alteration of consciousness level. Whilst inadequate analgesia may inhibit the patient's willingness to cough and take deep breaths, leading to accumulation of secretions and atelectasis, over-sedation as a result of high doses of opioid may equally impair the clearance of secretions and predispose to respiratory complications. Despite the fact that surgical techniques have evolved over the past decade that enable endoscopic procedures to be carried out within the thorax for diagnostic and therapeutic procedures, thus reducing post-operative analgesic requirements, it is necessary to be able to treat post-thoracotomy pain effectively, as most major thoracic procedures are still performed by the open route.

Increasing awareness of the inadequacies in the treatment of post-operative pain together with a better understanding of the pathophysiology of pain mechanisms has stimulated a more coherent utilization of existing techniques, both drugs and drug delivery systems, to revolutionize post-operative pain management. In many hospitals, acute pain teams have emerged to co-ordinate and facilitate the use of pain-relieving techniques, and a multimodal approach is becoming commonplace. Not all patients undergoing thoracic procedures will require sophisticated forms of post-operative pain relief, but many will.

Thoracotomy is more painful than most other surgical incisions because of the extensive innervation of the structures that are damaged during the operation, and because of continuous movement of the chest wall with respiration and coughing, which acts as a repetitive pain stimulus. The incision itself extends over several dermatomes (T2–T10), and in addition chest drains may be placed at a lower dermatomal level. During chest opening, muscles and ribs may be resected or retracted, periosteum stripped and intercostal nerves cut or crushed. Intra-operatively, the shoulder is retracted and the lung may be contused. During chest closure, intercostal nerves may be trapped by sutures. Nociceptive impulses are transmitted from these structures by the intercostal nerves, the phrenic nerve branches (the diaphragmatic pleura), the vagus nerve branches (the lung and mediastinal pleura) and cervical spinal nerves (the shoulder). Sympathetic nerves, which innervate visceral structures, may also play a part in pain mechanisms, though this function is still ill defined in humans.

Poorly treated severe post-operative pain will have several adverse consequences. These include increased effects of the stress response, limitation of early mobilization (resulting in reluctance to undertake essential physiotherapy treatment with consequential respiratory complications) and, in some cases, the possible development of a chronic post-thoracotomy pain syndrome.

Pain is a multidimensional experience and the outcome of treatment may be influenced by a variety of factors, such as the patient's age and sex, personality, nutritional and smoking status, and any previous experience of surgery, particularly if it has been bad. A better understanding of the sources of pain, the physiology of pain mechanisms, the pharmacology of the drugs available for pain relief and the techniques available to deliver those drugs will enable medical personnel to optimize pain-relieving treatments to ensure the patient's post-operative course is the most comfortable possible.

The pathophysiology of acute pain

The physiology of acute pain (nociception) has traditionally relied on ideas first conceived by Descartes in 1644. Clinically, we use this 'route map' concept successfully in pain treatments such as local anaesthetic blocks. However, work during the last 10–15 years has revealed its inadequacies in explaining peri-operative pain. Much more is occurring in the nervous system during the peri-operative period than the simple input of a pain signal. The nervous system, being dynamic, is capable of adaptive responses to tissue injury, and this central neuroplasticity has a considerable impact on the processing of nociceptive impulses.

The surgical incision causes what has been described as a biological nuclear reaction, where over 100 endogenous chemicals are released, forming a so-called sensitizing or inflammatory soup. There are essentially three tissue cascades involved in this process. The clotting cascade produces some of the most allergenic endogenous substances known to humans. The arachidonic acid cascade causes the release of neuropeptides, nerve growth factor, histamine, seratonin and cytokines. The tissue oxidation cascade causes the release of active oxygen radicals of hydrogen peroxide and nitric oxide. This inflammatory soup initiates the nociceptive impulses, which are conveyed centrally via the dorsal horn nuclei.

Various routes are available through the central nervous system for these nociceptive impulses, and the signals may be modified by facilitation/excitation or inhibition at synapses between individual neurones. Information transfer takes place across these synapses due to the release of neurotransmitters. There are over 200 of these, but they are basically divided into two classes; facilitatory/excitatory and inhibitory.

Table 17.1 Classification of nerves (after Ganong, 1981)

Fibre type		Diameter (μm)	Conduction speed (msec⁻¹)	Function
A	α	12–20	70–200	Proprioception, somatic motor
	β	5–12	30–70	Touch pressure
	γ	3–6	15–30	Motor to muscle spindle
	δ	2–5	12–30	Pain, temperature, touch
B		< 3	3–15	Pre-ganglionic autonomic
C		0.2–1.3	0.5–2.3	Pain, reflexes Pre-ganglionic sympathetic

Facilitatory/excitatory neurotransmitters are amino acids and short-chain peptides. The two most common amino acids are aspartate and glutamate, and these act primarily at the N-methyl-D-aspartic acid (NMDA) and α-amino-3-hydroxy-5-methyl-4-isoxazolepropionic acid (AMPA) receptors. Substance P, a neurokinin, is an example of a short-chain peptide excitatory neurotransmitter.

Inhibitory neurotransmitters include the endogenous opiates, enkephalins, β-endorphins, norepinephrine, serotonin (5HT), somatostatin, γ-amino-butyric acid (GABA) and glycine.

Peripheral nerves are composed of motor, sensory and autonomic nerve fibres (axons) arranged in bundles (fascicli). They vary considerably in size, and these differences are related to the differences in function (Table 17.1).

Central neuroplasticity clinically manifests itself in two forms:

1. *Allodynia*. This is defined as a painful response to a normal, innocuous stimulus. It is a phenomenon predominantly mediated by changes in large-diameter neurones, which are normally concerned with the transmission of innocuous stimuli (A-beta fibres). It is more relevant in neuropathic pain states.

2. *Hyperalgesia*. This is defined as an increased response to a normally painful stimulus. There are two forms; primary and secondary. Primary hyperalgesia is seen in the immediate area of tissue injury, and is due to primary afferent nociceptive sensitization. Following injury, a second zone of hyperalgesia develops around the area of injury and is a spinally mediated event due to the stimulation of a wide dynamic range of neurones. Jaggar and Rice have recently produced experimental evidence that visceral injury can also cause secondary hyperalgesia in animal models, producing persistent visceral pain.

As well as conducting nociceptive impulses, unmyelinated C fibres and myelinated A-delta fibres also conduct other information such as temperature and tactile sensation (Table 17.1). A-delta myelinated fibres are subdivided into Types I and II. Type II fibres respond to pressure and temperature, and discharge at pressures of 1.7 bar and temperatures of 43°C and over. Type II A-delta fibres are responsible for the early detection of tissue injury and adapt rapidly. The number of synapses to the brain are few and, when stimulated, result in the production of an almost instantaneous motor reflex withdrawal from the source of damage. They are responsible for the phenomenon known as 'first pain'. Because the A-delta Type II fibres have no opioid receptors, either pre- or post-synaptically, this 'first pain' is unresponsive to opioid treatment.

The unmyelinated C fibres are slow conducting compared to the A-delta fibres. The number of synapses to the brain is greater, and they have opioid receptors. They are associated with 'second pain', and their effect can be much attenuated by opioids. In the resting state, a proportion of the C fibres are not excited by natural stimuli and remain silent. However, following tissue injury, the excitation threshold of the fibres falls so that they are activated by noxious and physiological stimuli. In the inflammatory state, therefore, these silent nociceptors are recruited.

The nociceptive sensitization associated with primary hyperalgesia is thus the result of complex interactions between the immune and nervous systems. Nerve growth factor, bradykinin and cannabinoids are all involved, together with many other substances, in the hyperalgesic process. Low threshold A and B fibres maintain their nociceptive input and interact presynaptically with C fibres, resulting in central sensitization. Prolonged stimulation of all these fibres results in prolonged excitation of the dorsal horn nuclei. This involves activation of the NMDA receptors in the dorsal horn, and subsequent stimulation increases the duration of excitation and outlasts the stimulus, a condition known as wind-up. Once wind-up has been initiated, much larger doses of opioids are required to suppress the excitation response. Strategies for reducing central sensitization include blockage of C fibre activity by local anaesthetics, opioid agonists acting pre- and post-synaptically on nociceptor afferents and antagonists acting on the NMDA receptor itself.

Experimental evidence suggests, therefore, that pain will be more easily and readily treated if analgesia is administered before the initiation of the noxious stimulus – so-called pre-emptive analgesia. Further evidence would suggest that continuing treatment to reduce secondary hyperalgesia may have an additional beneficial effect on the development of chronic post-operative pain.

Chronic post-thoracotomy pain

Long-term pain appears to be a common sequel to thoracotomy, occurring in 40–55 per cent of patients 2 years after thoracic surgery.

Very little is known about those factors that mark the transition from time-limited pain to chronic pathological pain. However, current understanding of central sensitization and neuroplasticity indicates that acute post-operative pain intensity and longevity may be a predictor for long-term thoracotomy pain. Katz et al. (1996) tested this hypothesis and found a correlation between the intensity of acute post-thoracotomy pain and the development of chronic long-term pain. They postulate that intercostal nerve damage may be responsible, and recommend that aggressive management of acute post-operative pain will not only be of immediate benefit to the patient but may disrupt peripheral and central neural processes responsible for the transition to chronicity.

Management of post-thoracotomy pain

Our understanding of the pathogenesis of clinical pain enables us to make three important predictions regarding the treatment of surgical pain:

1. Adequate management of such pain requires techniques aimed at the changes that can occur in the central nervous system, instead of merely interrupting the flow of sensory signals. Thus the aim is not necessarily just to produce total analgesia, i.e. blocking physiological as well as pathological pain processes, but to depress or reverse afferent-induced excitability changes in central neurones. Opioids, administered at appropriate dosage and delivered to the correct site, can do this.
2. The most effective way to treat clinical pain is to design treatment plans that prevent the occurrence of neuroplasticity. An example (already referred to) is that the dose of morphine required to prevent C fibre-induced excitability changes is an order of magnitude lower than that required to suppress those changes once they have occurred.
3. Treatment of established pain will be most effective when attempts are made at returning a disordered nervous system to normality, not just by breaking the afferent limb that initiates the changes but also by breaking the sympathetic and visceral disturbances that perpetuate the hyperexcitable wound-up state.

In addition to the basic triad of analgesic management, i.e. local anaesthetics, opioids and NSAIDs, increased evidence indicates that the use of NMDA antagonists (such as ketamine), GABA agonists (such as baclofen and benzodiazepines) and alpha-2 agonists (such as clonidine) will all augment the actions of the basic triad of analgesics.

The effective management of post-operative thoracotomy pain is therefore based on two criteria:

1. Anti-nociceptive treatment started before surgery, which has proved to be more effective in the reduction of post-operative pain than treatment given on recovery from general anaesthesia (phenomena of pre-emptive analgesia in its narrowest sense).
2. The effective blockade of noxious stimuli generated during surgery and during the initial post-operative period (inflammatory phase) reducing subsequent post-operative pain (the phenomena of pre-emptive analgesia in its broadest sense).

Both aspects of management can be induced by neural blockade with local anaesthetics, by systemic and epidural opioids and by non-steroidal agents.

Clinically impressive effects are observed when the blockade of noxious stimuli is not only complete peri-operatively but also extends into the initial post-operative phase, thereby combining both aspects.

Regional anaesthetic blocks for thoracic procedures

Intercostal block

The classic technique of intercostal block is by separate injections of each nerve in its individual intercostal space. This can be done in the mid-axillary line or any more proximal site, including the paravertebral region.

Anatomy

Intercostal nerves consist of the ventral rami of the first to twelfth thoracic nerves. After exiting the vertebral foramen, the intercostal nerve lies tucked in the groove on the underside of each rib (Fig. 17.1). Cadaver studies show that expecting the intercostal vein, artery and nerve to be located in that precise order is unrealistic. The nerve may run a variable course.

Each intercostal nerve gives off four branches as it proceeds on its circuitous route anteriorly (Fig. 17.2):

- 1st – grey ramus communicans; passes anteriorly to the sympathetic ganglion.
- 2nd – the posterior cutaneous branch; supplies the skin and muscle in the paravertebral region.
- 3rd – the lateral cutaneous division: arises anterior to the mid-axillary line. This branch is of primary concern when blocking the intercostal nerves for pain relief, because it sends subcutaneous fibres anteriorly and posteriorly to supply the skin.

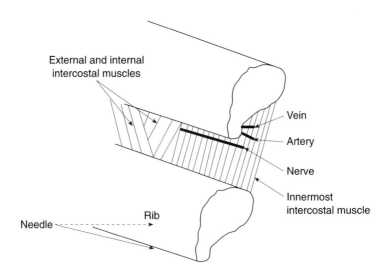

Figure 17.1 Conventional approach for intercostal block. The needle is advanced through the skin at the angle of the rib until bony resistance is encountered; it is then 'walked' off the lower edge of the rib, the tip angled caudally and advanced a few millimetres, taking care not to puncture the pleura. The needle is aspirated to exclude intravascular placement and local anaesthetic solution is then injected.

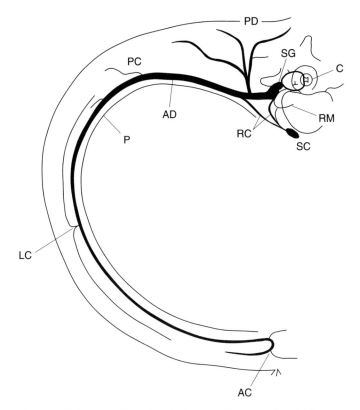

Figure 17.2 Schematic thoracic spinal nerve. AD = anterior division,
PD = posterior division, C = spinal cord, SG = spinal ganglion,
RM = recurrent meningeal, SC = sympathetic chain, RC = rami
communicantes, PC = posterior cutaneous, LC = lateral cutaneous,
AC = anterior cutaneous, P = pleura. Reproduced with permission from
J. Richardson and P. A. Lonnquist (1998). Thoracic paravertebral block. *BJA*,
81, 230–38.

- 4th – the terminal branch is the anterior cutaneous, which provides
  cutaneous innervation to the midline of the chest and abdomen.

Technique

The conventional approach

The intercostal block (Fig. 17.1) is performed posteriorly at the angle of the
ribs, just lateral to the sacrospinus group of muscles. At this point, the rib
thickness is about 8 mm. In most instances the block is easiest to perform
with the patient prone or sitting forward hugging a pillow. After patient
positioning, it is helpful to identify the inferior edge of the ribs with a
skin-marking pen. The lateral edge of the sacrospinus group of muscles is
identified, and can be marked as a vertical line. After the local anaesthetic
mixture is prepared, skin weals are raised at each junction of the sacrospinus
ligament and inferior border of the ribs with a 30 gauge needle. A 22 or

23 gauge short bevel needle is used to inject the local anaesthetic solution for the intercostal nerve blocks.

Starting at the lowest level, the needle is inserted until it comes into contact with the rib. If there is difficulty in contacting the bone, its depth and position should be redefined. While one hand maintains firm pressure/ contact between the rib and the needle, the other hand holds the hub and shaft between thumb, index finger and middle finger and 'walks' the needle off the lower edge of the rib. After negative aspiration for blood, 3–4 ml of local anaesthetic solution is injected. This process is repeated at all the intercostal spaces to be blocked.

If a long bevelled needle is used, the tip may easily be bent with repeated bony contacts during this block and can also increase the risk of bleeding and nerve damage.

The mid-axillary approach

The mid-axillary approach is more feasible in patients who cannot be turned supine or laterally, such as post-operative or trauma patients who experience severe pain on any movement. This approach might be more prone to pneumothorax and can miss anaesthetizing the lateral cutaneous branch of the nerve, as this takes off near the mid-axillary line and becomes superficial to innervate the skin of the antero-lateral chest wall. This can be overcome by injecting a few millilitres of local anaesthetic solution as the needle moves away from the rib cage to the skin.

Continuous intercostal block

At the completion of thoracotomy under general anaesthetic, the surgeon can peel back the parietal pleura from the ribs at the incision site and tunnel a 20 gauge epidural catheter (7–8 cm from the posterior midline) to the posterior intercostal space. Its position can be verified both visually and by palpation. In the same manner, a second intercostal catheter can be placed just above the incision. The remaining part of the catheter is tunnelled out through the chest wall and secured. This can be used for repeated intercostal injections or continuous infusion.

A test dose of 10 ml of 0.25 per cent bupivacaine with 1/200 000 adrenaline over 2–3 minutes should be given after negative aspiration for blood.

Intercostal catheterization has advantages over interpleural catheterization; there is no diffusion barrier of parietal pleura to overcome, and the local anaesthetic agent has direct access to the intercostal nerves without being diluted by the fluids in the pleural cavity.

Difficulties with catheter placement can arise with parietal pleural adhesions; torn parietal pleura will allow local anaesthetic leakage from the incision site and analgesic failure has been described.

Drugs and dosage

Excesses of volume or concentration of drugs may predispose to toxic effects. On the other hand, small volumes with lower concentrations will result in ineffectual block (Table 17.2).

Table 17.2 Drugs and dosages for intercostal blockade

Drug	Volume per intercostal space	Duration	Concentration (per cent)	Max. dosage (mg/kg)
Bupivacaine	3 ml	4–8 hours	0.25	2
Lignocaine	4 ml	1–2 hours	1	3–4
Bupivacaine with adrenaline	4 ml	4–8 hours	0.25	3
Lignocaine with adrenaline	4–5 ml	1.5–3 hours	1	7

Complications

- *Pneumothorax.* This is the most serious complication of an intercostal block. However, with proper technique the risk should be low, and the reported incidence is between 0.1 and 2.0 per cent.
- *Systemic toxicity.* This problem is most likely to occur if large volumes of concentrated drug are given or if the agent is injected intravascularly. Local anaesthetic agents can interfere with sodium channel conduction and cause hypotension and myocardial depression. Severe bradycardia and heart blocks can impede resuscitation. In performing multiple intercostal blocks, the maximum recommended dosage might be required. Blood levels of local anaesthetic agent are higher after intercostal block than after any other regional block. Addition of adrenaline to the solution will reduce systemic absorption.

Intrapleural block

This technique was first described by Kvalheim and Reiestad. They subsequently used it in 81 patients who had undergone breast surgery, renal surgery or cholecystectomy with subcostal incision. Complete analgesia was obtained in 78 out of 81 patients following injection of 20 ml of 0.5 per cent bupivacaine with adrenaline.

However, Rosenberg *et al.* has cast doubt on the efficacy of intrapleural blockade. They found that interpleural bupivacaine did not reduce the need for intramuscular opiates after thoracotomy. They postulated that loss of drug through suction tubing or restricted distribution over an operated lung might account for this.

The current explanation for the mechanism whereby analgesia is produced is that diffusion of local anaesthetic solution from the pleural cavity occurs across the endothoracic and subserous fascia and the innermost intercostal muscle to provide unilateral intercostal blockade.

Although intrapleural block provides satisfactory analgesia, it is inadequate for providing anaesthesia for even minor surgical procedures.

Technique

This involves percutaneous introduction of a catheter between the parietal and visceral pleura.

The open chest technique

The surgeon can insert an epidural catheter through the chest wall posterior and superior to the thoracotomy incision via a Tuohy needle. The catheter can then be sutured to the skin.

The closed chest technique

A Tuohy needle and a low resistance syringe are used. The needle is inserted in the mid-axillary line at the appropriate intercostal space and is 'walked off' the superior border of the rib with its bevel directed upwards (towards the parietal pleura). On entering the pleural space there is loss of resistance. When the syringe is removed, the hub of the Tuohy needle must be covered to prevent air from entering the pleural space. An epidural catheter is then advanced 6–10 cm intrapleurally.

Pleural puncture should be made at end-expiration in spontaneously breathing patients, and at the apnoeic end-expiratory period in mechanically ventilated patients.

Drug dosage

A bolus injection of 20 ml of bupivacaine 0.25 per cent or continuous infusion of bupivacaine 0.25 per cent with adrenaline 1 : 200 000 at a rate of 0.1–0.5 ml/kg per hour is suitable. Little difference has been observed between the analgesic potency of the different concentrations of bupivacaine for this block; hence, 0.25 per cent is recommended.

An average plasma concentration of 1.2 μg/ml bupivacaine has been observed after intrapleural administration of 100 mg bupivacaine with adrenaline.

Advantages/disadvantages

- In comparison with intercostal block, only a single needle puncture is required. Onset time and analgesia are comparable in both techniques.
- Distribution of an intrapleural infusion of local anaesthetic is posture-dependent. Its effectiveness thus depends on patients lying in the supine position.
- After thoracotomy, with the presence of intercostal drains, approximately 30–40 per cent of any dose administered is lost via the drains.
- Pneumothorax, lung laceration or bronchopleural fistula formation are possible.
- Pooling of the local anaesthetic agent over the diaphragm can cause phrenic nerve block. However, pulmonary function studies have indicated that a significant increase in FVC and FEV occur after administration of bupivacaine into the pleural cavity. The analgesia-related enhancement of respiratory effort probably outweighs any adverse effect on diaphragmatic function.

Extrapleural block

This block can be performed by the operating surgeon.

Technique

Before chest closure, the parietal pleura is peeled from the posterior wound margin and extended medially towards the vertebral bodies. The pocket thus created can be extended to involve two intercostal spaces above and below the incision.

A Tuohy needle is inserted percutaneously at a site close to the angle of the rib to emerge at the extrapleural pocket. An epidural catheter is threaded through the needle and positioned cranially, under direct vision, such that at least 3 cm of its length lies against the costovertebral joints in the extra-pleural pocket. The catheter is then affixed securely to the skin. The parietal pleura is reattached to the posterior edge of the wound before closure of the chest.

Drug dosage

After negative aspiration for blood or cerebrospinal fluid, a bolus dose of 0.5 ml/kg bupivacaine 0.5 per cent with or without adrenaline can be given.

A continuous infusion of 0.25 per cent bupivacaine at 0.2–0.4 ml/kg per hour will give satisfactory analgesia. Mean maximum serum bupivacaine at any time with this infusion is $2 \mu g/ml$.

Advantages/disadvantages

Extrapleural block has a high reported success rate with minimal compli-cations because of the placement of the catheter under direct vision at the optimal site for analgesic effect.

Paravertebral block

Paravertebral block can be used for the same indications as a thoracic epidural block. However, it has the advantage of producing a unilateral sympathetic block without the degree of hypotension seen with epidural blockade.

Anatomy

The paravertebral space is defined as a wedge-shaped cavity bounded above and below by the head and neck of adjoining ribs. The posterior wall is formed by the superior costo-transverse ligament, which runs from the lower border of the transverse process above to the upper border of the rib below. The base is formed by the postero-lateral aspect of the body of the vertebra, the intervertebral foramen and its contents. Antero-laterally the space is limited by the parietal pleura; medially it communicates with the epidural space via the intervertebral foramen, and laterally it adjoins the intercostal space.

The dura mater and the arachnoid mater fuse with the epineurium as the nerve exits the vertebral foramen. The intercostal nerves and their collateral branches (especially their posterior primary rami) and the thoracic sympa-thetic chain pass through the paravertebral space, making it an ideal site for nerve blocks. Each space communicates, superiorly and inferiorly, across the neck of the rib, with the spaces above and below it. Spread of solution into the epidural space has been demonstrated.

The paravertebral space contains loose connective tissue, with the nerve, intercostal artery and vein usually as singular structures. Since the needle passes into the loose alveolar tissue of the paravertebral space via muscle and superior costo-transverse ligament, it should be possible to elicit loss of resistance to identify the space.

To perform a paravertebral block, it is necessary to make contact with the transverse process of the appropriate vertebral body. In the mid-thoracic region (T4–T9), the angulation of the spinous processes is such that the tip of each spinous process is at the same level as, or just below, the transverse process of the vertebra below.

Technique

The patient is placed either in the lateral position with the side to be blocked uppermost, or sitting upright. Under full aseptic technique, a skin weal is raised with local anaesthetic solution about 3–4 cm from the midline and at a level with the cephaloid end of the spinous process of T5 or T6. A 20 gauge needle (or 16 gauge Tuohy needle if a catheter is to be passed for continuous infusion of local anaesthetic) is introduced through the skin weal perpendicular to the skin, and advanced until it hits the bony transverse process at a depth of 3–4 cm. The needle is then withdrawn slightly, redirected cephaloid and advanced 2–2.5 cm to pass above the transverse process. Loss of resistance can be used to identify the paravertebral space as the needle passes through the superior costo-transverse ligament into the loose alveolar tissue of the space (Fig. 17.3).

Drug dosage

At least four intercostal nerves may be blocked by 15 ml of 0.375 per cent bupivacaine given as a single shot. A continuous infusion of 0.25 per cent bupivacaine at 6–8 ml/hr can be used after a bolus of 10 ml.

Complications

- *Pleural tap and pneumothorax*. The risk is less with paravertebral block than intercostal block since the partial pleura is further away in the paravertebral space.
- *Vascular injury*. The artery and vein are usually singular structures in the paravertebral space. However, vascular injury can lead to haematoma formation and rapid absorption of local anaesthetic agent.
- *Epidural block and dural puncture*. These have both been reported.

Advantages/disadvantages

- In comparison to intercostal blocks, multiple intercostal nerves can be blocked by a single paravertebral injection and with a lesser risk of pneumothorax or lung injury.

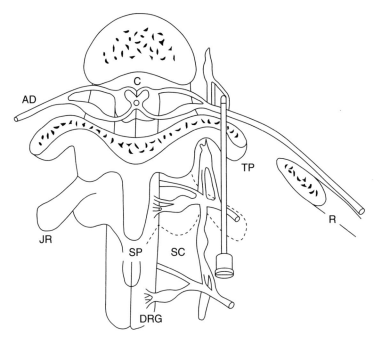

Figure 17.3 Optimal needle position in relation to the transverse process (TP) of the vertebra and the neural structures of the thoracic paravertebral space. R = rib, AD = anterior division, SP = spinous process, SC = sympathetic chain, DRG = dorsal root ganglion, C = spinal cord. Reproduced with permission from J. Richardson and P. A. Lonnquist (1998). Thoracic paravertebral block. *BJA*, **81**, 230–38.

- Epidural blockade is more reliable at producing satisfactory analgesia than paravertebral block, but is associated with greater potential for side effects.
- The success of paravertebral block can be enhanced by performing the block under radiological guidance. This is impractical, however, in the peri-operative context.

Thoracic epidural analgesia

The epidural technique was first used in 1901 when Sciard and Cattalin administered epidural analgesia via the caudal approach. In 1944, Vasconcellos reported the use of epidural anaesthesia for thoracic surgery.

In the 1950s, the use of a thoracic epidural as the sole anaesthetic technique for thoracic procedures was fashionable. This required co-operation between the surgeon, patient and anaesthetist. Current practice, however, is that thoracic epidural analgesia is used as an adjunct to, rather than a substitute for, general anaesthesia.

Anatomy of the thoracic spine

The spinous processes in the upper thoracic and cervical region (C1–T2) are almost horizontal. In the mid-thoracic region (T3–T9), the spinous processes are narrower and angulate more sharply and downwards, thus obscuring the interlaminar space. The inferior border of each spinous process lies just above the lamina of the vertebra below. The epidural space is also narrow. The spinous processes of the lower thoracic region (T10–T12) have only a slight downward angulation, and the anatomy is similar to that in the lumbar region (Fig. 17.4).

Technique of epidural blockade

The technique, together with its risks and benefits, should be discussed with the patient. Thoracic epidurals are preferably inserted in awake patients for immediate detection of impingement on nerves and confirmation of sensory blockade. However, depending on operator preference and experience, placement of the epidural after induction of anaesthesia is also widely practised.

The technique for localization of the epidural space is based on operator preference and previous experience with lumbar epidurals. Negative pressure is more consistently noted in the thoracic than the lumbar region; however, this is lost in patients with severe lung disease, and cyclical pressure changes may be transmitted from the pleural space in ventilated patients.

Thoracic epidurals can be performed with the patient lying on one side or sitting up with the spine flexed.

Anatomical landmarks that are helpful in proper placement of the epidural catheter at appropriate dermatomal levels are given in Table 17.3.

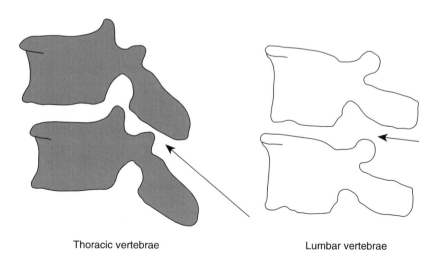

Thoracic vertebrae   Lumbar vertebrae

Figure 17.4 Diagram of thoracic and lumbar vertebrae showing the difference in angulation of the spinous processes and needle direction for midline approach to the epidural space.

Table 17.3 Anatomical landmarks and dermatomal levels for the placement of epidural catheters

Level	Anatomical landmark
C7	The most prominent spinous process palpable below the base of the neck
T3	The spine of the scapula
T7	The inferior angle of the scapula

Midline approach

This approach is more suitable for upper thoracic/cervical or lower thoracic/lumbar epidurals, but can be used for the mid-thoracic epidurals. Under full aseptic technique and after skin infiltration with local anaesthetic agent at the appropriate thoracic level, the epidural space is identified using a loss of resistance technique. If bony resistance is encountered by the needle, then its angulation should be altered. In the mid-thoracic region, due to the angulation of the spinous processes, the initial puncture with the Tuohy needle should be at a 45° angle to the skin.

Paramedian approach

Under full aseptic technique, the skin is infiltrated with local anaesthetic about 1 cm (a finger-width) lateral to the inferior border of the spinous process above the required thoracic level.

The epidural needle is inserted at an angle of about 45–50° to the skin and directed medially at about 25° to the midline. Little resistance is encountered until the ligamentum flavum is reached, since passage through the interspinous ligament is avoided. Loss of resistance is noted on passing through the ligamentum flavum.

With both approaches, the epidural catheter should thread up easily. Paraesthesia during identification of the epidural space or catheter insertion can readily be detected in an awake patient, and the needle or catheter moved to take pressure off nerves or nerve roots.

The thoracic epidural space is usually located 3–4 cm beneath the skin; sufficient length of catheter should be passed to leave 3–4 cm of catheter in the epidural space.

Physiology of thoracic epidural analgesia

Cardiovascular system

Cardiovascular effects of epidural blockade are due to direct consequence of blockade of the sympathetic cardiac fibres from the ventral roots of T1–T5, as well as potential modification of the adrenal medullary system via T6–L1. In humans, most clinical studies of thoracic epidural analgesia show a fall in heart rate, blood pressure and cardiac output. This depends on:

- The concomitant use of general anaesthesia
- The intravascular volume status
- The extent of sympathetic block.

Thoracic epidural analgesia (TEA) diminishes ischaemia and reduces the infarct size after acute coronary occlusion in dogs, with an increase in the endocardial/epicardial blood flow ratio. In humans, an improvement in ischaemic chest pain in patients with unstable angina can be obtained by TEA. Some argue that the use of TEA in patients with acutely ischaemic chest pain merely provides symptomatic relief and may mask the ongoing ischaemia. All the available data, however, suggest that ischaemia is diminished by TEA due to a decrease in myocardial oxygen demand. However, the potential hazard of TEA-induced hypotension, and hence reduced coronary perfusion pressure, must not be overlooked in patients with unstable angina whose coronary perfusion is more pressure-dependent than in patients without coronary artery disease.

Respiration
Most studies have demonstrated a modest reduction in FEV_1 and FVC in patients with high thoracic epidural block. These are significantly greater after a cervical block. This is presumably due to diaphragmatic dysfunction from phrenic nerve denervation.

Mid- and low thoracic epidurals probably improve respiratory function following thoracotomy as a result of diminishing the inhibitory effects of pain on deep breathing and coughing.

Hormonal effects
Thoracic epidural block that extends to L1 reduces stress-induced catecholamine release from the adrenal medulla in both humans and animal models. Cortisol levels are also blunted, which causes a reduction in the stress response. This may have a beneficial impact on post-operative outcome.

Safety of the technique

- Epidural infusion of a local anaesthetic agent, often in combination with an opioid, has gained increasing usage over the last 10 years. It provides excellent pain relief, improves mobilization and allows the patient to comply with physiotherapy. Increasing evidence suggests this improves the post-operative outcome.
- Whilst the technique is proven in its effectiveness, evidence is still required that it is safe in the normal ward environment.

Table 17.4 Literature reviews showing the incidence of trauma to the spinal cord after epidural

Study	No. of cases	Neurological complications and remarks
Lund et al. (1962)	10 000	Nine cases of neurological deficit. However, epidural catheter position, whether thoracic or lumbar, was not specified
Bonica et al. (1957)	3637	One case of cord trauma – block performed by a trainee
Dawkins et al. (1969)	4000	One case of permanent cord damage after thoracic epidural

- The potential danger of spinal cord injury during an epidural block is undeniable. Bromage recommends that these blocks should be performed by experienced anaesthetists and supervised trainees.
- Potential risks for the patient are associated with the insertion of a needle and catheter, the presence of an indwelling catheter in the epidural space and the use of continuous infusions of potentially harmful drugs.
- Dural puncture rate in most major teaching institutions is approximately 1 per cent. This can lead to post-dural puncture headache.
- Neuropathy occurs with an incidence of 0.002–1 per cent with epidural catheter placement (Table 17.4).
- Epidural haematoma seems extremely rare, and is estimated at an incidence of 1 : 150 000. This is most commonly linked to the use of anticoagulants or to pre-existing coagulopathy.
- Catheter migration within the epidural space or into an epidural vein and infection of the epidural space with long-term use can occur. The incidence is approximately 0.2 per cent.
- Epidural infection can lead to epidural abscess formation, although this is a rare complication.
- Infusion and injection of drugs into the epidural space permits drug errors to occur. Also, the life-threatening side effects of the agents used may occur:
  a. Local anaesthetics – hypotension, bradycardia and possible toxicity.
  b. Opioids – respiratory depression. Theoretically, a lipophilic opioid (fentanyl) reduces the risk of cephalad spread of the drug via the CSF.
- Urinary retention is markedly increased by the use of a thoracic epidural infusion.

Drugs and dosage guidelines

For thoracic epidural analgesia, either lipophilic opioid agents such as fentanyl, local anaesthetics or a combination of both are generally used.

The advantage of combined opioid/local anaesthetic mixtures is that the incidence of undesirable side effects of each agent can be reduced, as lower doses are required to achieve satisfactory analgesia. A suitable mixture is a solution containing 0.1 per cent bupivacaine and 10 μg/ml of fentanyl. A 10 ml bolus is given as a loading dose followed by a continuous infusion of 2–6 ml/hour. The loading dose and infusion rate should be reduced if the catheter is placed above T5.

Post-operative management

Ideally, the patient with a thoracic epidural should be nursed and monitored in a high dependency unit. In addition to regular cardiovascular and respiratory observations, the height of the block should periodically be checked using response to pinprick or cold (e.g. an ice cube). Mobility of the lower limbs should also be noted.

The nursing staff should be appropriately instructed, with a written protocol, as to the specific management of the epidural and potential complications.

Supplementary analgesia, if required, should consist solely of non-steroidal agents, avoiding parenteral opioids if opioids are being administered epidurally.

The epidural can safely be used for several days post-operatively, but it is usually no longer required after the second day, when alternative analgesia can be commenced satisfactorily and the patient becomes ambulant.

Opioid analgesia

Delivery methods

The traditional use of intermittent intramuscular opioids is now fortunately extremely rare. It produces peaks and troughs of pain relief, punctuated by periods of excessive sedation and hypoventilation. Over the last 20 years, the development of infusion pumps and patient-controlled analgesia devices in association with ward monitoring of pulse oximetry and blood pressure has brought about major advances in the relief of post-operative pain.

Continuous intravenous opioid infusions

Continuous intravenous opioid infusions have the following features:

- They can produce adequate analgesia
- They provide a stable therapeutic serum drug level
- They reduce the frequency of inadequate analgesia
- There is a risk of drug side effects because of patient variation in opioid need and drug clearance
- Close nurse supervision is necessary because of the side effects of hypotension, bradycardia and respiratory depression. Other side effects include pruritus, urinary retention and nausea and vomiting.

Patient-controlled analgesia (PCA)

PCA devices have been available now for about 20 years. PCA has the following features:

- Patients self-administer small intravenous doses of opioid
- Following good explanation of the technique, patient compliance and acceptability is high; easily understood explanatory leaflets are available
- Plasma opioid levels are maintained at relatively constant levels and side effects are low
- A loading dose can be administered peri-operatively or immediately post-operatively
- A lockout interval reduces the risk of overdosing

- A background infusion level may be provided in addition
- Nursing supervision levels may be reduced, but careful review is necessary, especially if a background infusion is in progress.

Drugs and dosage guidelines

The most commonly used drugs and dosages are as follows:

Drug	Concentration	PCA dose	Lockout interval
Morphine	1 mg/ml	1 mg	5
Diamorphine	1 mg/ml	0.5–1 mg	5
Pethidine	5 mg/ml	10–20 mg	5
Fentanyl	10 μg/ml	20–30 μg	4

Anti-emetics, usually cyclazine (3–5 mg/ml) or droperidol (0.05 mg/ml), may be added.

Non-steroidal anti-inflammatory drugs (NSAIDs)

The third component of the triad of analgesic drugs is the non-steroidal analgesic. These have both analgesic and anti-inflammatory properties, and may be used for mild to moderate pain. They have consistently been shown to reduce opioid requirements, and have the following features:

- They are as effective as opioids after minor surgery
- In the presence of severe post-operative pain, opioids will be necessary in addition to NSAIDs
- Concurrent use with opioids reduces opioid consumption post-operatively by between 17 and 70 per cent
- Cardiac and haemodynamic effects are absent
- Gastrointestinal toxicity is less with ibuprofen, indomethacin, ketorolac and diclofenac
- They cause platelet dysfunction, but no clinically significant increase in post-operative bleeding
- They reduce the renal blood flow and glomerular filtration rate, sodium retention and hyperkalaemia, and their use should be avoided in patients with cardiac failure, renal dysfunction, liver failure and sepsis
- Their use should be avoided in patients with a history of atopy and allergy.

Drugs and dosages

For drug dosage and route, see Table 17.5.

Table 17.5 Dosage and routes for non-steroidal anti-inflammatory drugs (NSAIDs)

Drug	Route	Adult daily dose (mg)
Ibuprofen	• Oral	600–1200
Diclofenac	• Oral • Suppository • Intramuscular injection	75–150
Ketorolac	• Oral • Intravenous injection	10–30
Indomethacin	• Oral • Suppository	50–200

Other forms of analgesia

Tramadol

Tramadol is a centrally acting analgesic drug indicated for the relief of moderate to severe pain. In addition to an opioid agonist effect, Tramadol seems to have significant anti-nociceptive activity mediated by inhibition of neuronal re-uptake of seratonin (5HT) and norepinephrine.

- It is effective in longer-term musculoskeletal pain
- It is effective when pain is no longer controlled by non-steroidals (NSAIDs)
- Sustained release preparations are more effective, and adverse effects are reduced
- Adverse effects include nausea, gastrointestinal intolerance, tiredness, dizziness and sweating
- There is a low potential for abuse and addiction
- There is less respiratory depression than with equi-analgesic doses of opioid.

Dosage

Oral preparation: a suitable dose is 50 mg three times daily. An increased dose of 100 mg three times daily gives slightly greater efficacy, but increases the incidence of unwanted adverse effects.

A sustained release oral preparation and an intravenous/intramuscular preparation (50 mg/ml) is also available.

Transcutaneous electrical nerve stimulation (TENS)

This is a non-invasive method of pain relief, which utilizes Melzack and Wall's gate theory of pain relief for its effect. There is also some evidence to suggest it may stimulate endogenous endorphin production.

- It is best used as an adjunct to other forms of analgesia, and some research suggests an opioid-sparing effect
- It is useful for the more chronic musculoskeletal type of pain
- It has no serious side effects
- It cannot be used in pace-maker dependent patients
- It may reduce the incidence of nausea and vomiting.

Monitoring the effectiveness of post-thoracotomy pain relief

Regular assessment of pain during the post-operative period is desirable for provision of adequate and safe pain relief. The best indicator of the effectiveness of pain management is an assessment of pain during coughing, deep breathing or movement (e.g. sitting up in bed). Objective assessment of pain is virtually impossible, but some degree of quantification can be achieved by using standardized scoring systems or scales.

Whatever method of acute pain management is undertaken in a hospital, a team approach is essential to good practice. This should involve nurses, physiotherapists, a pharmacist and medical staff, including advice from a senior member of the anaesthetic staff. Consideration should also be given to adequate and appropriate analgesia on discharge. Follow-up telephone contact with the patient can ensure that episodes of breakthrough pain are identified, and that appropriate treatment is sought early enough to prevent the potential transition to a chronic pain state.

KEY POINTS

- Thoracotomy is one of the most painful surgical procedures.

- Good post-operative pain relief is essential in preventing retention of secretions, atelectasis and chest infection.

- Chronic post-thoracotomy pain syndrome is relatively common.

- Pre-emptive analgesia and post-operative pain control may prevent the development of chronic post-thoracotomy pain syndromes.

- Multi-modal analgesia using the triad of local anaesthetic, opioid and NSAID is optimal. This approach may be further refined by the addition of an NMDA antagonist or α-2 agonist.

- Post-operative pain monitoring and an educated pain team may improve the outcome.

Bibliography

Bonica, J.J., Backup, P.H., Anderson, C.E. *et al.* (1957). Peridural block: analysis of 3367 cases and a review. *Anesthesiology*, **18**, 723–84.

Conacher, I.D. (1990). Pain relief after thoracotomy. *Br. J. Anaesth.*, **65**, 806–12.

Dawkins, C.J. (1969). An analysis of the complications of extradural and caudal block. *Anaesthesia*, **24**, 554–63.

Ganong, W. (1981). *Review of Medical Physiology*. Appleton & Lange.

Kane, R.E. (1981). Neurologic deficits following epidural or spinal anesthesia. *Anesth. Analg.*, **60(3)**, 150–61.

Katz, J., Jackson, M., Kavanagh, B. *et al.* (1996). Acute pain after thoracic surgery predicts long-term post-thoracotomy pain. *Clin. J. Pain*, **12(I)**, 50–5.

Kavanagh, B.P., Katz, J. and Sandler, A.N. (1994). Pain control after thoracic surgery. A review of current techniques. *Anesthesiology*, **81**, 737–59.

Kissin, I. (1996). Editorial view: Pre-emptive analgesia. *Anaesthesiology*, **84**, 1015–19.

Loan, W.B. and Morrison, J.D. (1967). The incidence of severity of post-operative pain. *Br. J. Anaesth.*, **39**, 695–8.

Lund, P.C. (1962). Peridural anaesthesia: A review of 10 000 administrations. *Acta Anaesth. Scand.*, **6**, 143–59.

Meyer, R.A., Campbell, J.N. and Raja, S.N. (1994). Peripheral neural mechanisms of nociception. In *Textbook of Pain* (P.D. Wall and R. Melzack, eds), pp. 13–44. Churchill Livingstone.

Rice, A.S.C. (1997). The pathophysiology of acute pain. In *Highlights in Pain Therapy and Regional Anaesthesia VI* (A. Van Zundert, ed.), pp. 222–47. ESRA Permanger Publications.

Rosenberg, P.H., Scheinin, B.M., Lepantalo, M.J. *et al.* (1987). Continuous intrapleural infusion of Bupivicaine for analgesia after thoracotomy. *Anesthesiology*, **67**, 811–13.

Royal College of Surgeons of England and the College of Anaesthetists. Commission on the Provision of Surgical Services (1990). *Report of the Working Party on Pain after Surgery*.

Woolf, C.J. (1991). Central mechanisms of acute pain. *Proceedings of the VIth World Congress on Pain* (M.R. Bond, J.E. Charlton and C.J. Woolf, eds), pp. 25–34. Elsevier Science.

Woolf, C.J. and Chong, M.-S. (1993). Pre-emptive analgesia: Treating post-operative pain by preventing the establishment of central sensitization (review article). *Anesth. Analg.*, **77**, 362–79.

18

Specialized modes of respiratory support in thoracic surgical patients

C. J. Bateman and B. F. Keogh

Introduction

The respiratory support of thoracic surgical patients may present difficult and complex problems due to pre-existing pulmonary disease, the impact of surgery and the presence of heterogeneous pathology in different lung regions. Optimum pulmonary support involves setting appropriate ventilatory targets, minimizing the risk of ventilation-induced trauma and achieving a balance of ventilatory effects on obstructive, restrictive and parenchymal pulmonary processes, all of which may co-exist in thoracic surgical patients.

Ventilatory practice following thoracic surgery

Following thoracic surgery, the majority of patients can be extubated at the end of the procedure or require a relatively short period of post-operative support. Such patients are commonly managed in the recovery area with very traditional ventilation modes, typically tidal volume preset, volume-cycled or time-cycled, mandatory flow-generated breaths. Patient interaction in synchronized intermittent mandatory ventilation or pressure–support modes may be used in the early post-operative phase, and may enhance patient comfort during emergence from anaesthesia or sedation.

A more difficult problem is posed by the small number of patients (less than 10 per cent of those undergoing major thoracic procedures) who require more prolonged support due to poor pre-operative lung function, extensive surgery, surgical complications or difficulties with pain control (particularly in bilateral or extensive reconstructive procedures). In such patients, the response to different ventilatory protocols will be variable, but can be predicted with knowledge of pre-operative pulmonary function and mechanics and of the likely effects of the surgery undertaken.

Principles of safe ventilatory practice

Ventilatory practice has evolved greatly since the mid-1980s, and is now based much more than previously on physiological foundations and lung protective practice. This evolution has been detailed in the 1993 report of

Table 18.1 Summary of recommendations of American College of Chest Physicians Consensus Conference on Mechanical Ventilation, 1993

Ventilatory protocols should encompass the following principles:

- Pathophysiology of disease varies within the course of illness
- Measures to minimize adverse effects of ventilation should be implemented whenever possible
- Physiological targets may not be in the normal range
- The pressure/volume cost of ventilation should be minimized and end-inspiratory plateau pressures not exceed 35 cmH$_2$O
- Dynamic hyperinflation should be recognized and avoided

a Consensus Conference on Mechanical Ventilation (Table 18.1). Such recommendations are based on experimental evidence and recent widespread changes in ventilatory philosophy.

Insights from animal studies

Recent animal studies have differentially assessed the traumatic effects of high airway pressure and tidal volume on pulmonary structures. These have demonstrated that alveolar over-distension, irrespective of airway pressure, is responsible for a form of structural lung damage. In addition, high inspiratory pressures are less likely to cause pulmonary damage if the associated lung volume change is small (e.g. in restrictive disease). At the other end of the spectrum, the repeated opening and closing of lung units at end-expiration can be shown to cause a different structural injury, primarily at the alveolar duct level. The shear forces thought responsible for this form of lung damage may be ameliorated by maintaining end-expiratory volume with either externally applied or intrinsic positive end-expiratory pressure (PEEP).

Such studies suggest that safe ventilatory practice invokes a narrow band of lung volume change, with specific avoidance of significant alveolar over-distension. In clinical practice, the effects of volume change and applied pressure can rarely be separated, so similar constraints can be proposed for a range of acceptable airway pressures. A plateau pressure of 35 cmH$_2$O has been recommended as a reasonable upper limit (the peak inspiratory pressure in pressure-limited modes). In most situations of compromised pulmonary function, some manipulation of end-expiratory volume with PEEP (total PEEP range 3–15 cmH$_2$O) will be appropriate. In patients with obstructive airways disease who exhibit high levels of intrinsic PEEP, lung damage associated with end-expiratory airway closure and re-opening is likely to be less relevant. Paradoxically, in pressure-limited ventilatory modes, titration of low levels of external PEEP (2–5 cmH$_2$O) may improve ventilatory mechanics in some patients with obstructive disease.

Oxygenation

Arterial blood gas targets have recently been liberalized in compromised patients. Recognition of the primacy of arterial saturation (SaO_2) as the relevant oxygenation parameter determining oxygen delivery (DO_2), as indicated by the following simplified equation, has resulted in acceptance of much lower oxygenation target values:

$$DO_2(ml/min/m^2) = \text{Cardiac index } (l/min/m^2) \times (Hb \times SaO_2 \times 1.34) \times 10$$

Hence, arterial saturation values of 88 per cent may be readily accepted in patients with compromised pulmonary function. Similarly, in those patients with preserved cardiovascular function, even lower values of arterial saturation may be accepted in order to avoid the deleterious effects of excessive pulmonary pressures or prolonged high inspired oxygen concentrations. Thus, although an SaO_2 of 80 per cent is by no means desirable, it remains compatible with survival and may, on rare occasions, be accepted on risk–benefit evaluation.

Such liberal goals are widely applied in severe pulmonary failure and are likely to be applied in surgical patients with severe parenchymal disease, in whom relatively minor surgical procedures such as lung biopsy or thoracoscopic intervention are somewhat peripheral to the primarily medical management of the underlying pulmonary process.

Carbon dioxide

The use of permissive hypercapnia (PH) in severe asthma was recommended by Perret in 1984, and in the adult respiratory distress syndrome (ARDS) by Hickling in 1990. The practice of PH has subsequently been incorporated into ventilatory protocols for patients with other diseases, and $Paco_2$ levels of 12–14 kPa are now commonly tolerated in the acute phase of severe respiratory illness. Thoracic surgical patients may already exhibit metabolic compensation for chronic respiratory acidosis, and this should be considered during ventilation and when assessing criteria for weaning off respiratory support.

Advances in monitoring and ventilatory optimization

Modern microprocessor ventilatory technology provides a wide range of monitoring software that can be used to optimize ventilator–patient interaction. Clinically useful options include pressure–volume loops, real-time inspiratory and expiratory flow profiles, measurements of intrinsic PEEP and trapped volumes, and analogue displays of expiratory capnography profiles. Measurements of pulmonary compliance and airways resistance are usually available, but their interpretation depends on the characteristics of the particular ventilatory mode employed.

Pressure–volume loops and intrinsic PEEP measurements have become increasingly popular and, although much can be learned from these two options, they are both subject to interpretation difficulties. Dynamic flow–volume loops are inferior to static assessments, and may specifically underestimate the lung volume at which the upper inflection pressure point is reached. Intrinsic PEEP measurements vary in method between different ventilators, and are at best semi-quantitative. Changes in frequency, tidal volume or inspiratory to expiratory (I:E) ratios inevitably change measured intrinsic PEEP values, which may then be used to direct lung volume recruitment and maintenance strategies. Disease progression or response to therapy can be inferred by intrinsic PEEP values, but such assessments are only truly valid if ventilatory parameters remain unchanged.

Conventional ventilatory options in the difficult thoracic surgical patient

The choice of ventilatory mode is influenced greatly by local factors, including available technology, familiarity and experience, and physician preference. Volume-preset ventilatory modes have long provided the foundation of ventilatory support, and have remained popular in North America. In Europe, there has been a definite swing towards pressure-preset or pressure-limited ventilatory strategies since the 1980s. A reflection of this change in philosophy is the emphasis on new pressure-oriented modes in the current European manufactured critical care ventilators.

Thoracic surgical patients pose potential difficulties that may confound attempts to optimize ventilation. The presence of unilateral and heterogeneous pathology, the high incidence of underlying chronic obstructive disease, regional differences in compliance and expiratory time constants, limited cardiopulmonary reserve and elements of pulmonary fibrosis are factors that complicate assessment of the appropriate mode. In such a varied group it is unlikely that any particular mode will be universally applicable, and the choice should be governed by safety principles, understanding of the subtle features of each mode and by an attempt to optimize ventilator–patient interaction.

The volume versus pressure ventilation discussion is likely to continue with eloquent arguments on both sides. The whole issue is greatly clouded by the lack of scientific data comparing different modes. The distinction between the two basic options is becoming less distinct as hybrid modes with features of each basic option have now been introduced. In the specific field of pulmonary failure in thoracic surgical patients, and in the context of protective ventilation and the acceptance of realistic blood gas targets, pressure-limited ventilation in one of its forms can be proposed as the more favourable option. Many of the favourable characteristics of pressure-preset ventilation have been outlined by Lachmann – admittedly in acute lung injury patients, but with physiological considerations relevant to different pulmonary conditions.

Volume-preset ventilation

Although the tidal volume guarantee of volume-preset ventilation may appear attractive, it is the least forgiving form of ventilation and may lead to high airway pressures, gas trapping and cardiovascular compromise. In addition, there is no added flow reserve to compensate for leaks and the relatively low inspiratory flow rates of a flow generator at standard settings (20–40 l/min) result in inhomogeneous ventilation and perpetuate existing ventilation–perfusion mismatch. In addition, there is no safe option for harnessing the lung volume recruitment capabilities of intrinsic PEEP.

Modification of the volume-preset mode by adding a pressure limit, increasing maximum inspiratory flow to > 100 l/min and setting high tidal volumes (a potential flow source for leak compensation) results in a safer and more flexible variant, but shifts the mode towards the pressure-preset spectrum. This mode is particularly attractive because it is essentially analogous to pressure control ventilation (PCV), but also provides a volume limit, which may be relevant in the situation of rapidly varying airways resistance. Another hybrid mode, pressure regulated volume control (PRVC), in which inspiratory pressure is minimized for a given preset tidal volume, confers added safety but is limited in its ability to compensate for large or variable leaks.

Pressure-preset ventilation

There are several advantages of pressure-limited modes in patients with heterogeneous pulmonary pathology. Most are pressure generator systems, and their high initial inspiratory flow rates result in distribution of gas according to local expiratory time constants. Lung units with low levels of intrinsic PEEP are preferentially ventilated early in inspiration, and those with higher levels receive lesser and later ventilation. The intrinsic pressure limit confers inherent safety and, combined with regional differences in inspiratory flow profiles, results in lung-protective ventilation and improved ventilation–perfusion matching. A decrease in pulmonary compliance or an increase in resistance will result in decreased tidal and minute ventilation, but this is acceptable and even desirable in the acute situation. The acceptance of permissive hypercapnia has removed many of the theoretical arguments opposing the use of pressure-limited modes.

Commonly used pressure-limited modes include pressure control ventilation (PCV) and its spontaneous variants, airway pressure release ventilation (APRV) and bilevel or biphasic positive airway pressure (BIPAP). The advantages of these modes include inherent pressure limitation, homogeneous distribution of ventilation, large flow reserve and the ability to harness favourable characteristics of intrinsic PEEP while limiting its deleterious effects. The use of PCV in inverse ratios (PC-IRV) of up to 3 : 1 provides excellent lung volume recruitment due to the development of intrinsic PEEP. PC-IRV has been applied extensively in the management of lung injury, and can be used safely even in the presence of differential compliance due to the dynamics of gas distribution in a pressure generator system.

BIPAP

Some confusion exists about the two acronyms used to describe variants of PCV that encompass spontaneous respiration. The initial description by Downs in 1987 of a system intermittently varying two levels of continuous positive airway pressure (CPAP) and with a very short expiratory time was termed APRV. BIPAP is the corresponding mode, which applies two levels of CPAP across the range of inspiratory : expiratory ratios and provides flow availability for spontaneous respiration throughout the respiratory cycle. BIPAP modes are increasing in popularity, and in many patients the additional efficiency of augmented spontaneous respiratory effort proves superior to mandatory ventilation. BIPAP can be used along a spectrum from total mandatory ventilation, through various intermittent mandatory and patient triggered options, to single level CPAP. This BIPAP spectrum was extensively discussed by Hormann in 1994. Favourable characteristics of BIPAP include inherent pressure limit, lung volume recruitment, excellent leak compensation, pressure-generator gas distribution profiles and a reported decrease in sedative requirements. BIPAP has been enthusiastically supported as an option in acute lung injury but, as is often the case, definitive data supporting this approach are lacking. One feature of BIPAP relevant to thoracic anaesthetic and critical care practice is that, on some ventilators, BIPAP more readily accepts extrinsic gas sources such as nitric oxide or volatile agents than other less flexible mandatory modes. Recent modifications include the ability to vary the rate of pressure rise from lower to higher CPAP levels, which may prove more comfortable for awake patients (and conceptually represents a move towards flow generator mechanics).

The role of BIPAP in thoracic surgical patients is as yet undefined. It is now being more widely applied, but there are few literature reports, and certainly none showing any superiority over other modes. In general it is well tolerated and has attractive features, but the occasional patient with severe gas trapping is encountered whose respiratory pattern becomes increasingly unco-ordinated in the BIPAP mode and who may require sedation or paralysis to break this gas-trapping cycle.

Adjunctive therapies in ventilatory support

The range of adjunctive techniques is considerable, and is outside the scope of this chapter. Of practical interest is the use of posture manipulation in these patients. Posture manipulation, and specifically the prone position, is regularly practised in acute lung injury patients and in other pathologies in the paediatric venue. Imaginative postural repositioning can influence ventilation–perfusion matching in heterogeneous pathology as well, and should always be considered due to its potential to enhance gas exchange and aid physiotherapy.

Selective pulmonary vasodilators such as inhaled nitric oxide and nebulized prostacyclin have been used in clinical practice since 1993. They can be delivered with almost any ventilatory mode, although the accuracy of dose delivered will depend on the mode used and the delivery systems employed. Despite favourable effects on arterial oxygenation, intrapulmonary shunt and pulmonary vascular resistance in up to 60 per cent of patients with severe pulmonary failure, the critical care community has so far been unable to show any outcome benefit from the use of nitric oxide. Although a controversial issue, this dilemma should not necessarily discourage the use of nitric oxide in severely hypoxic thoracic surgical patients. This is particularly true in the presence of pulmonary hypertension and in the current climate, where evidence for adverse effects of low doses of nitric oxide is not apparent. It will be a considerable time before the effects of nitric oxide on a variety of post-thoracic surgical conditions are properly assessed.

In the experimental venue, the search for a suitable and economically viable surfactant with reproducible effects is ongoing. Difficulties remain with determining the ideal surfactant, indications for its use in adults, effective dose and dosage schedule. Partial liquid ventilation (PLV), in which the lungs are filled with liquid perfluorocarbon to functional residual capacity and ventilated with tidal breaths above this volume, is receiving considerable attention. There are problems with PLV that are particularly relevant to thoracic practice. These include difficulties in predicting FRC values, loss of the discriminatory value of radiological imaging as the lung fields become completely opaque on chest radiographs and CT scans, and problems with tenacious secretions. PLV is also relatively contraindicated in the presence of air leaks, as perfluorocarbons are not well cleared from the pleural space. Although developments in this field are of great interest, it is difficult to predict a major impact of this therapy in thoracic surgical patients.

Independent lung ventilation (ILV)

The use of ILV in the post-operative phase, or in patients with asymmetric pulmonary pathology, is an obvious extension of the practice of one-lung anaesthesia. Double-lumen endobronchial tubes are the choice for ILV in critical care, although bronchial blockers and modified airway tubes have been used imaginatively to achieve lung separation. The original literature in this field is sparse, and is based mainly on case reports in the 1980s. The lack of more recent original information is probably a reflection of the rare instances in which this intervention is truly required.

Management of endobronchial tubes in ITU

The new generation of disposable polyvinyl chloride double-lumen tubes are more suitable for prolonged use than their red-rubber predecessors, principally because tracheal and bronchial cuffs are of low pressure and high volume design and the bronchial cuff profiles are ideally fashioned. Despite these advantages, high pressures (up to 80 mmHg) may be generated in these cuffs if they are over-inflated beyond sealing pressure. Even in apparently well managed endobronchial intubation, bronchoscopic visualization of the left main bronchus upon removal of the tube often reveals considerable mucosal oedema, abrasion and contact bleeding. Bronchial laceration and rupture is a rare but recurrent complication even with newer tubes and, indeed, tracheal rupture with such tubes has been reported. Although double-lumen tube management in the operating theatre is usually undertaken by experienced operators, this may not necessarily be the case in the intensive care unit. Comprehension of cuff management safety principles amongst the ICU staff must therefore be ensured.

Verification of ideal positioning of the double-lumen tube with fibre-optic bronchoscopy, repeated as required, is a vital component of effective ILV management. Fibre-optic bronchoscopy must be readily available, and tube selection should ensure that it is feasible. The tracheal intubating fibrescope (4 mm diameter) may be used for fibre-optic bronchoscopy in the smaller double-lumen tubes, but has a limited suction capability. Of the smaller adult tubes used in our institution, the intubating fibrescope will traverse the bronchial lumen of the 35 Fr Sher-i-bronch (Kendall Healthcare, Mansfield, MA, USA) and 35 Fr Bronchocath (Mallinckrodt Industries, Athlone, Ireland), but requires considerable force to traverse the small disposable Robertshaw (Phoenix Medical, Preston, Lancs, UK). A 3.6-mm paediatric bronchoscope may be used in this and smaller tubes, but the suction capability is much reduced.

The adult bronchoscope, typical diameter 4.9 mm, has a much more effective suction channel and will traverse the bronchial lumen of the medium Robertshaw tube, but neither 37 Fr versions of the Sher-i-bronch and Broncho-cath. It is obvious that bronchoscope sizes and available endo-bronchial tubes will vary between institutions. Pre-insertion testing of bronchoscope/double-lumen tube compatibility should ensure that fibre-optic bronchoscopy *in situ* is feasible, although if the bronchoscope fit is snug pre-insertion, distal acute angulation of the bronchial section, particularly when the tube is warm, can decrease the effective lumen diameter and cause obstruction to passage.

Stabilization of the double-lumen tube

The potential for double-lumen tube displacement in ongoing management is well recognized. Benumof has suggested that movements from the ideal position of 16–19 mm for left tubes and 1–8 mm for right tubes will disrupt ILV efficacy. Left-sided tubes should be chosen if possible, but in cases of left bronchial trauma, obstruction or stenosis, or following left lung transplantation, right-sided tubes are likely to be necessary despite the well-recognized positional difficulties with the right upper lobe bronchus.

Various methods of tube fixation are employed. Use of a combination of a cotton tie and adhesive tape (each system independently fixing the tube in position) and stabilization of the position after allowing time for slight distal migration of the tube as it warms *in situ* works well. Patients who require ILV should be heavily sedated, and are paralysed in many units. ILV is often required for a relatively short time (a few days), so complications from prolonged use of neuromuscular blocking agents may be avoided. Ventilator tubing should be independently supported, and great care taken to avoid kinks in the proximal aspects of the tube or the tube connectors. General nursing procedures, physiotherapy and radiographic imaging are all rendered much more labour-intensive by the need to ensure tube stability.

Detecting displacement of the double-lumen tube

Current ventilators provide varying levels of monitoring, which can be employed in continuous assessment of double-lumen tube position. Reductions in simple measurements such as tidal and minute volume or changes in calculated resistance or compliance should alert the user of tube mal-position. Minute ventilation or tidal volume alarms should be set at very discriminatory levels so that relatively small changes in expired minute ventilation will be highlighted. Leak measurements are available on some devices, and alerts can be programmed if leak increases. Airway pressure alarms are useful in volume-oriented ventilation, but are less discriminatory when pressure-preset ventilation is employed. Observation of pressure–volume loops, flow graphics or measurements of intrinsic PEEP are useful in identifying the nature of displacement, but are unlikely to provide a primary alert.

Expiratory capnography provides a valuable tool in the assessment of tube function. Absolute values are less relevant than trends, as end-tidal to arterial CO_2 gradients may be high in pulmonary disease. Expiratory CO_2 waveform analysis provides accessible information about airway obstruction, and waveforms are much preferred to digital values. A decrease in the slope of the early CO_2 exhalation waveform suggests an increase in expiratory obstruction and malposition.

Indications for ILV

The indications for ILV following thoracic surgery and in the ITU are reasonably self-evident, and can be classified on pathophysiological grounds.
They include:

- Airway protection in massive haemoptysis or in purulent disease
- Unilateral lung disease with marked disturbance of ventilation–perfusion matching, such as pneumonia, pulmonary haemorrhage, unilateral ARDS and refractory atelectasis
- Management of bronchopleural fistula
- Management of asymmetric pulmonary pathology following pulmon-ary transplantation
- Management of severe unilateral airway obstruction.

The effect of positive pressure ventilation can be surprisingly detrimental in some such cases. Differentials in airway resistance and pulmonary compli-ance between the two lungs enhance ventilation–perfusion mismatch. For example, lobar pneumonia in the presence of emphysema will predispose to severe hypoxia, due to shunting of blood away from hyperinflated, aerated zones to the consolidated areas of the contralateral lung. Applica-tion of PEEP or higher mean airway pressures in this context may further exacerbate the degree of intrapulmonary shunt and resultant hypoxia. The application of ILV allows each lung to be managed according to its indi-vidual pulmonary mechanics. Pressure–volume curves of each lung can be used to optimize individual lung ventilation.

Synchronous versus asynchronous ILV

The value of synchronization of delivered breaths is a recurrent question in ILV. Both synchronous and asynchronous approaches were reported more than 20 years ago. Synchronization may in theory prevent unfavourable mediastinal positional changes, but there is no evidence confirming this to be a problem in clinical practice. Synchronization of ILV with the cardiac cycle has also been proposed, but is of physiological interest rather than clinically relevant.

In practice, effective ILV usually involves out-of-phase ventilation. A grossly hyperinflated lung may receive only a few breaths per minute and require a very prolonged expiratory time, whereas a contralateral consolidated lung is likely to be ventilated in the normal frequency range. Some degree of synchronization can be achieved if the higher ventilatory rate is a product of the lower, but there is no evidence that this approach offers any advantage. Although synchronization is discussed in every review of ILV, scientific assessment of its value is essentially lacking. Synchronization between ventilators has previously involved additional technology at significant cost. At least one ventilator manufacturer, Draeger (Lubeck, Germany), has now included the synchronization facility within the standard software of new critical care ventilators. Extra cost implications are therefore limited to the ventilator linking cable. The availability of this option is of interest, but it remains unlikely that synchronization will be shown to be significantly superior to asynchronous ILV.

ILV in specific situations

Massive haemoptysis

Massive haemoptysis is distressing, and may be life-threatening. ILV is the emergency approach of choice, and will help to localize the origin of bleeding. In extreme circumstances, massive haemoptysis may be managed by clamping the endobronchial tube lumen dedicated to the bleeding lung. A tamponade effect may then arrest ongoing bleeding, allowing bronchoscopic assessment and further treatment in a more controlled fashion.

Single lung transplantation

Pulmonary transplantation presents unique challenges, which are considered in Chapter 15. The problem of differential lung mechanics is most evident in single lung transplantation (SLT). ILV was first reported in the post-operative management of SLT patients in 1991.

Experience in SLT has greatly increased within the last decade. Post-operative ILV may be applied in several scenarios. In acute graft dysfunction, ILV is indicated when lung volume recruitment techniques required in the transplanted lung prove incompatible with an emphysematous native lung. In another reported scenario of acute graft dysfunction, a patient underwent SLT for primary pulmonary hypertension and required ILV to wean from post-operative extracorporeal gas exchange after severe unilateral pulmonary oedema had developed in the transplanted lung. In severe pulmonary fibrosis, preferential hyperinflation of the transplanted lung may occur, but can usually be managed with conventional techniques.

The most common indication for ILV after SLT is gross hyperinflation of a severely emphysematous native lung. The transplanted lung is, by comparison, less compliant, and preferential ventilation further exacerbates native lung hyperinflation. Widespread atelectasis in the transplanted lung, gross mediastinal shift and cardiovascular collapse may all result

(a)

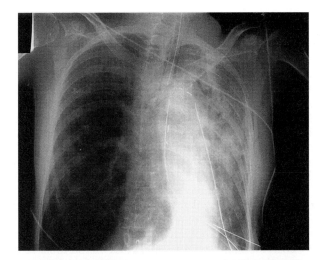

(b)

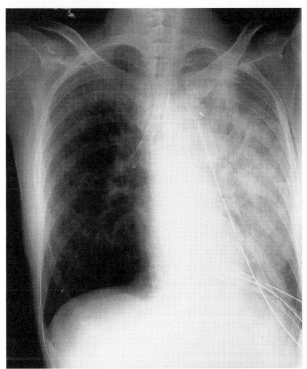

Figure 18.1

(a) Chest X-ray shows gross hyperinflation of the native right
  lung with massive mediastinal shift to the left after single
  lung transplantation.

(b) Chest X-ray follows insertion of a right-sided double-lumen
  tube with considerable decrease in volume of the right lung
  and central repositioning of the mediastinum. (X-rays courtesy
  of J. Mitchell and J. G. Farrimond, Harefield Hospital, UK.)

from intractable gas trapping in the native lung (Fig. 18.1). Institution of ILV with marked hypoventilation of the native lung allows normalization of mediastinal position and much improved cardiovascular parameters. In one large series from Harefield Hospital, UK, of more than 100 patients undergoing SLT for emphysema, more than 10 per cent of patients required this intervention.

Bronchopleural fistula (BPF)
The management of major air leaks is a well-recognized indication for ILV, and has been considered extensively in previous publications. The need for ILV has undoubtedly decreased in recent years due to improved conventional ventilatory options and a move away from volume-preset ventilation. Additional gas must be available to compensate for the large air leak and to maintain ventilation of the surrounding lung. Such new ventilatory strategies include pressure control ventilation, pressure-limited, high inspiratory flow generation and BIPAP, all of which provide considerable reserve in ventilatory flow. Application of these modes will, in most cases, stabilize gas exchange so that a considered decision about invasive or expectant management can be made.

This expectant approach is illustrated by Figure 18.2. This displays the chest radiograph of a 17-kg child, following acute viral pneumonia, who developed a massive air leak through the right lung in the presence of markedly different pulmonary compliance. ILV was never a realistic option due to her size and, despite unfavourable mechanical and ventilation–perfusion features, effective ventilation was achieved using a variant of pressure-control ventilation. During the acute phase of her illness, no emphasis was placed on reducing the volume of air leak and high mean airway pressures proved necessary to achieve barely acceptable oxygenation. On resolution of the illness, and with institution of weaning, the leak gradually decreased in volume and eventually sealed.

In some instances air leaks may prove unmanageable with conventional options, leaving ILV as the appropriate progression. Ventilation is then optimized on the unaffected side and various approaches applied to the damaged lung. In conventional management, peak and mean airway pressures are decreased, as are PEEP levels on that side. Some controversy exists about the use of PEEP in air leaks – although studies in the 1980s suggested that PEEP increases air leakage via a BPF, this needs to be balanced against the need to prevent atelectasis in the affected lung. High frequency ventilation (low-pressure philosophy as described below) on the affected side has been anecdotally and favourably reported on numerous occasions, and is theoretically attractive in this condition.

The authors are unaware of any clinical studies comparing different ventilatory options in the management of BPF, and it is their practice to adopt a very expectant approach to air leaks, using conventional technology with adequate flow reserve to compensate for large leak volumes. It is vital to ensure that intercostal drains are large enough to cope with the gas flow through the BPF and that they are ideally positioned. In this respect the authors have a very low threshold for transferring ventilated patients for computerized tomography (CT) of the thorax. CT is the definitive investigation for occult pneumothorax. Intercostal drain insertion can be guided

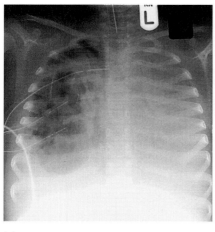

(a)

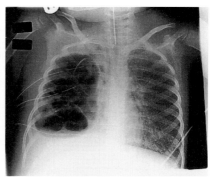

(b)

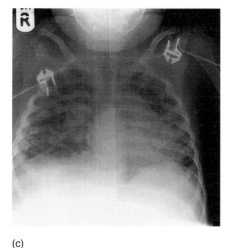

(c)

Figure 18.2

(a) Chest X-ray shows severe viral bronchial pneumonia with large air leaks from the right lung.
(b) Pneumonia has progressed to resolution of consolidation in the left lung, but residual pneumatocoeles with ongoing air leaks on the right side.
(c) Chest X-ray shows substantial resolution of pneumatocoeles after 1 month, and air leak had ceased.

directly by CT or indirectly by skin marking and later insertion, and can result in effective pleural space drainage, lung re-expansion and much improved pulmonary mechanics.

On rare occasions, air leaks can prove totally unmanageable and further options may need to be considered. Figure 18.3 shows the chest radiograph of a patient with severe emphysema who required cardiopulmonary resuscitation after bilateral lung volume reduction surgery. Ventilation subsequently proved extremely difficult due to large air leaks, particularly on the right. Despite exploring several ventilatory options, acceptable gas exchange proved difficult to achieve. Although further surgical intervention was a theoretical option, it was felt most unattractive in this patient. Extracorporeal gas exchange may be indicated in patients with uncontrollable air leaks, but represents a major therapeutic escalation. In this patient, escalation was thought inappropriate due to the severity of underlying disease and multiple organ insufficiency.

(a)

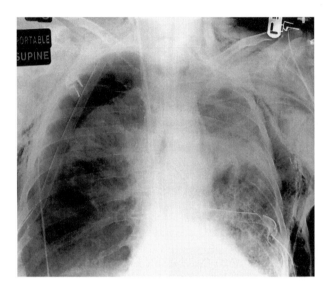

(b)

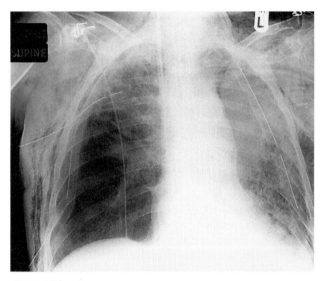

Figure 18.3

(a) Chest X-ray shows widespread surgical emphysema, left-sided
   endobronchial tube in position and collapse of the right lung
   despite an apparently well placed intercostal drain.
(b) Placement of a further intercostal drain resulted in some
   expansion of the right lung, but the massive air leak could
   not be controlled and arterial blood gases remained
   unacceptable.

High frequency ventilation (HFV)

High frequency technology has been utilized in thoracic and airway surgery since the early 1970s. Although well established in many centres for intra-operative management, the role of HFV in post-operative and critical care patients has remained undefined. A wide variety of HFV devices have been constructed, both locally and commercially, and have performed with variable (and at times disappointing) efficacy. Design features are crucial to the ventilatory performance of different HFV devices, and apparently small design alterations can greatly alter ventilator performance.

High frequency jet ventilation (HFJV)

The majority of HFV devices employed in adults and older children are jet ventilators, in which high pressure gas is accelerated during inspiration through a jet nozzle or the injector lumen of a modified endotracheal tube, or transtracheally via a variety of tracheostomy tubes. Gas entrainment enhances inspiratory pulse volume and exhalation is passive in this system. Adjustable ventilator settings are frequency (typical range 60–400 per minute), inspiratory time (I-time, 15–50 per cent) and driving pressure (variable depending on device, 1–3 atm), and some devices provide the option of adjustable external PEEP. Desirable monitoring features include peak, mean and minimum airway pressure and FiO_2.

Tidal volume cannot be accurately measured in HFJV, so traditional simple assessments of pulmonary mechanics are not available. Carbon dioxide clearance is most influenced by frequency and I-time, whereas oxygenation in atelectatic or oedematous lungs can be improved by increasing I-time or driving pressure (which increase mean airway pressure and hence lung volume). Ventilatory capacity is greatly influenced by the position of the jet source within the respiratory system. Patient selection and ventilatory strategies are both governed by knowledge of the technical and performance characteristics of the available HFJV device.

Positioning of the jet nozzle at the proximal end of the endotracheal tube provides an entrainment ratio of up to 200 per cent, resulting in a corresponding substantial increase in the jet pulse volume. Effective humidification of HFJV pulse gas is vital to ventilator safety in all but short operative procedures, and the high entrainment ratio in this configuration allows innovative humidification technology. In one commercial device, a bias gas, heated to 47°C and fully saturated with water vapour at this temperature, is delivered to an entrainment chamber containing the proximally sited nozzle. Mixing of heated, fully saturated bias gas with dry, room temperature nozzle gas results in the delivery of fully saturated humidified gas at patient temperature. Such effective humidification protects against airway mucosal trauma and mucous dessication during HFJV. Inadequate humidification or inadvertent failure of humidification can lead to necrotizing tracheitis with catastrophic sequelae.

Distal positioning of the delivered gas pulse within the trachea, via either a modified endotracheal tube or a fine catheter, results in a much lower entrainment ratio of approximately 25 per cent. This approach mandates

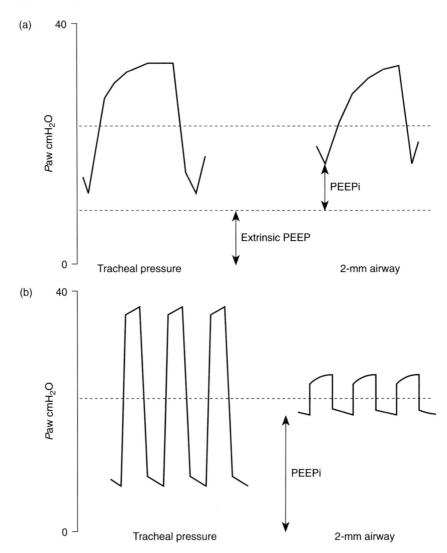

Figure 18.4 Schematic representation of airway pressure changes in central and peripheral airways:

(a) With pressure controlled-inverse ratio ventilation (PC-IRV), and
(b) with high frequency jet ventilation (HFJV).

In PC-IRV, intrinsic PEEP (PEEPi) can be generated with or without extrinsic PEEP. In HFJV, for a given mean airway pressure (dotted line) the increase in minimum alveolar pressure (by extrapolation) from central minimum pressure represents the level of PEEPi. Also of note is the difference in maximum alveolar pressures. For a given mean airway pressure, the alveolus is exposed to a considerably lower peak distending pressure in HFJV compared to PC-IRV. (Reproduced with permission from Keogh, B. and Evans, T.W. (1998). *European Respiratory Monograph*, **3(8)**, 490–510.)

direct humidification of the jet gas, which is technically difficult and of variable efficiency. This inefficiency may to some extent be offset by a much lower total ventilatory volume, and a correspondingly reduced humidification requirement in the proximal airways.

An interesting aspect of the use of HFJV is the associated degree of intrinsic PEEP. HFJV in its most potent form is conceptually analogous to pressure-controlled inverse-ratio ventilation (PC-IRV), although displaced considerably up the frequency spectrum (Fig. 18.4). When HFJV is applied with effective pulse volumes (i.e. proximal entrainment), frequencies > 150 per minute and I-time of > 35 per cent, considerable intrinsic PEEP is developed. At such settings, the minimum alveolar pressure approximates to the mean airway pressure and the difference between mean and minimum centrally measured airway pressure reflects the value of intrinsic PEEP. This degree of intrinsic PEEP can be of substantial benefit in pulmonary oedema or ARDS, but may be undesirable in those patients with obstructive airway disease. Some peak pressure limitation is provided in HFJV by a phenomenon known as 'blowback' (representing a balance between entrainment forces and their counteraction by airways resistance), but unlike pressure-control ventilation, peak pressure cannot be independently controlled. Recognition of the unique patient–ventilator interactions in HFJV suggests two quite different strategies in the post-operative management of thoracic surgical patients.

HFJV administered at low mean airway pressure

HFJV has been advocated for many years as an ideal ventilatory strategy in the management of bronchopleural fistulae, and can be shown to decrease gas leak through an experimental bronchopleural fistula. Inspiratory gas distribution in HFV is determined by airways resistance rather than compliance, hence lung units juxtaposed to a region of infinite compliance (i.e. a bronchopleural fistula) can be effectively inflated and ventilated during HFJV.

HFJV management of large air leaks ideally delivers small gas pulses into the airway so that peak and mean airway pressures are maintained at low levels. Exact settings depend on the device employed, but I-time is generally less than 25 per cent in order to limit the development of intrinsic PEEP. Clinical investigation has confirmed that 'tailoring' HFJV driving parameters to deliver short, low-volume pulses can result in intrinsic PEEP levels comparable to traditional forms of ventilation in patients with chronic obstructive airways disease. Paradoxically, clinicians may choose to apply small amounts of external PEEP in order to prevent large-scale end-expiratory collapse in the 'low-pressure' approach to HFJV.

Low-pressure HFJV may be applied in the management of tracheobronchial trauma, or following airway surgery. In these circumstances, pulmonary mechanics are often normal and HFJV provides effective ventilation without the need for an inflated tracheal cuff. HFJV may therefore be applied via a modified endotracheal tube, by a catheter or jet needle connected to a tracheostomy tube, or by connecting a proximal jet entrainment chamber directly to a tracheostomy tube. Humidification is vital whatever system is used, and it is the authors' practice to drip 5 ml of saline per hour into the trachea to enhance humidification.

In recent years, the Department of Anaesthesia at the Royal Brompton Hospital, UK, has moved away from HFJV back to conventional approaches in the management of tracheal trauma or surgery, particularly in patients with normal pulmonary compliance. Endotracheal tubes are employed, with the cuff either deflated or slightly inflated, in order to centralize the tube within the trachea and partially to control the leak. Alternatively, if a Montgomery tracheostomy tube is inserted, ventilation can be achieved without a cuff and even with an open tube system. In the presence of normal pulmonary compliance, proximal blocking of the laryngeal end of the Montgomery tube may not prove necessary, particularly if the patients are awake and can exercise some glottic control. If problems are predicted due to decreased compliance or to laryngeal pathology, the proximal end of the Montgomery tube can be plugged to minimize the proximal air leak. Ventilatory modes with flow reserve are employed, and are usually able to compensate for the degree of air leak. HFJV does represent an alternative and, usually, more effective option in those patients with decreased pulmonary compliance or in whom air leaks prove unmanageable.

HFJV has been used as an aid to weaning in patients with limited cardiopulmonary reserve. Features of HFJV relevant to weaning are the almost unlimited availability of gas flow, adjustable inspiratory support and negligible circuit resistance. Historically, such support has been delivered in various ways, and at one stage transtracheal ventilation was popular. Unfortunately, migration of transtracheal tubes has been reported and, with greatly improved ventilatory weaning options in the microprocessor age, the use of HFJV in this way is now rarely practised.

HFJV administered at high mean airway pressure

HFJV settings can be adjusted to generate substantial levels of intrinsic PEEP as part of a lung volume recruitment and maintenance strategy in acute lung injury or ARDS. In 1983 a prospective, randomized crossover comparison by Carlon et al. of HFJV and conventional ventilation in 309 patients with acute lung injury suggested that HFJV was as effective as conventional techniques but offered no clear advantage over the standard approach. This study resulted in waning enthusiasm for HFJV, but interpretation of the study took no account of the lack of lung volume recruitment or maintenance manoeuvres in either arm of the trial. More powerful HFJV devices have since been developed, which can provide effective ventilation in poorly compliant lungs and are capable of harnessing the lung volume recruitment potential of intrinsic PEEP. One such device was assessed in 90 patients with ARDS, and favourable improvements in oxygenation, CO_2 clearance and airway pressures were reported by Gluck in 1993. With the addition of further patients, it was observed that that those patients with severe ARDS who were switched to HFJV within 48 hours of ventilation achieved 76 per cent survival, as compared to the overall survival rate of 58 per cent. A report by Smith (1993) of HFJV in 29 paediatric patients demonstrated that survivors (69 per cent) spent significantly less time on conventional ventilation than non-survivors. Both these studies support the theoretical proposal that HFJV may limit ventilation-induced lung damage by decreasing alveolar over-distension and shear forces in poorly compliant lungs. In addition, if HFJV is thought appropriate, it should be applied early during the course of ventilatory support.

The relevance of this high-pressure approach to thoracic surgical patients lies in the management of acute lung injury following thoracic surgery. The new generation of potent HFJV ventilators is capable of lung volume recruitment in these poorly compliant patients. In addition, improvements in arterial oxygenation due to an increase in mean airway pressure, effective CO_2 clearance and effective ventilation even in the presence of large air leaks are features of HFJV performance in such patients. In this situation, oxygenation and lung volume stability are primary therapeutic goals, and the management of air leaks is a secondary issue. HFJV should be considered if acceptable oxygenation targets cannot be achieved in patients with acute lung injury following thoracic surgery.

High frequency oscillation (HFO)

High frequency oscillators incorporate an additional active expiratory phase, and hence are capable of operating at frequencies of up to 3000 per minute. Such devices have been employed successfully in the infant distress syndrome, but there are relatively few reports of success in older patients. The transition of HFO into the adult field has been hampered by technical difficulties; in particular, the massive heat generation associated with oscillating larger, adult-size gas volumes at such high frequencies.

HFO devices may be theoretically attractive in thoracic patients with heterogeneous pathology and gas trapping. Although dynamic airway collapse may negate the effect of the active expiratory phase in some patients, the option of having some control of this phase in the difficult patient is attractive. An adult version of an established neonatal ventilator has recently become available for clinical use (High Frequency Oscillator 3100B, Sensormedics, Yorba Linda, CA, USA). Although clinical assessment is very much at an early stage and the results of the initial studies of this device in lung injury are not yet available, the device may provide yet another versatile option in the difficult thoracic surgical patient.

External high frequency oscillation (EHFO)

A further option in high frequency technology is the Hayek Oscillator (Flexco Medical Instruments AG, Zurich, Switzerland), which is an external cuirass ventilator that encases the anterior aspect of the thorax and upper abdomen. The cuirass is connected to an oscillating pump, which generates a negative pressure baseline within the cuirass and oscillates active inspiratory and expiratory phases around this baseline. The frequency range extends to 999 per minute, but the device is usually deployed at frequencies less than 150 per minute. The ability of the device to achieve effective ventilatory capacity has been validated in normal subjects, and it can be shown to improve oxygenation and CO_2 clearance in patients with chronic airflow obstruction.

This EHFO device may have application in thoracic surgery, although effective device positioning is difficult in the presence of intercostal catheters. EHFO may provide a further option in the weaning of patients undergoing a protracted post surgical course, and it has been recommended as a weaning tool. In addition, the device has excellent sputum clearance characteristics and is used as an aid to physiotherapy in patients with cystic fibrosis, bronchiectasis and sputum retention. Although EHFO is not tolerated by all patients, it can contribute substantially to the care of the extubated patient who has difficulty in effectively clearing residual respiratory secretions.

Extrapulmonary options in gas exchange

Extracorporeal gas exchange (ECGE) for severe respiratory failure has been available since the early 1970s. Whilst this technology is now established in the neonatal venue, it is used infrequently and with variable success in older patients. Different forms of ECGE exist, but share the capacity to completely replace natural pulmonary function. Recent interest has also focused on partial support, either by modified ECGE systems or intracorporeal devices, in which native pulmonary function, particularly CO_2 clearance, is augmented but not entirely replaced.

Extracorporeal gas exchange (ECGE)

The use of ECGE in the critical care arena has been the subject of major controversy in the 1990s. ECGE in the non-neonatal setting is usually applied in catastrophic pulmonary failure, most commonly due to acute pneumonia or ARDS. ECGE is massively invasive, hugely labour intensive, expensive, and known to be associated with significant complications. In this context, justification of its use and agreement on appropriate criteria for implementing ECGE are major issues in the field of artificial organ support. Outcome information is now available in patients with ARDS, but little information is available concerning the use of ECGE following thoracic surgery.

Enthusiasm for ECGE in the 1980s was based on anecdotal reports of favourable survival rates of up to 66 per cent in severe ARDS. This was despite evidence from the earlier USA-ECMO study from which Zapol reported equally poor survival (8 per cent) in severe acute respiratory failure whether ECGE was applied or not. A recent prospective, comparative, protocol-controlled study reported by Morris et al. (1994) of conventional ventilation versus ECGE in severe ARDS showed similarly equivocal results, although survival in both arms of the study had improved to 35–40 per cent. This led these investigators to recommend that ECGE did not offer an advantage in the management of ARDS. The results of this study have not been universally accepted, and enthusiasts for ECGE have levelled criticism on several grounds – particularly the nature of ECGE technology used, the high incidence of severe haemorrhage (shown to be associated with an increased mortality in ECGE patients) and perceived delays in surgical intervention.

Proponents of ECGE suggest that percutaneous vascular cannulation, heparin-bonded oxygenators and circuitry, improved anticoagulation protocols and aggressive surgical intervention will lead to further improved outcome in ECGE. A report by Lewandowski in 1997 of 75 per cent survival in 122 severe ARDS patients managed with a criteria-defined clinical algorithm has further fuelled this debate. Survival in patients requiring ECGE on gas exchange criteria was 55 per cent, while 89 per cent of those who responded to so-called advanced therapy, and therefore did not require ECGE, survived. These results are impressive, but the data lacks the credibility of a comparative investigation in which the mortality of a patient group of matched illness severity to the ECGE patients, but who only received advanced conventional therapy, could also be defined.

The use of ECGE in thoracic surgical patients is an even more clouded issue. While it is possible to investigate outcome in a reasonably homogeneous group, such as patients with pneumonia or ARDS, no such easy option exists in thoracic surgical patients, who may require novel support for a variety of reasons. The potential requirement for ECGE in such patients is thankfully rare, but the need for ECGE as a life-saving manoeuvre, albeit possibly temporary, may be extremely acute. A recent review from a leading US ECGE centre of 100 patients requiring ECGE between 1990 and 1996 revealed 98 per cent of cases to be of a medical nature (53 per cent survival). The indications for ECGE were of a surgical nature in only two patients, reflecting the rarity of this indication. Both patients suffered tracheal obstruction and were successfully supported and weaned from ECGE (Kolla et al. 1997).

The occasional need for ECGE to facilitate the intra-operative surgical management of obstructive mediastinal tumours is well recognized, but it may be required for similar reasons in an emergency non-operative situation. Figure 18.5 shows chest radiographs of a patient presenting with a rapidly progressive mediastinal lymphoma, proven on mediastinal biopsy. Investigations showed that the mass compressed the lower trachea and left main bronchus and the right pulmonary artery much more than the left, resulting in a unique and potentially life-threatening ventilation–perfusion mismatch. Emergency ECGE was instigated with worsening compression and was maintained for 72 hours, during which time the combination of chemotherapy and corticosteroids resulted in tumour shrinkage, allowing weaning from ECGE. Similar anecdotal reports of the use of ECGE exist for a variety of conditions, including traumatic tracheobronchial disruption. The management of such cases is always difficult, and ECGE should always be considered if there is a treatable condition, a prospect of a favourable outcome within a realistic time frame and a lack of co-morbid disease likely to impact on the logistics of ECGE conduct or on outcome.

A relatively new indication for ECGE after thoracic surgery is the support of organ function following pulmonary transplantation. ECGE has been recently reported for successful immediate support of dysfunctional pulmonary grafts following bilateral single lung transplantation. A review by Macha et al. (1996) of 33 ECGE patients included 16 with primary graft failure within 7 days after pulmonary transplantation. In this group, 75 per cent were weaned from ECMO and 56 per cent survived to discharge.

(a)

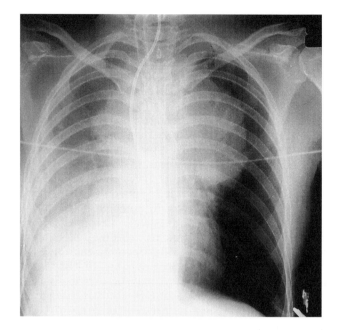

(b)

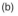
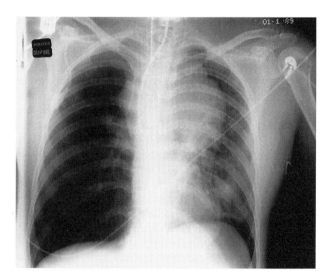

Figure 18.5

(a) Chest X-ray shows a large tumour compressing the lower
    trachea, left main bronchus and the right pulmonary artery
    more than the left. Positioning of left-sided double-lumen
    tube was extremely difficult. Collapse of the right lung was of
    little consequence as there was minimal blood flow to the
    right side. Soon after this X-ray was taken, gas exchange
    became unsupportable by conventional methods.

(b) Chest X-ray shows resolution after extracorporeal gas
    exchange, corticosteroids and chemotherapy.

The use of ECGE for late graft failure is much more questionable – in this paper, six such patients were treated with ECGE and none survived.

It is impossible to be dogmatic about the indications for ECGE in thoracic surgical patients. Potential indications are diverse, and the data to allow an objective assessment of the role of ECGE in these patients are lacking. Fortunately, most major thoracic surgical units are linked to cardiac centres so that the technology for ECGE should be readily available. A difficult question surrounds the issue of experience, technical expertise and the support infrastructure required to run a successful ECGE program. The implication from available ECGE data in medical patients is not surprising in that outcome is undoubtedly better in those units with an established programme and a reasonable volume throughput. This should not deter a surgical unit with available technology from instituting ECGE in an appropriate emergency situation. Indeed, transport ECGE systems are available in the USA that can be used to transport the patient to a referral centre after the situation is stabilized. A more difficult decision arises in a slightly less acute situation, when the benefits of transferring a patient to a unit with proven expertise are weighed against the potential risks in transfer of a patient in a precarious state.

Intravascular gas exchange (IVGE)

In 1990, the intravascular oxygenator (IVOX) commenced clinical trials in acute respiratory failure. The device is a miniaturized, hollow-fibre oxygenator, which is implanted via surgical venotomy and lies within the superior and inferior vena cavae (Fig. 18.6). Oxygen is drawn through the lumen of the device under vacuum, and oxygen and CO_2 exchange occurs across its non-thrombogenic, gas permeable outer membrane. The IVOX proved much less labour intensive than ECGE, and was attractive in its simplicity, low complication rate, limited anticoagulation requirement and potential for long-term implantation. From 1990–1993, 160 patients underwent implantation, the majority with pneumonia or ARDS (Conrad et al. 1994).

Despite the favourable safety profile of IVOX compared to ECGE, its gas exchange performance proved disappointing. Pre-pulmonary transfer of low volumes of oxygen invokes complex pulmonary physiology, but essentially the small increase in pre-pulmonary oxygen saturation that is generated by IVOX is overwhelmed by the deleterious effects on oxygenation of intra-pulmonary shunt. In addition, there is an inherent inefficiency in the net effect on systemic oxygenation of oxygen uptake into that volume of venous blood that subsequently perfuses effectively ventilated alveoli (this blood will be fully saturated in the left atrium regardless of any pre-pulmonary IVOX-related increase in oxygen content). Calculated oxygen uptake values were disappointing, ranging from 0–80 ml/min.

Carbon dioxide clearance exhibits no such inherent inefficiency. Clearance is a net effect, and typical values ranged from 40–80 ml/min of CO_2. The application of permissive hypercapnia increases the efficiency of CO_2 clearance, and favourable effects were seen in patients with CO_2 clearance difficulties, especially in severe asthma.

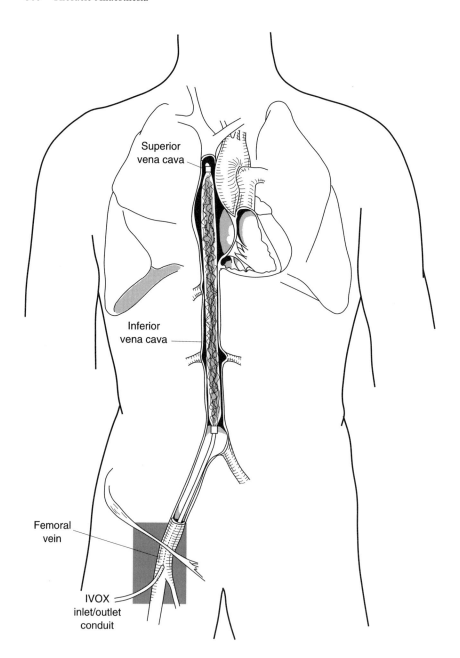

Figure 18.6 Schematic representation of IVOX in position. The device lies in both vena cavae and fibres pass into the right atrium, enhancing blood–device contact. (Reproduced with permission from J. D. Mortensen, Cardiopulmonics, Salt Lake City, USA.)

The fate of this pioneering technology was determined by its disappointing gas exchange potential, contributing at best 25 per cent of gas transfer requirements, and unfavourable survival statistics (43 per cent of patients survived to IVOX explantation, but only 25 per cent to hospital discharge). The IVOX was withdrawn from clinical practice in 1994. In retrospect, the CO_2 clearance potential of IVOX was essentially overlooked in the clinical study. The potential to modify ventilatory intensity, limit volutrauma, decrease minute ventilation requirements and enhance the progress from mandatory ventilation through the weaning process was never explored due to the nature of patient selection and specific orientation towards oxygenation.

Several of the IVOX recipients had undergone thoracic surgery. In the authors' series, two patients underwent lung biopsy prior to the institution of IVOX and the device allowed employment of an enhanced lung-protective ventilatory strategy. In one patient, with cryptogenic organizing pneumonitis, this ventilatory modification provided a major favourable contribution to clinical progress.

Evolving IVOX related technologies

The failure of IVOX has removed an attractive, medium intensity therapeutic option in the management of thoracic surgical and other patients with severe ventilation–perfusion mismatch. The IVOX-induced reduction in ventilatory requirements could be particularly beneficial in thoracic patients with limited pulmonary reserve or reduced ventilatory capacity related to disease of the chest wall or other mechanical components. Research in this area is ongoing and several prototypes have been produced, which are in various stages of non-clinical assessment.

The intravenous membrane oxygenator (IMO)

This device is the most developed IVOX successor, and has progressed through more than 15 prototypes. The IMO is similar to IVOX, is placed in the same intravenous position, and has various design modifications to improve gas mixing and exchange performance. A pulsatile balloon, similar to an aortic counterpulsation device, is incorporated to enhance mixing. *In vivo* gas exchange results are more than twice those of IVOX (oxygen 125–150 ml/min/m², CO_2 150–200 ml/min/m²) and, if reproduced in humans, these values represent more than 50 per cent of basal requirements.

Other design devices

Several other options remain under investigation. The intravenous pumping oxygenator (IVPO) is similarly placed, but has much larger, rhythmically inflating fibres, which enhance gas flux. The pumping artificial lung (PAL) is a miniature extracorporeal device with an integral pump. This may represent the first of the long proposed, compact gas exchange augmenting devices that could be readily attached to a patient in the post-operative or emergency situation and function with the simplicity of current haemofiltration systems. A more invasive option, the intrathoracic artificial lung

(ITAL), which is placed via sternotomy between the pulmonary artery and left atrium and hence may replace pulmonary function completely, has received media attention but the investigators envisage a considerable delay before clinical investigation is a reality.

Future prospects for IVGE

The lessons from IVOX suggest that, despite a favourable risk–benefit ratio and success in individual patients, IVGE devices will not make an impact on respiratory therapy unless their gas exchange potential is considerably enhanced. Several promising devices are in development, but the time of evolution from design and development to human trials is inevitably long and is influenced greatly by the intense scrutiny expected of device regulatory bodies. Success for future devices is much more likely if patient selection is tailored to device characteristics. Specifically, the CO_2 clearance potential of IVGE may prove very useful in the acute management and weaning of thoracic surgical patients with poor pulmonary mechanics and ongoing, troublesome broncho-pulmonary air leaks. IVGE devices should not be seen as alternatives to ECGE, but as providing a less labour-intensive and safer option in patients who have sufficient native pulmonary function to require only partial support.

The dilemma of post-pneumonectomy pulmonary oedema

One of the most vexing conditions encountered in thoracic surgical practice is the phenomenon described in the North American literature as post-pneumonectomy pulmonary edema (PPE). Recent reviews by Slinger (1995) and Williams (1996) have considered the aetiology of this florid condition, a form of acute lung injury, and fluid balance issues, along with the impact of one-lung anaesthesia, have been extensively considered. It is also clear that the same pathophysiological process may be seen in more limited lung resections. Although there are limited data, it appears that approximately 5 per cent of lung resection patients suffer some degree of acute lung injury and that the mortality associated with the most severe form (ARDS) is high. In a series from the Royal Brompton Hospital only two of 17 patients with ARDS following thoracic surgery survived, whereas five of seven patients who developed the less severe form of acute lung injury survived (Hayes et al. 1995).

The ventilatory management for such patients is similar to patients with ARDS from other causes. Pulmonary compliance and functional lung volume are markedly reduced, so aggressive lung volume recruitment and maintenance techniques should be immediately applied. Pulmonary air leaks may complicate management, but should not distract attention from the fundamental pulmonary abnormality and the need to recruit accessible functional alveoli. Following a short stabilization period, it is the authors' practice to transfer all patients for thoracic CT imaging, both to assess disease severity and identify therapeutic directions.

The authors have employed HFJV techniques in the high-pressure mode with some success, particularly in those patients who required high (>20 cmH$_2$O) values of total PEEP. In recent years, with improved conventional technology, patients have usually been managed with variants of pressure-controlled inverse-ratio ventilation. Liberal oxygenation targets are applied, and permissive hypercapnia is almost routine in such patients. Ideally, the aim is to limit peak airway pressure to less than 30 cmH$_2$O, and mean airway pressures typically lie within the range of 20–25 cmH$_2$O. Total PEEP is often in the region of 15 cmH$_2$O and, with I:E ratios of 3:1, this comprises both external (5–10 cm) and intrinsic (4–7 cm) PEEP components. These settings are designed to be lung protective, and inspired oxygen concentration is reduced to the arbitrary figure of 60 per cent if possible. Ventilatory settings are influenced by semi-quantitative assessments of pulmonary mechanics, the validity of which may be further obscured by air leaks. Prone or lateral repositioning is usually undertaken, particularly if CT scan suggests regional differences amenable to postural therapy. Selective pulmonary vasodilators such as nitric oxide are attractive in such patients due to commonly increased pulmonary vascular resistance, and usually result in some improvement in oxygenation. As in other conditions, the influence on outcome of nitric oxide therapy remains uncertain.

The use of ECGE in this condition is a difficult dilemma. Knowledge of the pro-inflammatory effects of cardiopulmonary bypass and the incidence of acute lung injury (1–3 per cent) associated with its use in cardiac surgery suggests that ECGE may further exacerbate post-surgical lung injury. ECGE does, however, provide the opportunity for short-term stabilization of unacceptable gas exchange, during which time fluid balance and hydrostatic forces across the lung may be manipulated by haemofiltration and cardiovascular pharmacology. Figure 18.7 displays chest radiographs of a patient following resection of an extensive right Pancoast tumour requiring pneumonectomy and large volume transfusion. Florid pulmonary oedema developed within hours in the remaining lung, emergency veno-arterial ECGE was instituted and the patient was successfully weaned within 72 hours following fluid balance manipulation and lung volume recruitment.

The therapy of PPE has evolved considerably in the 1990s, along with therapy for acute lung injury associated with other conditions. The application of support principles described earlier in this chapter has resulted in improved survival in acute lung injury. Survival rates of 70 per cent or more are now being reported from specialist referral centres. It remains to be seen whether similar improvements in outcome will be seen in this particularly difficult sub-group of lung injury patients.

(a)

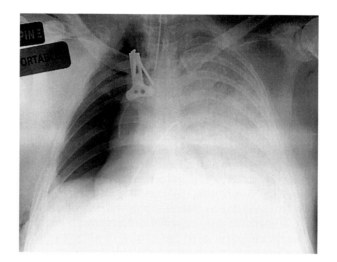

(b)

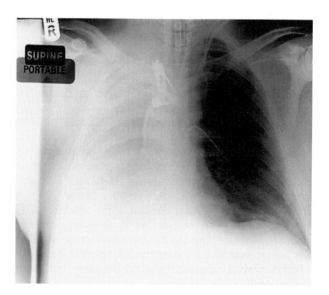

Figure 18.7

(a) Chest X-ray shows florid post-pneumonectomy pulmonary oedema requiring ECGE.

(b) Chest X-ray shows almost complete resolution of ARDS a week following surgery, and filling of the right pneumonectomy space.

KEY POINTS

- Developments in ventilatory technology have greatly improved respiratory support options in difficult thoracic surgical patients. Such patients often present with heterogenous pathology and markedly deranged ventilation–perfusion matching, and may undergo very extensive and prolonged surgical procedures.

- Ventilatory strategies must be protective to functional pulmonary structures and applied in the context of realistic and often liberal blood gas targets.

- In conventional ventilatory options, pressure-preset techniques provide intrinsic safety and greater flexibility, flow reserve and leak compensation, rendering them superior to volume-oriented ventilatory modes in these difficult patients.

- Independent lung ventilation (ILV) in unilateral disease may be life saving in massive haemoptysis and in single lung transplantation. Prolonged ILV is a difficult undertaking and, in other situations of unilateral disease, advanced conventional options may now provide an effective and simpler alternative.

- Extrapulmonary gas exchange is an option in the extreme situation. Intravascular gas exchange remains under development, and is of uncertain efficacy. Extracorporeal gas exchange is regularly reported as a life-saving option in thoracic emergencies. Although complications are high, the risk–benefit ratio may be considered favourable in a treatable condition in which the duration of artificial support is not likely to be unduly prolonged.

Bibliography

Carlon, G.C., Howland, S.W., Ray, C., Miodownik, S. and Griffin, J.P. (1983). High frequency jet ventilation. A prospective randomised evaluation. *Chest*, **84**, 551–9.

Conrad, S.A., Bagley, A., Bagley, B. and Schaap, R.N. (1994). Major findings from the clinical trials of the intravascular oxygenator. *Artif. Org.*, **18**, 846–63.

Gluck, E., Heard, S., Patel, C., Mohr, J. and Calkins, J. (1993). Use of ultrahigh frequency ventilation in patients with ARDS. A preliminary report. *Chest*, **103**, 1413–20.

Hayes, J.P., Williams, E.A., Goldstraw, P. and Evans, T.W. (1995). Lung injury in patients following thoracotomy. *Thorax*, **50**, 990–1.

Hormann, Ch., Baum, M., Putensen, Ch. *et al.* (1994). Biphasic positive airway pressure (BIPAP) – a new mode of ventilatory support. *Eur. J. Anaesthesiol.*, **11**, 37–42.

Kolla, S., Awad, S.A., Rich, P.B. *et al.* (1997). Extracorporeal life support for 100 adult patients with severe respiratory failure. *Ann. Surg.*, **226**, 544–66.

Lachmann, B. (1992). Open up the lung and keep the lung open. *Intens. Care Med.*, **18**, 319–21.

Lewandowski, K., Rossaint, R., Pappert, D. *et al.* (1997). High survival rate in 122 ARDS patients managed according to a clinical algorithm including extracorporeal membrane oxygenation. *Intens. Care Med.*, **23**, 819–35.

Macha, M., Griffith, B.P., Keenan, R. *et al.* (1996). ECMO support for adult patients with acute respiratory failure. *ASAIO J.*, **42**, M841–4.

Morris, A.H., Wallace, C.J., Menlove, R.L. *et al.* (1994). Randomized clinical trial of pressure-controlled inverse-ratio ventilation and extracorporeal CO_2 removal for adult respiratory distress syndrome. *Am. J. Resp. Crit. Care Med.*, **149**, 295–305.

Slinger, P.D. (1995). Peri-operative fluid management for thoracic surgery. The puzzle of post-pneumonectomy pulmonary edema. *J Cardiothorac. Vasc. Anesth.*, **9**, 442–51.

Slutsky, A.S. (1993). Mechanical ventilation. ACCP Consensus Conference. *Chest*, **104,** 1833–59.

Smith, D.W., Frankel, L.R., Derish, M.T. *et al.* (1993). High frequency jet ventilation in children with the adult respiratory distress syndrome complicated by pulmonary barotrauma. *Paediatr. Pulmonol.*, **15,** 279–86.

Williams, E.A., Evans, T.W. and Goldstraw, P. (1996). Acute lung injury following lung resection: is one-lung anaesthesia to blame? *Thorax*, **51,** 114–16.

Zapol, W.M., Snider, M.T., Hill, J.D. *et al.* (1979). Extracorporeal membrane oxygenation in severe acute respiratory failure. A randomised prospective study. *JAMA*, **242,** 2193–6.

19

Controversies in thoracic anaesthesia

J. Gothard and H. Porter

Introduction

In a comprehensive text of this nature, there is bound to be some overlap of chapter contents. This is particularly likely in a chapter where controversies and conflicting areas of opinion are to be discussed. Of necessity, the authors assume the reader will have gained background knowledge in the specific areas concerned from the expert descriptions in previous chapters. Where appropriate some of this information will be briefly repeated, but the main intention is to discuss controversial aspects of anaesthetic management for thoracic surgery.

The authors' views are bound to be somewhat personal and therefore biased to a degree, but these views are balanced by other opinions within this comprehensive book. It is not their intention, however, to act as devil's advocate; as clinicians, they firmly believe patient safety is of paramount importance, particularly in the modern world, where medical staff are expected to deal with a high through-put of surgery in ever shortening periods of time.

Bronchial blocker versus double-lumen endobronchial tube

Children and small adults are too small to accept standard sizes of double-lumen tubes. The smallest double-lumen endobronchial tube currently manufactured is a 28 Fr left-sided Bronchocath (Mallinckrodt). This is too big for most patients under approximately 30–35 kg, and has impractically small ventilation lumina. Bronchial blockade is therefore a practical way of achieving one-lung ventilation in children. In this unit, a Fogarty embolectomy catheter is currently used as a bronchial blocker in this age group. This is placed through the anaesthetized child's nose, and advanced into the larynx and upper trachea under direct vision using a standard laryngoscope and Magill's forceps. Once the blocker is within the trachea, it is advanced into the appropriate bronchus with the aid of a rigid paediatric bronchoscope. Following inflation of the Fogarty balloon, the rigid bronchoscope is withdrawn and a small endotracheal tube is then inserted orally alongside the stem of the catheter. Conventional positive pressure ventilation can then be instituted.

A blocker of this type can be used to facilitate one-lung anaesthesia if it is inserted into the main bronchus of either lung. It can also be placed in such a way to block specific lobes if, for example, there is the possibility that infected material will spread from lobe to lobe in the presence of bronchiectasis.

In adult practice, it is conventional to separate the two lungs by using a double-lumen endobronchial tube. Lobar blockade is not possible with a conventional double-lumen tube, and this remains the main advantage of a bronchial blocker in both adults and children. Bronchial blocking techniques had, however, fallen out of favour in adult practice until the early 1980s. The introduction of a disposable endotracheal tube combined with a moveable bronchial blocker (Univent tube) by Inoue and co-workers in 1982 changed this situation.

Univent tube (bronchial blockade) compared with double-lumen endobronchial intubation

The Univent tube is made in a variety of sizes for use in adults. It comprises a tracheal tube with a channel through the anterior internal wall, which holds a moveable blocker with a low-pressure, high-volume cuff or balloon. The tube is placed in the trachea in the usual way, and the blocker advanced, preferably under fibre-optic bronchoscopic control, to occlude the appropriate main or lobar bronchus. In the absence of commercial alternatives, the Univent tube is now the standard type of bronchial blocker used in adult practice. As previously stated, a blocker allows specific lobes to be isolated. In bronchiectasis, the remaining lobe or lobes on the operative side are unprotected from the spread of secretions if a double-lumen tube is used. In addition, infected secretions can seep past the endobronchial cuff into the opposite, dependent lung. Repeated suction to both lungs limits this contamination, although with good pre-operative preparation this may not be a great problem.

The main drawback of blocking techniques is that, if they fail (e.g. by dislodgement), all protection from the spread of secretions is lost. Should ventilation suddenly become a problem during surgery when a blocker is in use, it is probable that the blocker has moved from its original position. Deflation of the balloon should rapidly restore adequate ventilation if this is the case. One other real advantage of the Univent tube over double-lumen tubes is its ease of use for a difficult laryngeal intubation. If intubation is particularly difficult, the Univent tube is likely to be easier to pass through the larynx in comparison with a bulky double-lumen tube, particularly if it is necessary to use a bougie or fibre-optic bronchoscope.

The main disadvantage of a Univent tube is that it is less versatile than a double-lumen tube, particularly if a lung resection such as pneumonectomy or right upper lobectomy is planned, or a sleeve resection is to be undertaken. In these circumstances, it is preferable to place a double-lumen tube in the lung contralateral to the surgery in order to give the surgeon a clear field. If a Univent tube is employed for these procedures, the blocker is initially placed in the surgical lung to facilitate one-lung anaesthesia.

It is therefore necessary to deflate and withdraw the blocker into the trachea to allow the surgeon to fashion bronchial anastomoses. This is likely to hinder surgical access at a crucial stage of the operation.

Summary

The advantages and disadvantages of the Univent tube (compared with double-lumen tubes) are summarized below. The real advantages of the Univent tube apply to the very few situations when lobar blockade is required or when a patient is difficult to intubate. It is difficult to see, therefore, the Univent tube being used in preference to a double-lumen tube for the majority of thoracic operations. Indeed, it has not achieved a great deal of popularity in the UK since its original description. Finally, the Univent tube is currently approximately three times the cost of a disposable double-lumen tube. Presumably the cost would decrease if more were used, but this appears unlikely at present.

KEY POINTS
Advantages of the Univent tube

- Lobar blockade is possible.

- It is easy to use for difficult laryngeal intubation.

- Tube change at the end of surgery if post-operative ventilation is required is eliminated.

Disadvantages of the Univent tube

- It is less versatile than the double-lumen tube (e.g. the problems of pneumonectomy, lobectomy and sleeve resection, where the blocker will need to be withdrawn from the operative site).

- Inflation/deflation of the operative lung is more difficult (due to the small lumen of the suction port to the blocker).

- The blocker can migrate.

- It is more expensive than the double-lumen tube.

Routine use of fibre-optic bronchoscopy to check positioning of double-lumen tubes

Smith *et al.* (1986) were the first authors to highlight that checking the position of left-sided double-lumen tubes clinically was inaccurate. In a subsequent study, McKenna *et al.* (1988) reported that, with right-sided double-lumen tubes, the ventilation slots of 10 per cent of Robertshaw tubes and 90 per cent of Bronchocath tubes were not opposed to the right upper lobe orifice when checked by fibre-optic bronchoscopy (FOB). This was despite the fact that they were thought to be in the correct place on the basis of the usual clinical criteria. There is no doubt that the use of the fibre-optic bronchoscope has revolutionized the management of endobronchial intubation. The slim fibre-optic bronchoscopes/laryngoscopes developed for anaesthesia (e.g. Olympus LF-2) are robust and relatively inexpensive. The LF-2 has a tip of 3.8 mm, and can be passed down the lumen of endobronchial tubes as small as the 35 Fr Bronchocath, provided the internal plastic moulding is smooth. It will not, however, pass down a small Robertshaw tube. Newer anaesthetic paediatric fibrescopes are now being introduced, however, and these can be inserted down the smaller double-lumen tubes.

The fibre-optic bronchoscope can be used to place the endobronchial tube under direct vision from the outset in patients who are difficult to intubate, or if the tube cannot be positioned blindly in the appropriate bronchus. In the latter situation, it is a relatively simple task to insert a double-lumen tube into the trachea, locate the appropriate main bronchus with a fibre-optic bronchoscope passed down the tube, and then 'rail-road' or slide the tube into position over the bronchoscope.

In the majority of cases, the fibre-optic bronchoscope will be used to check the position of tubes following blind placement. This check will need to be repeated after positioning of the patient, as double-lumen tubes can easily be displaced when the patient is turned from the supine to the lateral position.

Whether the fibre-optic bronchoscope should be used routinely in every case is still a point for discussion. There is everything to be gained and little to be lost if it is used each time a double-lumen tube is placed. If the tube position is satisfactory, this is reassuring. If the position has to be readjusted, fibre-optic bronchoscopy will optimize ventilatory management and also provide useful information if the tube migrates intra-operatively. The constraints of time taken to undertake the procedure and sterilize the instrument between cases are the only minor drawbacks to this approach.

Analysis of flow–volume and pressure–volume loops during two-lung and then one-lung ventilation has been described as an alternative or complementary approach to the diagnosis of tube malposition during thoracotomy. This analysis is, perhaps, a more sophisticated and objective version of the anaesthetist's 'feel' of the reservoir bag during manual ventilation. This and changes in, or loss of, the end-tidal carbon dioxide trace can also warn of tube malposition. Fibre-optic bronchoscopy remains superior to these other methods in detecting tube malposition, but its use intra-operatively can be difficult. This may further interfere with ventilation, and will certainly distract the singe-handed anaesthetist from the important task of monitoring the patient. The authors initially try to manage a displaced double-lumen tube on clinical grounds, taking into account the information gleaned at the initial fibre-optic bronchoscopy. The surgeon can also palpate the position of a double-lumen tube once the bronchi have been dissected out, and this will provide further information. If these methods fail and it is essential to provide one-lung anaesthesia, they then resort to the use of the fibre-optic bronchoscope, taking care that the patient is adequately monitored and that oxygenation is not further impaired.

Summary

In ideal circumstances, a fibre-optic bronchoscope should be used to check the position of endobronchial tubes before and after positioning of the patient. Whether the routine use of the fibre-optic bronchoscope in these circumstances improves patient outcome, however, remains unknown.

There is a greater margin of safety in placing left-sided double-lumen tubes because of the increased length of the left main bronchus compared with the right. It is probably acceptable, therefore, to rely on clinical checking procedures after the placement of left-sided double-lumen tubes in tall patients. It is not uncommon, however, for a left-sided double-lumen tube to block off the left upper lobe orifice in short patients; hence the findings of Smith et al. (1986).

The fibre-optic bronchoscope is an invaluable aid in siting the double-lumen tube if there is distorted bronchial anatomy or if the tube cannot be placed blindly, even in the presence of normal anatomy. Finally, it may also be of use on the very rare occasion when a bronchopleural fistula occurs after lung resection (particularly pneumonectomy) and it is essential to place the double-lumen tube accurately at the first attempt.

KEY POINTS

- If the clinical assessment of a double-lumen tube position is inaccurate, fibre-optic bronchoscopy is the most effective way of checking its position.

- Other methods of checking tube position (e.g. spirometry or end-tidal carbon dioxide analysis) are less accurate than the use of fibre-optic bronchoscopy.

- Fibre-optic bronchoscopy enables certain placement of a double-lumen tube when blind methods fail.

- The only minor (and relative) drawback to the use of the fibre-optic bronchoscope is the increase in anaesthetic time.

- Intra-operative use of the fibre-optic bronchoscope is more difficult. It distracts the anaesthetist's attention and may exacerbate ventilation problems.

Total intravenous anaesthesia (TIVA) versus inhalational agents in terms of effect on hypoxic pulmonary vasoconstriction

Paralysis and intermittent positive pressure ventilation (IPPV) are used during thoracotomy to overcome the problems of the open pneumothorax created by surgery. The compliance of the non-dependent lung remains higher than that of the lower lung during IPPV, so that preferential ventilation continues to the upper lung and may be further accentuated when the chest is opened.

One-lung ventilation is employed at various times during lung resection, primarily to improve surgical access to the upper non-ventilated lung. This eliminates preferential ventilation, but creates a far more serious problem of ventilation–perfusion mismatch.

Physiology of one-lung anaesthesia – brief resumé

Venous admixture

Pulmonary blood flow continues to the upper lung during one-lung anaesthesia, creating a true shunt in a lung where there is blood flow to the alveoli but no ventilation. This shunt is the major cause of hypoxaemia during one-lung ventilation, although the alveoli with low ventilation–perfusion ratios in the dependent lung contribute to some extent. The blood to the upper lung cannot take up oxygen, and therefore retains its poorly oxygenated mixed venous composition. This mixes with oxygenated blood in the left atrium, causing venous admixture and lowering arterial oxygen tension (Pao_2). Total venous admixture can be calculated from the shunt equation (Nunn, 1993), which estimates what proportion of the pulmonary blood flow would have bypassed ventilated alveoli to produce the arterial blood gas values for a particular patient. In published work on one-lung anaesthesia, the terms venous admixture and shunt (Qs/Qt) are used synonymously.

Venous admixture increases from a baseline value of approximately 10–15 per cent during two-lung ventilation to a level of 30–40 per cent during one-lung ventilation. The Pao_2 can be maintained in the safe range of 9–16 kPa with an inspired oxygen concentration between 50 and 100 per cent in the majority of patients. In individual patients, however, the Pao_2 may fall considerably lower than this, despite a high inspired oxygen concentration. This variation is hardly surprising considering the number of inter-related physiological factors that come into play.

The role of hypoxic pulmonary vasoconstriction

Hypoxic pulmonary vasoconstriction (HPV) is a homeostatic mechanism whereby pulmonary blood flow is diverted away from hypoxic areas of lung, thereby optimizing oxygenation of the arterial blood (Eisenkraft, 1994). The major stimulus for HPV is hypoxia, both in the alveoli (low Pao_2) and blood perfusing the lungs (low mixed venous oxygen). The precise mechanism of HPV remains unknown, but it appears to be produced by each smooth muscle cell in the wall of the pulmonary artery responding to oxygen tension in its vicinity. The smooth muscle in the wall of the arteries depolarizes and develops spontaneous electrical activity in response to hypoxia. Nitric oxide production may be inhibited by hypoxia, so this could also be implicated in the mechanism of HPV.

HPV is not related to innervation of the lung, as it occurs after lung transplantation. It is inhibited in a variety of pulmonary pathologies, including adult respiratory distress syndrome (ARDS) and pneumonia.

Many other factors inhibit HPV. These include pulmonary vasodilator drugs, high pulmonary vascular pressure, alkalosis, acidosis, hypothermia, positive end expiratory pressure (PEEP), volatile anaesthetic agents and handling of the lung.

HPV – volatile agents versus TIVA

In vitro experiments have clearly shown that volatile anaesthetic agents inhibit HPV, but in *in vivo* studies it has been difficult to demonstrate inhibition. This is because, although volatile agents do depress HPV directly, they also enhance HPV indirectly by reducing cardiac output (as cardiac output drops there is an enhancement of the HPV response). There is, therefore, an apparent unchanged HPV response in the presence of volatile anaesthetic agents during one-lung anaesthesia.

Intravenous anaesthetic agents do not inhibit HPV, but the majority of studies have failed to demonstrate a significant benefit, in terms of arterial Pao_2 when they are used to provide anaesthesia during one-lung ventilation.

A study by Kellow et al. (1995) demonstrated that propofol did not inhibit HPV during one-lung anaesthesia. These authors concluded that propofol could be considered as an alternative to volatile agents for use during thoracotomy but they pointed out that, in their study, propofol depressed right ventricular function to a greater degree than isoflurane. Reid et al. (1996) compared the effects of propofol–alfentanil versus isoflurane anaesthesia on arterial oxygenation during one-lung ventilation. Their study does not support the theory that total intravenous anaesthesia decreases the risk of hypoxaemia during one-lung ventilation.

Summary

HPV seems, on current evidence, to play little role in reducing hypoxaemia during the time it takes to complete the average lung resection. It must also be remembered, when reading the literature, that handling of the lung reduces HPV, and this may have a very significant effect in clinical practice. Potent inhaled anaesthetic agents such as isoflurane are not contraindicated during one-lung ventilation, and may even be desirable because of their bronchodilator properties and ease of use. Significant inhibition of HPV is more likely with halothane and therefore this drug, although now rarely used in adult practice, should be avoided altogether during lung resection.

Finally, despite the comments above there may be some cases where, if Pao_2 is very low during one-lung ventilation, it is worth changing from an inhalational anaesthetic to an intravenous technique. In practice, this probably means substituting an isoflurane based anaesthetic with a total intravenous anaesthesia (TIVA) technique using propofol, and monitoring its effect on arterial oxygenation.

KEY POINTS

- Inhalational agents depress HPV directly.
- Inhalational agents also enhance HPV because of a reduction in cardiac output.
- As a result of the above, there is an unchanged response in HPV when inhalational agents are used during one-lung ventilation.
- The present consensus concerning inhalational agents for one-lung anaesthesia is that they are not contraindicated and may be beneficial in some patients because of their ease of administration, bronchodilatation effect and rapid elimination.
- Some patients (e.g. those with generalized lung disease) may benefit from a change to intravenous agents. A clearcut advantage with propofol has, however, not yet been demonstrated.

High frequency jet ventilation (HFJV) versus one-lung ventilation

High frequency jet ventilation (HFJV) was originally developed, mainly in Scandinavia, for ventilation during tracheal surgery. It has also been used with some success during thoracotomy via either an endobronchial double-lumen tube or an endotracheal tube. El-Baz *et al.* (1982), using a single-lumen endobronchial tube, demonstrated a reduction in shunt fraction and an improvement in arterial oxygen concentration when HFJV was employed during one-lung ventilation. This improvement, compared with conventional positive pressure one-lung ventilation, was particularly marked when the bronchial cuff was released, thereby creating a CPAP in the surgical non-dependent lung.

Despite studies showing that HFJV is satisfactory during thoracotomy, it has not been widely accepted and is currently used by individual enthusiasts. Jenkins *et al.* (1987) reported that, although surgical conditions and gas exchange were satisfactory during HFJV, it was difficult to assess adequacy of ventilation. Howland and co-workers (1987) found that surgical access was hindered by over-distension of the upper lung during HFJV. Neither group recommended the technique for routine clinical practice.

The role of HFJV in more specialized circumstances

HFJV has been advocated for the management of patients with a bronchopleural fistula, and for use during a number of operative procedures including bilateral bullectomy, sleeve resection of the right upper lobe, and airway surgery.

A number of authors have reported favourably on the use of HFJV in patients with a bronchopleural fistula. Roth *et al.* (1988), however, found that, despite a reduced peak airway pressure, the air leak through a bronchopleural fistula can increase with HFJV, particularly if chest drain suction is employed. Animal experiments carried out to quantitate the effect of HFJV on the air leak through a bronchopleural fistula have also produced conflicting results.

High frequency jet ventilation has been advocated for the intra-operative management of bullectomy and excision of lung cysts. Obligatory end-expiratory pressure is produced by many jet ventilation systems, however, so pneumothorax remains a complication of their use. A more conventional approach is to separate the two lungs with a double-lumen tube and ventilate the lung contralateral to surgery, omitting nitrous oxide and using low inflation pressures. Conacher (1997) has, more recently, issued a note of caution concerning the use of HFJV during lung volume reduction surgery (LVRS) because of the likelihood that 'high, occult PEEP is generated'.

HFJV, via relatively fine catheters, can be used to provide gas exchange during airway surgery such as carinal resection or tracheal resection. Soiling of the lungs is a potential problem with this mode of ventilation, however, and many experienced anaesthetists prefer to use small cuffed endotracheal tubes in the distal airway to prevent the spread of secretions. Finally, if a catheter is passed distal to an obstruction when this mode of ventilation is commenced, it is vitally important to ensure that provision is made to allow egress of gas from the lungs.

Summary

Despite the potential benefits, HFJV has not become the norm during thoracic surgery. The mechanical simplicity of endobronchial tubes combined with the use of sophisticated intensive care type of ventilators within the operating theatre provides satisfactory, safe ventilation, even for the grossly abnormal lungs of patients undergoing LVRS or lung transplantation. There has been no compelling reason to embrace the technology of HFJV for intra-operative use, although individual clinicians have done so successfully. HFJV remains a useful option for post-operative ventilation in patients who develop acute respiratory distress syndrome (ARDS), and in certain specialized circumstances discussed above.

KEY POINTS
Disadvantages of high frequency jet ventilation

- There is obligatory PEEP with most systems.

- Anaesthetic gas delivery is difficult, although this is easily overcome with use of TIVA.

- It is noisy.

- There is the potential for lung distension.

Advantages of high frequency jet ventilation

- Peak airway pressures are low.

- It can be delivered via an endotracheal tube for thoracotomy.

- It may be useful for airway surgery, lung cysts and bronchopleural fistula.

Use of pulmonary vasodilators to improve oxygenation during one-lung ventilation

Ventilation is the main parameter to which changes are made in order to reduce hypoxia during one-lung ventilation. Increasing interest is being shown in the pharmacological manipulation of pulmonary blood flow during one-lung ventilation, but this is at an early stage of investigation. As with the use of pulmonary vasodilators in other spheres of medicine, a major problem is to create a selective effect with a pulmonary vasodilator drug. In the case of one-lung ventilation, this needs to be in the dependent ventilated lung, not in the non-ventilated lung and preferably not in the systemic circulation.

The pulmonary vasodilator prostaglandin E_1 has been selectively infused into the pulmonary artery of the ventilated lung in adult patients undergoing one-lung ventilation (Chen *et al.* 1996). This has been found to reduce venous admixture/shunt fraction (Qs/Qt), improve arterial oxygenation and lower pulmonary vascular resistance.

Selective infusion into one single pulmonary artery is relatively difficult to achieve, and other workers have studied the effects of inhaled nitric oxide (NO) into the dependent, ventilated lung during one-lung ventilation for thoracic surgery. One of the first studies of this type (Wilson *et al.*, 1997) failed to show any benefit from this technique in adult patients. A previous study by Rich *et al.* (1994) carried out in cardiac surgical patients did, however, show that inhaled nitric oxide selectively decreases pulmonary vascular resistance in patients with pre-existing pulmonary hypertension undergoing one-lung ventilation. This effect did not impair or enhance oxygenation in the pulmonary hypertensive patients, nor did it improve oxygenation in patients with a normal pulmonary vascular resistance who were studied.

A further study by Moutafis *et al.* (1997) has taken matters a step further by investigating the effects of inhaled nitric oxide and its combination with intravenous almitrine on oxygenation during one-lung ventilation. Almitrine, a peripheral chemoreceptor agonist, appears to enhance hypoxic vasoconstriction in isolated lungs and has been used, somewhat controversially, to improve oxygenation in ventilated patients with ARDS. In the study by Moutafis and co-workers, inhaled nitric oxide did not improve arterial oxygenation during one-lung ventilation when used alone. The introduction of intravenous almitrine, however, in combination with inhaled nitric oxide during one-lung ventilation, did ameliorate the fall in arterial oxygenation.

The NO synthase inhibitor nitro-L-arginine methyl ester (L-NAME) has also been used (Freden *et al.* 1996) intravenously and in nebulized form in animal experiments to block the production of NO and decrease blood flow to hypoxic areas of lung. This approach could potentially be used to reduce blood flow to the non-ventilated lung during one-lung anaesthesia. This form of treatment is, however, at a very early stage of investigation.

Summary

It is an attractive concept to use pulmonary vasodilators and related drugs in order to improve oxygenation during one-lung ventilation. Intravenous drugs have systemic effects, and it is relatively difficult to selectively infuse drugs into a single main pulmonary artery. The use of inhaled NO during one-lung ventilation provides an attractive method of improving blood flow to the ventilated lung without the above problems. Initial studies of the use of inhaled NO during one-lung ventilation in humans, however, have not demonstrated an improvement in oxygenation. The combination of inhaled NO with intravenous drugs such as almitrine may prove to be beneficial in the future, but all of these studies are at a very early stage. In conclusion, it is too early to draw definite opinions from these early studies, and there are no firm indicators that pulmonary vasodilators should be used on a routine basis during one-lung ventilation at the present time. This situation could change rapidly.

KEY POINTS

- Pulmonary vasodilators need to be delivered selectively to the ventilated lung.
- Infusion of drugs into the pulmonary artery is impractical for routine use.
- Inhaled nitric oxide has not been proven to improve oxygenation during one-lung ventilation.
- Combination of inhaled nitric oxide and intravenous almitrine may be useful.
- Clinical research into the use of pulmonary vasodilators during thoracotomy is at a very early stage.
- The use of drugs to enhance HPV in the non-ventilated lung is a possible alternative approach.

Should patients be nursed in an intensive care unit following routine thoracic surgery?

In the immediate post-operative period, the main concerns following lung resection are to establish a satisfactory respiratory pattern, haemodynamic stability and good analgesia. This is best accomplished in a high dependency unit (HDU) or recovery unit with full monitoring and ventilation facilities and, most importantly, trained nursing staff. This does not mean that all patients require intensive care following thoracic surgery, as the majority of patients nursed in an operating theatre recovery unit will be fit to return to a ward high dependency unit by the evening of surgery.

The majority of patients will be extubated in the operating theatre once spontaneous respiration has been established. Certain patients will, however, require a period of mechanical ventilation.

Some patients may require a short period of mechanical ventilation whilst the effects of anaesthetic agents and opioids (intravenous or epidural) are allowed to 'wear off', rather than be abruptly antagonized with naloxone. In this group of patients, ventilation via the double-lumen tube, with the bronchial cuff deflated and/or the tube partially withdrawn into the trachea, is a suitable option.

A further subset of patients, particularly frail elderly patients with poor lung function who have undergone extensive surgery, benefit from elective post-operative ventilation. In this latter group, the double-lumen tube should be changed to an endotracheal tube at the end of surgery and the patient transferred to the intensive care unit for a period of post-operative ventilation (often overnight). This period of ventilation allows re-warming, correction of fluid and acid–base balance, optimum recovery from intra-operative atelectasis, and the establishment of adequate analgesia to be carried out in a controlled environment. Intermittent positive pressure ventilation (IPPV) is established and optimized in the usual manner. Most competent surgeons do not worry unduly about the effect of positive pressure or suction on their bronchial stump anastomoses following lung resection, but an attempt is made to keep inflation pressures within the normal range. If necessary, pressure limited ventilation can be used.

Requirement for intensive care

From the above discussion, it is evident that the majority of patients undergoing thoracotomy do not require management in an intensive care unit (ICU). They do, however, require initial management in a well-equipped and appropriately staffed recovery or high dependency area close to the operating theatre. Subsequent management should also be carried out in a high-grade HDU environment.

A number of patients will be transferred to the ICU immediately following surgery, and others will also be admitted if they fail to progress from the operating theatre HDU or if they develop major post-operative complications on the ward. The former group of patients with planned admission to the ICU will include the elderly frail patients discussed above, plus cases such as lung volume reduction surgery, lung transplantation, major chest wall surgery, thoraco-abdominal laparotomy and omental or muscle flap repairs to chronic bronchopleural fistulae. Routine lung resection for primary malignant tumour continues to have a significant morbidity and mortality, however, and a number of these patients will require ICU care. In the Society of Cardiothoracic Surgeons Annual Return for 1995–96 (UK Thoracic Register), there was an operative mortality of 2.9 per cent for lobectomy and 8.2 per cent for pneumonectomy. The mortality rates for many units will be lower than these figures, but there will nevertheless always be a significant mortality while surgical resection offers the only long-term cure for lung cancer. The major cause of death after lung resection, not surprisingly, is respiratory failure, followed closely by cardiac events such as myocardial infarction, cardiac failure and cardiac arrest. Many deaths occur in the ICU following prolonged treatment of multi-system failure.

The patients who develop respiratory and cardiac complications in the post-operative period are often elderly smokers with pre-existing lung disease, poor pulmonary function and myocardial ischaemia. Occasionally pulmonary complications occur in relatively fit patients, and this serves to highlight the multifactorial aetiology of post-operative respiratory failure. The spectrum of respiratory problems following lung resection ranges from mild sputum retention to the acute respiratory distress syndrome. These are briefly discussed below.

Sputum retention

Problems of sputum retention after thoracic surgery can be considered the norm in smokers. Smoking induces mucus gland hyperplasia and mucosal metaplasia, together with impaired cilial function. Sputum retention is, therefore, to be expected after surgical trauma to the lungs is superimposed on these physiological and functional defects.

Patients with poor lung function, and particularly those whose FEV_1 is less than 1 l post-operatively, cannot cough effectively to clear secretions. In addition, a radical lung resection may involve section of the recurrent laryngeal nerve, leaving the larynx incompetent and preventing an adequate rise in intrathoracic pressure prior to the explosive act of coughing. Similarly, phrenic nerve damage results in paradoxical diaphragmatic movement. This also reduces the force of coughing, but can be offset to some extent by plication of the diaphragm on the side of surgery. Finally, chest wall resection can cause a degree of paradoxical respiration, even after the insertion of a rigid chest wall prosthesis. Secretions are likely to accumulate, therefore, in the inadequately ventilated areas of lung underlying this area.

Physiotherapy is, in the presence of adequate analgesia, an effective method of clearing retained sputum. This is largely a mechanical problem, but retained secretions are likely to become infected and appropriate antibiotic cover is instituted on the basis of sputum cultures.

If these simple measures fail to solve the problem of sputum retention, a mini-tracheostomy tube can be inserted through the cricothyroid membrane as a direct route for bronchial suction. This procedure, carried out under local anaesthesia, is theoretically straightforward. In unskilled hands it can lead to disaster as a result of bleeding into or around the trachea, which can only further impair arterial oxygenation.

Continuing difficulties with sputum clearance, despite the above measures, usually leads to endotracheal intubation and mechanical ventilation. Formal tracheostomy may be required later to aid weaning from ventilation in this small group of patients.

Respiratory failure

There is restricted ventilation and an altered pattern of breathing following thoracotomy (Entwistle, 1991). The characteristic mechanical abnormalities result in a reduction in vital capacity, tidal volume and FEV_1, as well as the reduction in functional residual capacity associated with anaesthesia.

Pain is the principal inhibitor of chest wall movement, but obesity, the supine position and interstitial oedema of damaged tissue all have a restrictive effect on ventilation. As a result, post-operative hypoxaemia is almost inevitable following thoracotomy, and it is out of proportion to the quantity of lung removed or collapsed. Patients who are hypoxaemic pre-operatively, not surprisingly, are more likely to be so post-operatively. Measures that can be adopted to minimize hypoxaemia and pulmonary complications are listed in Table 19.1.

In addition to hypoxia, carbon dioxide retention is also a problem following thoracotomy. During the first few hours after surgery, hypercarbia is common. As satisfactory analgesia is established in the patient awakening from anaesthesia, serial blood gas analyses are undertaken to monitor oxygenation and possible carbon dioxide retention. A raised $Paco_2$ is not initially of great concern, provided that the trend of serial estimations is downwards and the patient is awake with a satisfactory respiratory pattern. In this department, the patient is not transferred to a ward high dependency area until the $Paco_2$ is approximately 7.0 kPa or less, with a downward trend in measured values. If carbon dioxide levels are towards the upper end of this limit, the arterial line remains *in situ* and arterial blood gas values continue to be monitored on the ward HDU.

Chronic obstructive pulmonary disease (COPD) is a frequent finding in patients presenting for thoracic surgery, although this is unlikely to be severe in those scheduled for lung resection (but not lung volume reduction

Table 19.1 Measures to reduce pulmonary complications and hypoxaemia post-operatively

---

- Provision of adequate analgesia with minimal respiratory depression
- Erect or semi-erect upper body position to increase FRC
- Humidified oxygen therapy to reduce tenacity of secretions
- Regular physiotherapy
- Incentive spirometry
- Continuous positive airway pressure (CPAP) intermittently by face mask

---

surgery). Carbon dioxide retention and hypoxaemia secondary to alveolar hypoventilation is nevertheless a particular risk in this group. Patients should therefore be monitored carefully whilst breathing a known, fixed, low concentration of oxygen. The bicarbonate level in a pre-operative arterial blood gas sample will provide a further guide as to what level of arterial Pa_{CO_2} can be expected in these patients.

Acute lung injury and post-pneumonectomy pulmonary oedema

From the above discussion concerning sputum retention and respiratory failure after thoracic surgery, it will be appreciated that lung surgery combines many of the elements involved in the aetiology of acute respiratory distress syndrome (ARDS).

Lung injury has been recognized as a potential complication of lung resection for many years, and has been termed post-pneumonectomy pulmonary oedema (PPE). In its extreme form, PPE represents one cause of the acute respiratory distress syndrome (ARDS), although many patients not meeting the diagnostic criteria for ARDS fulfil those for the less severe acute lung injury (ALI). Despite the terminology, PPE is not confined to pneumonectomy patients, but also occurs following lobectomy. PPE complicates 4–7 per cent of pneumonectomies and 1–7 per cent of lobectomies, with a very high associated mortality of 50–100 per cent. These statistics do not, however, take into account the incidence of ALI following lung resection. Figures for ARDS and ALI following lung resection at the Royal Brompton Hospital are summarized in Table 19.2. These figures reinforce the fact that, whilst ICU is not required for the majority of thoracic surgical patients, it is essential for some.

It is becoming increasingly evident that ischaemia–reperfusion injury mediated by reactive oxygen species is implicated in the aetiology of pulmonary injury following lung resection (Williams *et al.*, 1996).

During one-lung ventilation, relative ischaemia of the non-dependent lung being operated upon is followed by re-expansion and reperfusion of the remaining lung tissue after lobectomy, and by hyperperfusion of the ventilated lung after pneumonectomy. It is therefore likely that all patients undergoing lung resection and one-lung ventilation are subjected to conditions under which there is an increased risk of developing lung injury. Factors that determine the degree of endothelial damage in ALI and the release of vasoactive substances such as nitric oxide (NO) and their influence in modulating HPV have yet to be elucidated. Whether further work in this

Table 19.2 Lung injury following lung resection: a retrospective study. Royal Brompton Hospital 1991–1994. All cases of ALI/ARDS identified using criteria of Bernard *et al.* (1994)

	No. of cases	ARDS (n = 17)	ALI (n = 7)
Pneumonectomy	103	5 (4.8 per cent)	2 (1.9 per cent)
Lobectomy	231	12 (5.2 per cent)	5 (2.2 per cent)
Wedge resection	135	0	0
Total no. cases	469	17 (3.6 per cent)	7 (1.5 per cent)
Total no. deaths (overall)	–	15	2
Deaths (percentage of total)	–	3.4	0.5

Lung injury (ALI + ARDS) occurred in 5.1 per cent of patients; mortality for ARDS (once established) was 88 per cent; mortality for ALI was 29 per cent.
Data: Courtesy of T. Evans and E. Williams, Royal Brompton Hospital, London.

field can lead to management strategies that will decrease the incidence of ALI following lung resection is also open to question.

As stated above, reperfusion injury has been implicated in the aetiology of ARDS after lung resection, but a number of other factors are associated with this problem. Possible causes of, and contributing factors to, PPE are listed in Table 19.3. The effects of some of these factors – particularly fluid overload, hyperinflation and right ventricular failure – can be ameliorated by specific management strategies.

Fluid overload has certainly been incriminated as a cause of PPE in many studies, but by no means all. It is recommended, therefore, that fluid overload is avoided peri-operatively (Slinger, 1995) and that a total positive fluid balance should not exceed 20 ml/kg for the first 24 hours (including the operative period). Blood and fluid loss at operation is often difficult to estimate, however, and some patients may already have an element of renal dysfunction, which will deteriorate further in the face of dehydration.

Hyperinflation of the lung during one-lung ventilation has also been incriminated as a factor contributing to PPE. It may be that conventional tidal volumes of 10 ml/kg during one-lung ventilation approach the levels that can cause volutrauma. This is particularly so after right pneumonectomy, where damage to the left lung lymphatic drainage also has a role to play. Using lower tidal volumes in patients with high inflation pressure or abnormal pressure–volume loops may limit ventilatory damage intra-operatively. Care should be taken not to over-inflate the lung when testing for lung air leaks and bronchial stump competence.

Table 19.3. Factors contributing to post-pneumonectomy pulmonary oedema

- Fluid overload
- Damage to lymphatic drainage (surgical)
- Hyperinflation of lung intra-operatively ('volutrauma')
- Right ventricular dysfunction
- Reperfusion injury
- Cytokine release
- Oxygen toxicity

Right ventricular dysfunction, caused by an increased afterload as the cardiac output is channelled through a smaller pulmonary vascular bed, is common following thoracotomy. Patients following pneumonectomy have an increase in pulmonary vascular resistance of up to 30 per cent on exercise, and this is accompanied by desaturation. Post-thoracotomy patients also have an increase in right ventricular pressure in the early post-operative period, which coincides with the withdrawal of supplemental oxygen. Hypercarbia contributes to an increase in pulmonary artery pressure. In high-risk patients, oxygen therapy should be continued until satisfactory saturations are sustained continuously on room air. If overt right ventricular failure is suspected clinically, and is confirmed by central venous pressure measurements and echocardiography, then inotropic and pulmonary vasodilator therapy is indicated.

Cardiovascular complications following lung resection

Moderate hypotension, hypertension and even mild myocardial ischaemia can be treated adequately in an HDU rather than an ICU in the post-operative period. The chronic dysrhythmias that may occur in the later post-operative period can, in the majority of circumstances, also be treated and monitored on the ward HDU. Acute blood loss will almost certainly require surgical re-exploration and subsequent admission of the patient to ICU. Severe ischaemia leading to myocardial infarction and myocardial failure will, again, require admission of the patient to ICU and aggressive treatment if there is to be a reasonable chance of survival. These scenarios are briefly discussed below.

Hypotension

Hypotension is not uncommon in the early post-operative period. As the patient is fully re-warmed and analgesia is established, peripheral vasodila-tation occurs. A standard fluid regimen of, for example, dextrose/saline solution 1 ml/kg per hour (with potassium supplementation) is therefore inadequate at this stage. Transfusion of colloid is required in order to 'fill' the circulation. An artificial plasma expander (such as a starch solution) may be used if the haemoglobin level is satisfactory, and infused on the basis of the central venous pressure and clinical condition of the patient. It may be necessary to transfuse up to a litre or more of colloid, but above this level a careful reappraisal of the patient's clinical status is required to avoid over-transfusion.

If hypotension persists despite presumed adequate volume replacement, and blood loss into the drains is not excessive, hidden blood loss should be sought. Considerable amounts of blood can accumulate in a pneumo-nectomy space, for example. This may or may not be revealed if the chest drain is briefly unclamped, but a chest X-ray showing a rapidly filling space is an indication that active blood loss is continuing in those with or without a drain. Similarly, a chest X-ray may reveal sequestered clot after lobectomy.

If hypotension persists despite adequate filling, it may be necessary to initiate inotropic therapy, particularly in those patients known to have pre-existing myocardial dysfunction. A urinary catheter should also be inserted at this stage if one is not already in place. If a relatively low dose of an inotrope such as dopamine or dobutamine fails to improve blood pressure, cardiac output and urine output, then investigation and treatment of the hypotension should be escalated. Placement of a Swan–Ganz catheter will allow measurement of left-sided cardiac filling pressures and cardiac output. This, combined with echocardiographic assessment, will guide further management. In practice these latter steps are rarely indicated, but, if they are, admission of the patient to ICU is mandatory.

Hypertension and myocardial ischaemia

Thoracic surgical patients often have concomitant cardiovascular disease. Anti-anginal therapy should always be continued up to and including the day of surgery, and should be recommenced post-operatively. In the immediate post-operative period hypertension can occur, particularly if analgesia is sub-optimal and the patient is hypercarbic. Intravenous nitroglycerine is used to control hypertension below an arbitrary value of approximately 150 mmHg (depending on pre-operative blood pressure) whilst analgesia is established. Control of blood pressure with nitroglycerine reduces post-operative blood loss and lessens the risk of myocardial ischaemia due to its additional coronary vasodilator effect. Sublingual nifedipine (in the absence of a suitable intravenous calcium antagonist) is also useful in controlling hypertension.

If medical management of myocardial ischaemia proves difficult or inadequate, the patient will require admission to ICU for monitoring and further treatment. This is particularly so if myocardial failure becomes an issue or if respiratory and renal function also deteriorate (as is often the case).

Summary

The majority of patients can be adequately managed in an HDU rather than an ICU environment following routine thoracic surgery. A small subset of patients will certainly require admission to intensive care. The majority of this latter group of patients, but not all, can be identified from the extent of their surgery and their pre-operative condition. Once major complications develop following thoracic surgery, intensive therapy provided by an experienced medical and nursing team is mandatory.

KEY POINTS

- The majority of thoracic surgical patients can be managed in an HDU post-operatively.

- A minority of patients will require admission to an ICU from the outset (e.g. elderly frail patients with poor lung function, plus cases such as lung volume reduction, lung transplantation, thoraco-abdominal laparotomy, major chest wall surgery and surgery for major airway fistulae).

- Mortality remains significant after lung resection for carcinoma.

- High-risk patients in the above group, plus those that develop major complications, will also require admission to ICU.

Optimal techniques of analgesia post-thoracotomy

Pain control following thoracic surgery is discussed elsewhere in this book, and it is not the intention to repeat this material. Preferred methods of pain relief will certainly differ from unit to unit, and will depend on a number of factors. These include surgical case mix, medical and nursing expertise, seniority of medical staff, time available and level of recovery/HDU facilities. The practice of pain relief in this unit has evolved over a number of years, but is relatively simplistic, using techniques that have proven to be effective with a minimum risk to the patient. Different techniques may be equally effective and safe in the hands of others. The authors' approach to post-operative analgesia and their views on the use of epidural analgesic techniques are set out below.

Choice of analgesic technique

Patients scheduled for lung resection and oesophageal surgery are encouraged to accept epidural analgesia. High-risk patients are advised that this is the most suitable form of analgesia for them, unless there are specific contraindications. Those undergoing lesser procedures, such as video-assisted thoracoscopic surgery (VATS) and mediastinoscopy, are usually managed with intravenous opioid drugs unless their operation is likely to be particularly painful (e.g. pleurectomy). Patients who decline epidural analgesia and those in whom epidural block is contraindicated or difficult to establish are also managed with intravenous opioids. These are administered as a continuous infusion or via a patient-controlled delivery system. The group managed with intravenous opioids may also require supplementation of their analgesia with non-steroidal anti-inflammatory drugs (NSAIDs) or alpha-2 adrenoreceptor agonists. Alternatively, a local anaesthetic block or infusion technique can be used in conjunction with intravenous opioids (Table 19.4).

Epidural analgesia

Thoracic epidural analgesia with local anaesthetic agents was, at one time, considered to be the best form of analgesia following thoracotomy. A high block is required to produce satisfactory analgesia, however, and the ensuing sympathetic blockade causes a number of cardiovascular side effects. These include a decrease in cardiac output, reduction in heart rate, decreased systemic vascular resistance and a drop in mean blood pressure. These cardiovascular complications limit the usefulness of thoracic epidural analgesia with local anaesthetic agents alone, and increasing interest has therefore been shown in the use of epidural opioid drugs. Epidural opioids can be administered by the thoracic or lumbar route, and are often combined with a low concentration of a local anaesthetic agent. This improves the quality of analgesia without causing cardiovascular side effects. The main complications associated with the use of epidural opioids include respiratory depression, nausea, pruritus and urinary retention.

Table 19.4 Regional anaesthetic techniques for thoracic surgery

---

Intercostal nerve block:
- Relatively simple to perform intra-operatively. Main disadvantages are short duration of action (unless indwelling intercostal catheters are sited) and failure to ameliorate pain from the diaphragmatic pleura, mediastinal structures and areas supplied by the posterior primary rami

Cryoanalgesia intercostal block:
- Application of extreme cold (−20 to −60°C) under direct vision to the intercostal nerves. Produces disruption of impulse transmission lasting several months. Decline in popularity due to poor analgesic results and possible association with chronic post-thoracotomy pain. Late post-operative pain is not uncommon following thoracotomy, however, and this causal relationship is not definitely established

Intrapleural block:
- Local anaesthetic agent is infused between the visceral and parietal pleura via an indwelling catheter. Analgesic action is due to widespread intercostal nerve block. This does not spread to the intercostal space. Analgesia is unpredictable due to variable loss of drug into the chest drains, binding with blood in the thorax, and rapid systemic absorption

Paravertebral block:
- Percutaneously inserted catheter at one site allows considerable spread of drug between adjacent paravertebral spaces. Provides good analgesia of both anterior and posterior primary rami. Main disadvantages are problems of accurate siting and easy displacement

Epidural block:
- Thoracic epidural block with local anaesthetic agents provides excellent analgesia, but side effects with extensive sympathetic blockade limit the usefulness of this technique. Epidural block with opioids combined with low-dose local anaesthetic agents is now more popular by either the thoracic or lumbar route

---

There is now a substantial amount of literature on the use of epidural opioids for post-operative analgesia (Kavanagh, 1994). This seems to suggest that lipophilic opioids such as fentanyl are more effective when placed in the epidural space at a level corresponding to that of the surgery (the segmental effect). Conversely, satisfactory analgesia can be achieved if lipophobic opioids, such as morphine, are placed in the epidural space some distance from the site of surgery. The low lipophilicity of morphine, however, means that drug present in the cerebrospinal fluid (CSF) is likely to migrate rostrally with CSF flow. This may result in delayed respiratory depression (Green, 1992).

Contrary to the discussion above, the authors currently use diamorphine (which has a relatively high lipid solubility) via the lumbar epidural route to provide analgesia post-thoracotomy. Diamorphine has a rapid onset of action but shows a variable duration of action, which may exceed morphine. This is probably due to its initial uptake into the spinal cord as diamorphine and continued action through hydrolysis to its active metabolites of mono-acetyl morphine and morphine. Diamorphine is commonly used by the epidural route in the UK, but is unavailable in many other countries.

The authors prefer to administer epidural diamorphine via a high lumbar route, and combine this with a low concentration of a local anaesthetic agent. Thoracic opioid epidural analgesia may be optimal, but it has a number of disadvantages that they believe outweigh the advantages.

The main questions pertaining to the use of the thoracic epidural route involve its safety, ease of cannulation and whether it holds significant advantages over the lumbar route. Reports of neurological damage associated with thoracic epidurals are rare, although serious complications have occurred. The true incidence is likely to be higher than that reported in the literature due to the medico-legal implications. Thoracic epidurals can be established with the patient awake or anaesthetized. It is safer for the patient to be awake so that the sign of shooting pain from cord puncture is not obscured by general anaesthesia. Bromage (1989) has stated that thoracic epidurals should only be established in the awake patient.

It is more difficult to identify the thoracic space than the lumbar space due to the steeper angulation of the thoracic spinous processes. In addition, the epidural space is shallower in the thoracic region, making dural tap more likely. Failure to identify the thoracic space is also reported at a rate of 2–10 per cent, and this reflects anatomical difficulty, level of operator experience and reluctance to persevere when the likely complications are of a very serious nature.

It is perhaps not surprising from the above discussion that the authors elect to use opioid drugs combined with low-dose bupivacaine administered via the high lumbar route. This regime provides effective analgesia with minimal complications. Ropivacaine may prove to be a more suitable local anaesthetic drug to use in this situation, however, because it produces less motor block than bupivacaine and is less cardiotoxic.

Summary

Thoracic epidural analgesia provides the most satisfactory pain relief following thoracotomy, and is the gold standard of analgesia after thoracic surgery. There is a degree of practical difficulty in establishing a thoracic epidural, however, and this is certainly operator related. The complication rate of thoracic epidural cannulation is reported to be low, but this is in expert hands. The authors prefer to compromise and use the high lumbar route for epidural analgesia, using an opioid in combination with a low-dose local anaesthetic agent.

KEY POINTS

- Thoracic epidural analgesia is probably the most effective form of analgesia post-thoracotomy.
- A high lumbar epidural provides satisfactory analgesia (with opioids), and does not have the practical difficulties of the thoracic route.
- Intravenous opioids are satisfactory for many operations, but often need supplementation with other drugs or with local anaesthetic techniques.

Bibliography

Bernard *et al.* (1994). The American–European Consensus Conference on ARDS. *Am. J. Resp. Crit. Care. Med.*, **149**, 818–24.

Brodsky, J.B. (1988). Con: proper positioning of a double-lumen endobronchial tube can only be accomplished with endoscopy. *J. Cardiothorac. Anesth.*, **2**, 105–9.

Bromage, P.R. (1989). The control of post-thoracotomy pain. *Anaesthesia*, **44**, 445–6.

Chen, T.-L., Lee, Y.-T., Wang, M.-J. *et al.* (1996). Endothelin-1 concentrations and optimization of arterial oxygenation and venous admixture by selective pulmonary artery infusion of prostaglandin E_1 during thoracotomy. *Anaesthesia*, **51**, 422–6.

Conacher, I.D. (1997). Anaesthesia for the surgery of emphysema. *Br. J. Anaesth.*, **79**, 530–38.

Ehrenwerth, J. (1988). Pro: proper positioning of a double-lumen endobronchial tube can only be accomplished with endoscopy. *J. Cardiothorac. Anesth.*, **2**, 101–4.

Eisenkraft, J.B. (1994). Anaesthesia and hypoxic pulmonary vasoconstriction. In *Recent Advances in Anaesthesia and Analgesia* (R.S. Atkinson and A.P. Adams, eds), vol 18, pp. 103–22. Churchill Livingstone.

El-Baz, N.M., Kittle, C.F., Faber, L.P. *et al.* (1982). High-frequency ventilation with an uncuffed endobronchial tube. *J. Thorac. Cardiovasc. Surg.*, **84**, 823–8.

Entwistle, M.D., Roe, P.G., Sapsford, D.J. *et al.* (1991). Patterns of oxygenation after thoracotomy. *Br. J. Anaesth.*, **67**, 704–11.

Freden, F., Berglund, J.E., Reber, A. *et al.* (1996). Inhalation of a nitric oxide synthase inhibitor to a hypoxic or collapsed lung lobe in anaesthetized pigs: effects on pulmonary blood flow distribution: *Br. J. Anaesth.*, **77(3)**, 414–18.

Garcia-Aguado, R., Mateo, E.M., Onrubia, V.J. and Bolinches, R. (1996). Use of the Univent system tube for difficult intubation and for achieving one-lung anaesthesia. *Acta Anaesthesiol. Scand.*, **40**, 765–7.

Gayes, J.M. (1993). Pro: one-lung ventilation is best accomplished with the Univent endotracheal tube. *J. Cardiothorac. Vasc. Anesth.*, **7**, 103–7.

Green, D.W. (1992). The clinical use of spinal opioids. In *Anaesthesia Review* (L. Kaufman, ed.), vol. 9, pp. 80–111. Churchill Livingstone.

Howland, W.S., Carlon, G.C. and Goldiner, P.L. (1987). High-frequency jet ventilation during thoracic surgical procedures. *Anesthesiology*, **67**, 1009–12.

Inoue, H., Shotsu, A., Ogawa, J. *et al.* (1982). New device for one-lung anaesthesia: endotracheal tube with movable blocker. *J. Thorac. Cardiovasc. Surg.*, **83**, 940–1.

Jenkins, J., Cameron, E.W.J., Milne, A.C. and Hunter, R.M. (1987). One-lung anaesthesia. Cardiovascular and respiratory function compared with conventional and high frequency jet ventilation. *Anaesthesia*, **42**, 938–43.

Kavanagh, B.P., Katz, J. and Sandler, A.N. (1994). Pain control after thoracic surgery. A review of current techniques. *Anesthesiology*, **81**, 737–59.

Kellow, N.H., Scott, A.D., White, S.A. and Feneck, R.O. (1995). Comparison of the effects of propofol and isoflurane anaesthesia on right ventricular function and shunt fraction during thoracic surgery. *Br. J. Anaesth.*, **75**, 578–82.

McKenna, M.J., Wilson, R.S. and Bothelho, R.J. (1988). Right upper lobe obstruction with right-sided double-lumen endobronchial tubes: a comparison of two tube types. *J. Cardiothorac. Anesth.*, **2**, 734–40.

Moutafis, M., Liu, N., Dalibon, N. *et al.* (1997). The effects of inhaled nitric oxide and its combination with intravenous almitrine on Pao_2 during one-lung ventilation in patients undergoing thoracoscopic procedures. *Anaesth. Analg.*, **85**, 1130–5.

Nunn, J.F. (1993). *Applied Respiratory Physiology* (4th edn). Butterworth Heinemann.

Reid, C.W., Slinger, P.D. and Lenis, S. (1996). A comparison of the effects of propofol–alfentanil anesthesia on arterial oxygenation during one-lung ventilation. *J. Cardiothorac. Vasc. Anesth.*, **10(7)**, 860–3.

Rich, G.F., Lowson, S.M., Johns, R.A. *et al.* (1994). Inhaled nitric oxide selectively decreases pulmonary vascular resistance without impairing oxygenation during one-lung ventilation in patients undergoing cardiac surgery. *Anesthesiology*, **80**, 57–62.

Roth, M.D., Wright, J.W. and Bellamy, P.E. (1988). Gas flow through a bronchopleural fistula. Measuring the effects of high-frequency jet ventilation and chest-tube suction. *Chest*, **93**, 210–13.

Slinger, P. (1993). Con: the Univent tube is not the best method of providing one-lung ventilation. *J. Cardiothorac. Vasc. Anesth.*, **7**, 108–12.

Slinger, P.D. (1995). Perioperative fluid management for thoracic surgery: the puzzle of post-pneumonectomy pulmonary edema. *J. Cardiothorac. Vasc. Anesth.*, **9**, 442–51.

Smith, G.B., Hirsch, N.P. and Ehrenwerth, J. (1986). Placement of double-lumen endo-bronchial tubes. Correlation between clinical impressions and bronchoscopic findings. *Br. J. Anaesth.*, **58**, 1317–20.

Williams, E.A., Evans, T.W. and Goldstraw, P. (1996). Acute lung injury following lung resection: is one-lung anaesthesia to blame? *Thorax*, **51**, 114–16.

Wilson, W.C., Kapelanski, D.P., Benumof, J.L. *et al.* (1997). Inhaled nitric oxide (40 ppm) during one-lung ventilation, in the lateral decubitus position, does not decrease pulmonary vascular resistance or improve oxygenation in normal patients. *J. Cardiothorac. Vasc. Anesth.*, **11(2)**, 172–6.

Index